D1557724

Handbook of Medicine
in
Developing Countries
Second Edition

Dennis Palmer, D.O.
and
Catherine E. Wolf, M.D.

The Paul Tournier Institute is the educational divison of the Christian Medical & Dental Associations. The Paul Tournier Institute sponsors conferences and creates resource tools developed to help physicians, dentists, and other healthcare professionals investigate and discuss how the world of faith can be integrated with the world of biomedicine.

The Christian Medical & Dental Associations is a professional society of physicians, dentists, and allied helthcare professionals. It also provides a variety of ministries to the healthcare professional including student ministries, marriage growth conferences, short-term domestic and foreign missionary opportunities, medical ethics statements, and personal mentoring. The aim of CMDA is to change the face of healthcare by changing the hearts of doctors. For more information about CMDA call 1-423-844-1000 or write CMDA at P.O. Box 7500, Bristol, TN 37621.

Library of Congress Control Number: 2002112438
ISBN # 0-9706631-1-0

Table of Contents

FOREWORD

The first edition of the Handbook of Medicine in Developing Countries was well received by thousands of healthcare personnel around the world. Many took the time to not only express their appreciation, but to give ideas and suggestions for the next edition. Their contributions, along with the input and critique of an editorial board of missionary docs, have added 100 plus pages of superb information to this second edition. The authors have also updated the entire volume with the latest scientific advances in diagnosis and treatment.

If you have the first edition, you need this update. If you practice overseas or take care of patients that travel the world, you need this book in your reference library. Why? Because what I related in the first edition foreword still holds true:

"The retired Canadian cardiologist next to me had embarked on the adventure of a lifetime. He had signed up to serve as part of a medical relief team I was leading into Somalia in the midst of a devastating civil war and famine. Compassion had motivated him, but this was his first medical experience overseas, and he was noticeably apprehensive. As we began to taxi down the Nairobi runway in the back of a U.N. C-130, he leaned over to confess, "The last time I practiced general medicine was 40 years ago." With a chuckle I responded, "Good-that's exactly where health care is in Mogadishu!"

For many doctors from progressive countries, practicing medicine in developing countries is like entering a time warp. Medicine choice is limited. Few if any laboratory or other diagnostic tests are available. Health care providers are forced to depend largely on patients' history and a physical exam.

At the same time, you are confronted with a wide variety of unfamiliar and often advanced diseases that inflict hordes of people desperate for your care. If managed care means rationing limited resources and using the least costly diagnostic and therapeutic modalities, then it was birthed in developing countries.

After residency, I practiced overseas for 11 years as the medical director of a 130-bed hospital. When I first arrived, I served as the third doctor in the primary facility for 300,000 people. We couldn't have survived if it hadn't been for 20-30 doctors a year who donated a few weeks to a month of their time to help through World Medical Mission. The challenge we faced was teaching those volunteer doctors how to practice in a radically different medical environment, an environment where they would take care of 50 in-patients and dozens of out-patients each day-with a few deliveries and surgeries thrown in for good measure. At the time, there was no comprehensive and convenient reference specifically designed for health care personnel working short-term or long-term in developing countries. I would have given anything to have a resource like this handbook to put in the hands of those volunteer doctors.

From experience, I know that in the midst of a very busy day, you need something clear, concise and well-indexed-a convenient resource you can carry with you in your pocket for quick reference. With limited and varied therapeutic choices, it needs to list a good range of treatment options, emphasizing the drugs recommended on the World Health Organization-approved drug list. It needs to be written by doctors with years of experience in a variety of developing countries since disease patterns differ widely around the world. This book fits that bill.

With more students, doctors and healthcare professionals traveling overseas each year, this book will be the first thing they pack. Some will go to share their skills and others just for a vacation. All of them will know they have an important resource to give them guidance when they need it. Expatriate and national health care providers will find this book essential as they take care of patients in rural hospitals and bush clinics. It's been designed to hold up under the harsh conditions where they labor. With more and more people traveling internationally, this book will also serve as a handy diagnostic reference for U.S. doctors as they provide care for people on their return. It will help them think outside the box of U.S. medicine and help them diagnose diseases they may have never seen before.

It has been my pleasure to encourage the authors as they researched and wrote. Their hard labor will ease our burden, inform our decisions and most importantly, save lives."

I trust this new edition will be as helpful to you as it has been to me. Dr. Wolf and Dr. Palmer have done a superb job. As always, contact us with your ideas, critiques or stories of how this handbook has helped you.

David Stevens, M.D., M.A. (Ethics)
Executive Director
Christian Medical & Dental Associations

CONTRIBUTORS

Cheryl Cowles, MD - Private practice in obstetrics and gynecology. Formerly, at Tenwick Hospital, Kenya.

Philip R. Fischer, MD, DTM&H - Consultant at the Mayo Clinic and Professor of Pediatrics at the Mayo Medical School in Rochester, Minnesota. He has been with the Africa Inland Mission since 1984 (six years in central Africa, currently Medical Ministries Consultant).

John Hall, MD - Private Practice, Dermatology, Kansas City, Mo; Lecturer in Medicine, UMKC School of Medicine; Teaching Staff, Department of Dermatology, Children's Mercy Hospital.

Karen McClean, MD, FRCPC, FACP - Associate Professor of Medicine and Microbiology, Program Director, Internal Medicine Residency Training Program, University of Saskatchewan. Overseas experience includes Chitokoloki Mission Hospital, Northwest Province, Zambia: Medical Officer (1985-1989); Loloma Mission Hospital, Northwest Province, Zambia: Visiting Consultant (1995-2002).

Allan Ronald, OC, MD,MACP - Distinguished Professor, Emeritus, University of Manitoba.

James D. Smith, MD - Professor Emeritus, Otolaryngology Head and Neck Surgery Oregon Health Science University, Portland, Oregon; Visiting Professor, Department of Otolaryngology, National University of Singapore, Singapore.

Doug Soderdahl, MD, FACS - Clinical professor of Public Health and Epidemiology, University of Hawaii School of Medicine, Honolulu, Hawaii; Honorary Professor of Urology, Shaanxi Provincial People's Hospital, Xi'an, Shaanxi Province, China; Medical Education International team leader for China; Urologist and Executive Director of Global Medical Missions.

Paul G. Steinkuuler, MD - Ophthalmologist, Christian Blind Mission International, Fianarantsoa, Madagascar. Formerly: Chief of Ophthalmology, Texas Childrens Hospital, Baylor College of Medicine, Houston, Texas. Formerly: Ophthalmologist, International Eye Foundation, Blantyre, Malawi. Formerly: Ophthalmologist, International Eye Foundation, Nakuru, Kenya.

John Tarpley, MD - Professor of Surgery, Vanderbilt University School of Medicine; Chief, General Surgery, Veteran's Affairs Medical Center, Nashville, Tennessee. Long term medical missionary at the Baptist Medical Center in Ogbomoso, Nigeria.

Alva B. Weir III, MD - Private Practice Hematology/Oncology, Clinical Professor of Medicine University of Tennessee. Missionary Experience: Eku, Nigeria 1983-1985, Tirana, Albania 8 trips 1995-2001.

PREFACE

Many physicians, residents and medical students are involved each year in short-term international health experiences. Most are asked to work outside their area of training and expertise. Many physicians who routinely practice medicine in the western "developed" world have difficulty adjusting to the lack of technology and pharmaceutical resources commonly found in the "developing" or Third World. It is in both crossing from the "developed" world into the "developing" world and in crossing from one's own specialty to other specialties that problems arise due to lack of knowledge or experience. It is in an effort to meet this need that the *Handbook of Medicine in Developing Countries* has been written.

We have attempted to summarize key aspects of clinical evaluation and management of the most common medical, surgical, pediatric and obstetric problems encountered in developing countries. Since infectious diseases continue to constitute the majority of cases seen, we have emphasized this area. The treatment guidelines we have developed use basic radiology, diagnostic lab studies and therapeutic recommendations from the essential drug formulary since these will most likely be consistently available. We mention more sophisticated diagnosis and management as secondary information. The diagnostic and therapeutic guidelines outlined here are not exhaustive or comprehensive. The information is not designed for use in the parts of the world where the latest in technology and pharmaceuticals are available.

In this second edition of the *Handbook*, we have had the assistance of a dedicated group of specialty trained physicians who also have extensive experience working in hospitals in developing countries. Their expertise has enhanced the depth of the information presented here. We greatly appreciate their efforts in revising this material. We have also benefited from the evaluations of many physicians who have used the book in the field. Their candid comments have been very helpful. We have incorporated many of their suggestions into the material.

We are extremely grateful to the many patients we both helped care for in our respective years as overseas medical missionaries. Their medical problems provided the basis for the clinical material presented here, and their patience, strength, and perseverance in the midst of the adversities of daily life provided the inspiration to undertake such a task as this. We trust that they will reap the benefit of this effort.

We have taken great care to check these guidelines against other reliable sources, however we cannot guarantee that the text is error free. These are guidelines only. As always, treatment of each patient must be individualized, and adapted to the specific clinical situation. Decisions regarding the management of patients must rest with the prescribing clinician.

Finally, we consider this to be a work in progress. Feedback regarding the material presented here is very much appreciated.

Dennis D. Palmer, D.O.
Catherine E. Wolf, M.D.

CHAPTER 1

INFECTIOUS DISEASES

Drugs of Choice for Bacterial Infections

Diagnosis	Etiology	Drug of Choice
BONE		
	Staph aureus	Cloxacillin; Clindamycin
Osteomyelitis	*Salmonella*	Ciprofloxacin (for Gram negatives - in adults)
	Children < 8 yrs: above plus *H. influenzae*	Chloramphenicol*
	other Gram (-) rods	Cefuroxime; Ceftriaxone
	N. gonorrheae	Ceftriaxone
Septic arthritis	*Staph aureus*, Group A strep, Gram (-) rods	Cloxacillin; cefazolin; ciprofloxacin for Gram negative
	Children: *Salmonella, H. influenzae*	Cefuroxime, ceftriaxone, chloramphenicol*
BREAST		
Mastitis/abscess	*Staph aureus*, anaerobes	Cloxacillin; clindamycin
CNS		
Meningitis < 1 mo old	Group B or D Strep, *E. coli* and other gram negatives, *Listeria*	Ampicillin + Cefotaxime IV (or Gentamicin)
1 mo- < 8 yrs	*H. flu, S. pneumonia, N. meningitidis*	Ampicillin + Cefotaxime IV (or Chloramphenicol*)
adults	*S. pneumonia, N. meningitidis*	Cefotaxime + Ampicillin; chloramphenicol*
adults >50 yrs	*S. pneumonia, N. meningitidis, Listeria*	Cefotaxime + Ampicillin; high dose IV penicillin G; chloramphenicol*
GI		
Gastritis	*Helicobacter pylori*	Bismuth + tetracycline (or Amoxicillin) + metronidazole If available: omeprazole + amoxicillin + clarithromycin
Diarrhea Noninflammatory	*Enterotoxigenic E. coli* (common cause of Traveller's Diarrhea)	Treatment generally not required; ciprofloxacin may be used in adults; azithromycin in children
	Vibrio cholera	Tetracycline, Trimethoprim/sulfa if < 8 years
	Clostridium difficile	Metronidazole; PO vancomycin
	Shigella species	Trimethoprim/sulfa; ampicillin; ciprofloxacin, Nalidixic acid (check local susceptibilities)

Drugs of Choice for Bacterial Infections (continued)

Diagnosis	Etiology	Drug of Choice
GI (continued)		
Diarrhea Inflammatory	Enterohemorrhagic *E. coli* (O157)	No treatment- may precipitate hemolytic uremic syndrome
	Campylobacter jejuni	Erythromycin
	Vibrio parahemolyticus	None
	Salmonella enteritidis	Treatment can prolong carrier state - generally not recommended unless accompanied by systemic symptoms Trimethoprim/sulfa; chloramphenicol*
Diarrhea Penetrating	*Salmonella typhi*	Chloramphenicol;* ampicillin; trimethoprim/sulfa; ciprofloxacin
	Yersinia enterocolitica	Chloramphenicol;* tetracycline; trimethoprim/sulfa; ciprofloxacin
GENITOURINARY		
Urethritis, Cystitis	Gram (-) rods, *Staph saphrophyticus*	>5 wbc or + leukocyte esterase: Trimethoprim/sulfa; amoxicillin; 1st generation cephalosporin; ciprofloxacin, nitrofurantoin
Pyelonephritis	Gram (-) rods	Trimethoprim/sulfa; 1st or 3rd generation cephalosporins; ciprofloxacin; severe: ampicillin + gentamicin IV
Epididymitis	*N. gonorrheae, Chlamydia,* Gram (-) rods	Rx for GC and non-GC urethritis (ceftriaxone plus doxycycline) or Trimethoprim/sulfa (in older males)
Prostatitis	Gram (-) rods	Trimethoprim/sulfa; tetracycline; ciprofloxacin
Gonorrhea (assume penicillin and TMP/SMX resistance)	*N. gonorrheae* (usually treated syndromically to include *N.gonorrheae* and *C. trachomatis*)	Ceftriaxone; ciprofloxacin; cefixime plus tetracycline (ofloxacin and some newer quinolones can be prescribed as single drug regimen)
Disseminated gonorrhea	*N. gonorrheae*	Ciprofloxacin; ceftriaxone
Nongonococcal urethritis	*Chlamydia, Ureaplasma*	Tetracycline; erythromycin
Endometritis	Bacteroides, Group B or A Strep, Gram (-) rods	Ampicillin + gentamicin + metronidazole; piperacillin; clindamycin + gentamicin
PID	*N. gonorrhea, Chlamydia,* anaerobes	Ceftriaxone + doxycycline; ofloxacin; piperacillin

Diagnosis	Etiology	Drug of Choice
GENITOURINARY (continued)		
Syphilis	*T. pallidum*	Benzathine penicillin
Congenital syphilis	*T. pallidum*	Penicillin G (crystalline penicillin)
Herpes genitalis	Herpes simplex type II	Acyclovir; famciclovir
Anogenital warts, condylomata accuminata	Human papilloma virus	Podophyllin; bi-trichloracetic acid; surgical excision
Chancroid	*Haemophilus ducreyi*	Erythromycin; ciprofloxacin; ceftriaxone
Granuloma inguinale	*Calymmatobacterium granulomatis*	Doxycycline; trimethoprim/sulfa; erythromycin; ciprofloxacin
Lymphogranuloma venereum	*Chlamydia trachomatis*	Doxycycline; erythromycin
	Candida	Nystatin; clotrimazole vaginally; fluconazole orally
Vaginitis	*Trichomonas vaginalis*	Metronidazole; tinidazole:
	Bacterial vaginosis	Metronidazole; clindamycin intravaginally
UPPER RESPIRATORY		
Otitis media	*S. pneumoniae, H. influenzae, Moraxella catarrhalis* "Sterile"	Amoxicillin; trimethoprim/sulfa; amoxicillin/clavulanic acid for failures
External Otitis	*Pseudomonas*	Antibiotic / steroid otic drops (gentamicin-hydrocortisone etc.) acetic acid drops Severe-ciprofloxacin
Sinusitis acute purulent	*S. pneumoniae, H. influenzae,* Group A strep	Amoxicillin; trimethoprim/sulfa; amox/clav.acid
Dental infection	Oral microflora, *Bacteroides*	Penicillin V; penicillin G + metronidazole; clindamycin
Exudative pharyngitis	Group A strep	Benzathine penicillin; penicillin V; erythromycin; cephalexin
Croup Epiglottitis	Viral *H. influenzae*	Intubation . Parenteral antibiotics initially: cefotaxime, chloramphenicol Amoxicillin/clav acid; TMP/SMX; ciprofloxacin (in adults)

3

Drugs of Choice for Bacterial Infections (continued)

Diagnosis	Etiology	Drug of Choice
LOWER RESPIRATORY		
Bronchiolitis	Viral	None
Bronchitis	Viral, *Mycoplasma*, *S. pneumoniae*, *H.influenzae flu*, *M. catarrhalis*	Usually no therapy; erythromycin, amoxicillin, trimethoprim/sulfa if evidence of bacterial infection
Pertussis	*Bordetella pertussis*	Erythromycin to reduce infectiousness; not effective for altering course
Pneumonia Younger adult	*S. pneumoniae*	Penicillin IV or amoxicillin; CAF; new quinolones
	Mycoplasma, viral, *Chlamydia*	Erythromycin; tetracycline
Smoker or child	Above + *H. influenzae*, *M. catarrhalis*	Amoxicillin; trimethoprim/sulfa; new quinolones
Older adults with underlying illnesses, or seriouslly ill	*S. pneumoniae*, viral, *H. influenzae*, Gm- bacilli, *Staphylococcus*, *Legionella*	Outpatient: erythromycin (clarithromycin or azithromycin); trimethoprim/sulfa; newer quinolones; tetracycline
		Hospitalized: erythromycin+CAF; chloramphenicol; newer quinolones
Aspiration/lung abscess	Mixed aerobic and anaerobic bacteria	Clindamycin; or high dose penicillin G+ metronidazole
SEPSIS		
Neonate	Group B or D Strep, Gm - rods, *Listeria*	Cefotaxime + Ampicillin Ampicillin + gentamicin
Child	*H. influenzae* (< 8 years of age) *S pneumonia*, *N. meningitidis*	Cefotaxime, cefuroxime, chloramphenicol*
Adult	Gm + cocci, Gm - rods, anaerobes	Cefotaxime; cloxacillin + metronidazole; Clindamycin+gentamicin; piperacillin/tazobactam
Urinary tract source	Gm - rods	Ampicillin + gentamicin; ciprofloxacin
Intra-abdominal or pelvic infections	Gm - rods, *Enterococcus*, anaerobes	Ampicillin + gentamicin + metronidazole or clindamycin; Piperacillin/tazobactam; imipenem
Biliary tract	Gm - rods, *Enterococcus*, anaerobes, *Clostridia* sp.	Ampicillin + gentamicin + metronidazole; piperacillin/tazobactam

Diagnosis	Etiology	Drug of Choice
SKIN		
Acne (inflammatory)	*Propionibacterium acnes*	Tetracycline
Anthrax	*Bacillus anthracis*	Penicillin, erythromycin, tetracycline, ciprofloxacin
Buruli ulcer	*M. ulcerans*	Surgical debridement Rifampicin + amikacin or streptomycin
Cellulitis	Group A strep, *Staph aureus*	Cloxacillin; cephalexin
	Buccal or periorbital cellulitis in children: *H. influenzae, S. pneumoniae*	Cefuroxime, Amox/clav, Chloroamphenicol
Fever blisters	Herpes simplex type I	Acyclovir; famciclovir (in resource limited settings reserve for shingles, or genital HSV)
Impetigo	Group A strep, *Staph aureus*	Cloxacillin; clindamycin, cephalexin
Lymphadenitis	Group A strep, *Staph aureus*	Cloxacillin; clindamycin, cephalexin
Pyomyositis	*Staph aureus*	Cloxacillin, cephalexin, aggressive drainage
Shingles	Herpes zoster	Acyclovir, or famciclovir
WOUNDS		
Traumatic	Group A strep, *Staph aureus*	Cloxacillin; cephalexin; clindamycin
Bites	Oral flora; anaerobes and unique organisms	Amox/clav.acid; clindamycin and ciprofloxacin; piperacillin

* Chloramphenicol carries risk of aplastic anemia and should be reserved for serious infections where other options are not available.
N.B. Tetracycline and Doxycycline should not be used in children < 8 years, ciprofloxacin and other quinolones should not generally be used in children

Drugs of Choice for Parasitic Infections		
Infection	**Drug**	**Dosage**
Amebiasis - cyst passers	Iodoquinol	650 mg tid x 20 days (30 mg/kg/day)
	or Paromomycin	10 mg/kg tid x 7 days
	or Diloxanide	500 mg tid x 10 days (30 mg/kg/day)
Amebiasis - dysentery	Metronidazole	750 mg tid x 10 days (35-50 mg/kg/day)
	or Tinidazole	1 gm bid x 3 days (50-60 mg/kg/day) followed by iodoquinol, paromomycin or diloxanide
Amoebic liver Abscess	Metronidazole	750 mg tid x 10 days (35-50 mg/kg/day)
	or Tinidazole	600-800 mg tid x 5 days (50-60 mg/kg/day followed by iodoquinol, paromomycin or diloxanide

Drugs of Choice for Parasitic Infections (continued)

Infection	Drug	Dosage
Ascaris	Mebendazole	100 mg bid x 3 days (child - same)
	or Albendazole	400 mg as single dose (child - same)
	or Pyrantel pamoate	11 mg/kg (max 1 gram) daily x 3
	Piperazine - for biliary or intestinal obstruction	150 mg/kg stat then 65 mg/kg q12h x 6 doses
Cryptosporidium	Paromomycin	25-35 mg/kg/day (tid) x 5-10 days with meals (limited efficacy)
Cutaneous larva migrans (dog or cat hookworm)	Thiabendazole	50 mg/kg/day (bid) x 2-5 days (max 3 gm/day)
	or Ivermectin or Albendazole	150-200 mcg/kg once 200 mg bid x 3 days
Cyclospora	TMP/SMX	160mg TMP / 800 mg SMX (1 DS tab) bid x 7-10 days Children: 5 mg TMP / 25 mg SMX per kg bid x 7- 10 days
Dracunculus (guinea worm)	Metronidazole	250 mg tid (30 mg/kg/day) x 10 days
	or Thiabendazole	50-75 mg/kg/day in two doses x 3 days.
Echinococcus (Hydatid disease)	Albendazole	15 mg/kg/day in 2 doses (max 400 mg bid) x 28 days (repeat at 2 week intervals x 3). Use as an adjunct to surgical or percutaneous drainage.
Enterobius vermicularis (pinworm)	Mebendazole	100 mg as single dose, repeat after 2 weeks, pediatric dose - same
Filariasis Lymphatic	Diethylcarbamazine	5-6 mg/kg in divided doses for 2-3 weeks. Begin at low dose, 25-50 mg/day, and increase to full dose over 3-5 days - see text.
Onchocerciasis	or Ivermectin	200 - 400 mcg/kg as a single dose (+/- albendazole 400 mg)
	Ivermectin	150 mcg/kg (usually two tablets in adults) as a single dose, with water, on an empty stomach. Repeat at 6-12 months intervals
	or Diethylcarbamazine	25 mg daily for 3 days, then 50 mg daily for 3 days, then 100-150 mg daily for 10 days
Flukes - liver and intestinal	Praziquantel	75 mg/kg/day in three doses x 1-2 days

Infection	Drug	Dosage
Giardiasis	Metronidazole	250 mg (15 mg/kg/d) tid x 5 days
	or Tinidazole	2 gm as single dose; child: 50 mg/kg as single dose
	or Albendazole	400 mg qd x 5 days
	or Furazolidone	100 mg qid x 7-10 days (6 mg/kg/d in 4 doses x 7-10 days)
Hookworm (Ancylostoma)	Mebendazole	100 mg bid x 3 days
	or Albendazole	400 mg as single dose
Isospora belli	Trimethoprim/sulfa	Non-HIV infected: TMP/SMX 160/800 mg bid x 10 days (10/50 mg/kg/day).
	1 double strength tablet = 160 mg TMP / 800 mg SMX)	HIV infected: TMP/SMX 160/800 mg qid x 10 days then 160/800 mg bid x 3 weeks. (20/100 mg/kg/day in 4 doses x 10 days then 10/50 mg/kg/day in 2 doses x 3 weeks)
		HIV infection: long term suppressive Rx required (1 DS tab 3x weekly)
Lice	Lindane shampoo	Apply to dry hair, then lather, and rinse
	Ivermectin	200 mcg/kg x one dose
Leishmaniasis	Meglumine antimonate or Sodium Stibogluconate	20 mg antimony/kg/d (preferably as 2 divided doses) x 3-4 weeks
	Amphotericin B Liposomal Ampho B	0.5-1.0 mg/kg IV daily or every other day for up to 8 weeks3 mg/kg/d on days 1-5 then days 14 and 21
Malaria simple	Chloroquine Fansidar	10 mg/kg of base initially, then 5 mg/kg in six hours, then 5 mg/kg/d x two days Infant 6 wks-1 yr.　　¼ tablet Child 1 yr-3 yrs　　½ tablet Child 4 yrs-8 yrs　　1 tablet Child 9 yrs-14 yrs　　2 tablets Adult　　　　　　3 tablets
Malaria resistant	Quinine	25-30 mg/kg/day in divided doses q 8 hrs for 7 days (combine with tetracycline, doxycycline, clindamycin, fansidar or TMP/SMX)
	Mefloquine	20 mg/kg (up to 1.5 gm) as a single dose or divided into two doses 6-8 hrs apart
	Malarone (250 mg atovaquone / 100 mg proguanil)	4 tablets daily x 3 days 11-20 kg: one tablet daily x 3 days 21-30 kg: two tablests daily x 3 days 31-40 kg: three tablets daily x 3 days

Drugs of Choice for Parasitic Infections (continued)

Infection	Drug	Dosage
Malaria severe	Quinine	20 mg/kg IV over 4 hours as loading dose, then 10 mg/kg over 2-4 hours every 8 hours until pt can take PO
	Artemisinin compounds	dose depends on the specific compound available. Treatment durations of < 7 days may have a higher rate of recurrence. Combine with Mefloquine. See text.
Malaria prophylaxis	Mefloquine	250 mg weekly < 15 kg: 5 mg/kg weekly 15-19 kg: ¼ tablet weekly 20-30 kg: ½ tablet weekly 31-45 kg: ¾ tablet weekly
	Malarone	One tablet daily 11-20 kg: ¼ tablet daily 21-30 kg: ½ tablet daily 31-40 kg: ¾ tablet daily
	Doxycycline	100 mg daily (2 mg/kg/d for children > 8 years)
	Primaquine	30 mg base daily (0.5 mg/kg base daily) NB: Check for G6PD deficiency first
	Chloroquine +/- proguanil	5 mg/kg base per week (proguanil: 200 mg / day)NB: efficacy poor in most areas - reserved for use where there is not chloroquine resistance or no other options
	Not Suitable for Prophylaxis	Artemisinin compounds Fansidar Halofantrine Quinine
P. vivax / P. ovale (prevent relapses)	Primaquine	15 mg (base) / day x 14 days or 45 mg (base) weekly x 8 weeks0.3 mg (base) / kg/day x 14 days
Paragonimiasis	Praziquantel	25 mg/kg tid x 2 days
Scabies	Lindane lotion	Apply topically to entire body except head, wash off after 6 hours
	Benzyl benzoate	Apply topically over entire body except head, repeat in 24 hours without bathing
	Sulfur 5-10% in Petrolatum	Apply topically daily x 3 days
	Ivermectin	200 mcg/kd x one dose
Schistosomiasis	Praziquantel	40-60 mg/kg/day in 2-3 doses x 1 day

Infection	Drug	Dosage
Strongyloides	Thiabendazole	50 mg/kg/day in two doses x 2 days (max 3 gm)
	or Ivermectin	200 mcg/kg as single dose x 1-2 days
	or Albendazole	400 mg once daily x 3 days
Tapeworm	Niclosamide	All species: single dose of 2 gms (11-34 kg - single dose of 1 gm) chewed well
	or Praziquantel	*T. saginata* or *T. solium*: 10 mg/kg x 1 dose (see text for other species)
Neurocysticercosis	Praziquantel	50 mg/kg/day in 3 doses x 15 days
	or Albendazole	15 mg/kg/day in 2 doses (max 400 mg bid) x 3-30 days
Toxoplasmosis	Pyrimethamine	25-100 mg/d x 3-4 weeks
	+Sulfadiazine	1-2 gm qid x 3-4 weeks
Vaginal Trichomoniasis	Metronidazole	2 gm once or 250 mg tid x 7 days (15 mg/kg/day)
	or Tinidazole	2 gm once (50 mg/kg)
Trichinosis	Mebendazole	15 mg/kg bid x 10-14 days
	or Albendazole	400 mg bid x 14 dayscover with steroids for severe symptoms
Trichuris (Whipworm)	Mebendazole	100 mg bid x 3 days
	or Albendazole	400 mg as single dose
Trypanosomiasis *T. cruzi*	Nifurtimox	Adults: 8-10 mg/kg/d in 4 doses x 90 - 120 d 1-10 years: 15-20 mg/kg/d in 4 doses x 90 days 11-16 years: 12.5-15 mg/kg/d in 4 doses x 90 days
	Benznidazole	Adults: 5-7 mg/kg/d in 2 doses x 30-90 days 1-12 years: 10 mg/kg/d in 2 doses x 30-90 days
African trypanosomiasis Hemolymphatic	Suramin	100-200 mg test dose IV, then 1 gm IV on days 1, 3, 7, 14 and 21 Children: 20 mg/kg on days 1, 3, 7, 14 and 21
CNS disease	Melarsoprol	2-3.6 mg/kg/d IV x 3 days, after 1 wk: 3.6 mg/kg/d x 3 days, repeat in 10-21 d Children: initial dose 0.36 mg/kg IV increase dose gradually to maximum of 3.6 mg/kg with doses at 1-5 day intervals for a total of 9-10 doses (total dose of 18-25 mg/kg over 1 month)

Drugs of Choice for Parasitic Infections (continued)		
Infection	**Drug**	**Dosage**
Visceral larvae migrans (Toxocariasis)	Diethylcarbamazine	6 mg/kg/day in three doses x 10 days
	or Mebendazole	100-200 mg bid x 5 days
	or Albendazole	400 mg bid x 3-5 days

I. BACTERIAL INFECTIONS
A. Anthrax
1. **General**
   a. Agent: *Bacillus anthracis*, a large Gm + spore-forming rod.
   b. Spread by contact with infected animals and animal products. There is recent concern that the agent could be used in bio-terrorism.
   c. Incubation period is 12 hours - 7 days.
   d. Cutaneous disease is most common (95%). Begins as a pruritic papule, usually at the site of skin injury, which develops into an ulcer with surrounding vesicles. Black necrotic central eschar develops in 5-7 days. Brawny edema of the infected area frequently occurs.
   e. Inhalation anthrax is characterized by a brief flu-like prodrome and rapid progression to severe dyspnea often with nonproductive cough and stridor. The chest x-ray may show widening of the mediastinum and pleural effusions. Parenchymal infiltrates may or may not be present. Early treatment is essential. Isolation is not required.
   f. Gastrointestinal anthrax results from ingestion of contaminated meat and may present with fever, abdominal pain, vomiting and diarrhea (often bloody) with rapid progression to generalized sepsis. It may also present with ulceration in the oropharynx accompanied by extensive local edema.
2. **Management**
   a. Cutaneous anthrax - PCN G 4 million units IV q4h (children < 12 years: 50,000 units/kg q6h) for 2-4 days until edema subsides, then oral Pen VK for total of 7-10 days.
   b. Alternative drugs include ciprofloxacin (400 mg IV q12h, children: 10-15 mg/kg q12h), doxycycline (100 mg q12h, children > 8 years: 2 mg/kg q12h), tetracycline (2 gm/d), chloramphenicol (12.5-25 mg/kg q6h, max. 2-4 gm/d).
   c. If edema of the neck interferes with breathing, steroids may be helpful (hydrocortisone 100-200mg/d IV).
   d. Inhaled or GI anthrax has high mortality. Treat with PCN G 4 million units IV q4h (children < 12 years: 50,000 units/kg q6h). Some recent sources recommend use of at least two antibiotics (ie: ciprofloxacin or doxycycline plus penicillin). Step-down to oral penicillin to complete 60 days.

B. Brucellosis (Undulant fever)
 1. General
  a. Etiology
   (1) Small Gm (-), intracellular coccobacillus.
   (2) Four species are known to cause human disease.
   (3) Infection usually occurs through exposure to animal carcasses or unpasturized dairy products in endemic area.
   (4) Distribution is world wide, but is especially common in the . Middle East, India, and Central and South America.
  b. Clinical presentation
   (1) Onset may be abrupt or over weeks.
   (2) Major symptoms are fever (FUO), malaise, fatigue, anorexia, weight loss.
   (3) Focal symptoms develop in 1/3 of patients - bone pain, back pain.
   (4) Minimal physical findings are present - lymphadenopathy and occasionally hepatosplenomegaly may be present.
  c. Diagnosis
   (1) Requires a high index of clinical suspicion.
   (2) Difficult to culture even under ideal conditions.
   (3) Serological testing is helpful (if locally available).
 2. Management
  a. Doxycycline 1-2 mg/kg/dose bid x 4-6 wks if > 8 years old.
  b. TMP/SMX 10 mg trimethoprim/kg/day po x 4-6 wks if < 8 yrs old.
  c. Consider adding rifampin 15-20 mg/kg po daily to decrease risk of relapse.
  d. Consider adding streptomycin (10/mg/kg/dose im bid) or gentamicin (1.6 mg/kg/dose IV or IM q8h) for first week for severe complicated disease.
  e. The flouroquinolones are not as effective as these regimens and are usually not the agents of first choice.
  f. Sometimes an empirical trial of a tetracycline(doxycycline) or TMP/SMX is necessary in patients with a persistent febrile course and no other explanation. A response should occur within a week.
C. Relapsing Fever
 1. General
  a. Relapsing fever is caused by spirochetes in the genus *Borrelia*. *Borrelia recurrentis* causes louse-borne relapsing fever (LBRF), *Borrelia duttoni* (and multiple other species) cause tick-borne relapsing fever (TBRF).
  b. *Borrelia* are visible on blood smears with common tissue and microbiologic stains (Giemsa, Leishman, Field stains).
 2. Clinical syndromes

a. Louse-borne relapsing fever typically occurs in displaced populations living in overcrowded conditions. Man is the only host. Lice are infected by feeding on spirochetemic patients during febrile episodes and infection is transmitted to another host when lice are crushed on the skin during scratching. Transplacental transmission can infect the fetus. Transmission by blood transfusion has been reported.

(1) Severity of clinical illness is highly variable from asymptomatic parasitemia to a severe, sometimes fatal, febrile illness.

(2) Incubation period is 2-10 days.

(3) Typical cases present with sudden onset of fever and chills, severe headache, myalgias and arthralgias. Cough, dyspnea, nausea and vomiting are frequent symptoms. Hepatosplenomegaly, jaundice and bleeding manifestations (petechial rash, conjunctival hemorrhages and epistaxis) are common on examination.

(4) The initial febrile episode lasts 5-7 days, with irregular (typically sustained) fever throughout the episode. The febrile episode ends in a crisis, spirochetes disappear from the bloodstream and the patient gradually recovers. Approximately 2/3 of patients will experience a relapse 5-9 days after the first attack subsides. Clinical manifestations are milder than during the initial attack and rash is usually absent. Some patients will experience multiple relapses, but rarely more than four.

(5) Complications include iridocyclitis, meningitis, cranial nerve palsies, pneumonitis, myocarditis, splenic rupture.

b. Tick-borne relapsing fever is transmitted by a variety of species of soft ticks. These ticks typically live in crevices in walls and floors of dwellings and are transient, nocturnal feeders. Transmission occurs rapidly once the tick begins to feed, often within the first minute of feeding. Patients with TBRF often have no recognized history of tick bites.

(1) Severity of clinical illness is typically less than LBRF but fatal cases can occur.

(2) Incubation period is 1-14 days.

(3) The initial febrile episode begins abruptly with high fever, headache and myalgias. Hepatosplenomegaly is common but jaundice is infrequent. Hemorrhagic manifestations are less common than in LBRF. Pneumonic symptoms are relatively common in TBRF.

(4) The initial febrile episode lasts 4-5 days. Subsequent episodes occur at intervals of several days to several weeks. Relapses are more numerous than in LBRF. Typically 3-6 relapses occur, but as many as 11 have been reported in untreated patients.

(5) Neurological complications are more frequent in TBRF than in LBRF. Cranial nerve palsies (especially facial palsy) are the most

common neurologic complication. Focal neurologic signs include hemiplegia, aphasia and peripheral nerve palsies. Other neurologic complications include lymphocytic meningitis, subarachnoid hemorrhage, encephalitis, iritis and optic atrophy. Neurologic abnormalities usually resolve completely, without long-term sequelae.

(6) TBRF in pregnancy may cause premature labour, stillbirth and spontaneous abortion. Relapsing fever in pregnant patients is more severe than in non-pregnant women.

3. Diagnosis

a. During febrile episodes, *Borrelia* can be seen in the blood on thick or thin blood films (wavy filaments located extracellularly).

b. Organisms tend to be numerous in LBRF but can be difficult to find in TBRF.

4. Treatment

a. Both louse-borne and tick-borne relapsing fever can be treated with any of the following antibiotics: penicillin, tetracycline, erythromycin, or chloramphenicol. Single dose therapy with tetracycline or procaine penicillin has proven effective in LBRF but is less well established in TBRF. The recommended duration of treatment for TBRF is 7 days.

Treatment of Relapsing Fever			
Medications		Louse-borne RF	Tick-borne RF
Oral	Erythromycin	500 mg stat (10 mg/kg)	500 mg q6h (10 mg/kg q6h)
	Tetracycline	500 mg stat (10 mg/kg > 8 yrs)	500 mg q6h (10 mg/kg q6h > 8 years)
	Doxycycline	100 mg stat (2 mg/kg stat > 8 years)	100 mg q12h (2 mg/kg q12h > 8 years)
	Chloramphenicol	500 mg stat (12.5-25 mg stat)	500 mg q6h (12.5-25 mg q6h)
Parenteral	Chloramphenicol	500 mg stat (12.5-25 mg stat)	500 mg q6h (12.5-25 mg q6h)
	Procaine Penicillin IM	600,000 units (< 12 years: 25,000 - 50,000 units)	600,000 units q24h (< 12 years: 25,000 - 50,000 units q 24 h)

b. Jarisch Herxheimer reactions frequently occur following the administration of the first dose of treatment. Reactions are common in LBRF and uncommon in TBRF. The Jarisch Herxheimer reaction is initiated by a rigor, followed by a sudden rise in temperature. Pulse, blood pressure and respiratory rate all increase initially. This is followed by a period of flushing, profuse sweating and hypotension. Steroids neither prevent nor ameliorate symptoms. Treatment is supportive, with fluid replacement to counteract hypotension. Meptazinol (a partial opioid agonist) can reduce the severity of the reaction.

5. Prevention

    a. Louse-borne relapsing fever - delousing, (avoid crushing of lice) and treatment of clothing with insecticide powder (lindane 1%, malathion 1%) or heat sterilization is effective in preventing infection. In high-risk settings, adequate water for washing clothing and maintaining good hygiene is important in preventing outbreaks. In outbreak settings, mass treatment with single dose doxycycline will terminate transmission.

    b. Tick-borne relapsing fever - avoid sleeping in abandoned buildings and on floors. Buildings inhabited by infected patients should be treated with insecticide to prevent transmission to other household members. Ticks are relatively resistant to DDT. Insecticide-impregnated bed nets should be effective in preventing transmission since ticks are nocturnal feeders.

D. Sepsis

  1. General

    a. Choice of drugs should be based on probable source of infection, Gram-stained smears of appropriate clinical specimens and immune status of the patient.

    b. When evaluating a patient for possible sepsis, it is important to look for other causes of fever and toxicity appropriate to your setting. If no source of bacterial infection is apparent, consider the possibility of malaria, typhoid fever, tuberculosis, or HIV disease.

    c. Malaria treatment should always be considered for febrile patients with no obvious bacterial source of infection.

    d. Typhoid fever should be considered in patients with prolonged fever and GI complaints, especially if accompanied by delirium. In children, GI symptoms may be absent - typhoid should be considered in any unexplained fever.

    e. Recurrent *Salmonella* bacteremia can occur in patients with sickle cell anemia, schistosomiasis and HIV infection.

    f. Patients with signs of chronic disease and cachexia should be evaluated for tuberculosis and HIV disease. These patients may have bacterial sepsis in addition to their chronic underlying disease, and can be quite toxic.

  2. Antibiotic therapy (give for 10-14 days)

Empiric Treatment of Sepsis	
Clinical situation	**Empiric antibiotic therapy**
Neonate	Ampicillin IV/IM + gentamicin IV/IM
Child	Ampicillin IV + chloramphenicol IV or po 3rd gen. Cephalosporin (cefotaxime, ceftriaxone)
Adult, non-compromised	Ampicillin + gentamicin + chloramphenicol or metronidazole or clindamycin 3rd generation cephalosporin + aminoglycoside
Urinary tract source	Ampicillin + gentamicin
Intra-abdominal or pelvic infections	Ampicillin + gentamicin + anaerobic agent (chloramphenicol or metronidazole or clindamycin) Ciprofloxacin + metronidazole
Biliary tract	Ampicillin or 1st gen. cephalosporin + gentamicin + chloramphenicol or metronidazole
Skin / Soft tissue source	Cloxacillin or clindamycin First generation cephalosporin

E. Tetanus
1. General
a. Caused by *Clostridium tetani*. Spores contaminate wounds and on germination produce a neurotoxin (tetanospasmin), which interferes with normal neuronal transmission. This produces the characteristic muscle rigidity and spasms of tetanus.

b. A history of penetrating injury is common, but 10-20% have no history of trauma. Tetanus may also occur in association with pregnancy, surgery, burns, injections, ulcers, bites and umbilical stump infections in newborns.

c. Incubation is from 1-55 days. 80% have onset within 14 days. Overall mortality is 30-55% with high mortality being associated with short incubation (near 100% mortality if the incubation period is 1-2 days).

2. Symptoms
a. Trismus and spasm of facial muscles are usually the first signs, followed by dysphagia. Generalized spasms follow within 72 hours in 60% of patients. Once established, generalized spasms are usually stable for one week, then decline over several weeks.

b. Severe sympathetic nervous system hyperactivity may be seen, including labile hypertension, tachycardia, sweating, and vasoconstriction.

3. Treatment
a. Decrease external stimuli including light, noises, and procedures.

b. Maintain an adequate airway. The cause of death is usually respiratory arrest. Use oral feedings cautiously. Tracheostomy may reduce airway obstruction from spasms. Intubation, ventilation, and paralysis with neuromuscular blocking agents may be necessary in severe cases, if available.

c. Tetanus antitoxin (equine) 25,000 units IM or IV after a test dose. Human tetanus immunoglobulin (HTIG) 500 units IM is preferred, if available.

d. Sedation - diazepam 40-200 mg per day IV in divided doses (0.25mg/kg/dose). May be combined with chlorpromazine 25 mg IV every 3-4 hours (1mg/kg/dose).

e. Antibiotics - PCN G 4-6 million units IV q6h x10d is usually given, however newer recommendations are to use metronidazole 500 mg IV q 6 hours x 7-10d (children: 7.5 mg/kg/dose q6h).

f. Propranolol may be used to control sympathetic hyperactivity.

g. Wound debridement may eliminate the site of toxin production. Should be performed immediately at the time of presentation.

h. Tetanus toxoid - clinical tetanus does not confer immunity. Give a series of three injections one month apart beginning at time of discharge.

i. Recovery is gradual, requiring 4-6 weeks in severe tetanus.

4. Tetanus prophylaxis

a. Clean, minor wounds - need tetanus toxoid if immunization history is uncertain, or if > 10 years since last booster. Either diphtheria tetanus (Td) or tetanus toxoid (TT) may be used.

b. Major wounds

(1) If a complete primary immunization series is reliably documented, and > 5 years since last booster, Td alone is required. (If < 5 years no booster required).

(2) If a complete primary immunizations series is uncertain, both tetanus toxoid and TIG (Human Tetanus Immune Globulin) are required. Equine anti-toxin can be used if human TIG is unavailable. A test dose should be given first.

(a) TIG: 250-500 units IM   - or -

(b) Equine anti-toxin after skin test: 3,000-5,000 units IM.

(c) Td at another site, same time.

c. Patients with uncertain immunization histories need to complete the full series of Td or TT vaccination (3 doses 1-2 months apart). If the first dose is given with wound treatment, these patients need follow-up appointments to complete the series.

F. Diphtheria

1. General

a. Diphtheria is caused by *Corynebacterium diphtheriae*, a gram-positive bacillus.

b. Virulent strains of *C. diphtheriae* produce an exotoxin that inhibits protein synthesis. The toxin affects all types of cells but its effects are most prominent in the myocardium (myocarditis), neurons (demyelination) and kidneys (tubular necrosis).

c. Humans are the only known source for infection with *C. diphtheriae*. Infection is transmitted by respiratory droplets or by direct contact with respiratory secretions or exudate from skin lesions. Asymptomatic carriers are important sources of infection.

2. Clinical manifestations

  a. Local signs of infection occur in the upper respiratory tract or skin.

    (1) Nasal diphtheria - serosanguinous or seropurulent discharge with whitish membrane on nasal septum.

    (2) Tonsilar diphtheria - malaise, sore throat, gray membrane with patches of green or black necrosis. In early cases the membrane may have a glossy white appearance. Marked cervical adenopathy produces the characteristic "bull neck" in severe cases.

    (3) Laryngeal and tracheal diphtheria: hoarsenss, dyspnea, stridor, brassy cough. Accessory muscle use, retractions and cyanosis indicate obstruction and the need for tracheostomy.

    (4) Cutaneous diphtheria - common in the tropics. Chronic, non-healing ulcers with dirty gray membrane. Group A strep and *Staphylococcus* are often present on culture. The ulcer is indolent and non-progressive and rarely associated with systemic complications. It is an important source for transmission to others.

  b. Systemic manifestations include cardiac or neurologic toxicity caused by systemic absorption of toxin.

    (1) Cardiac toxicity - symptoms of myocarditis usually appear 1-2 weeks after onset, as respiratory disease is improving. ST changes and first degree A-V block are early signs and may progress to complete heart block and other arrhythmias. Signs and symptoms of congestive heart failure may appear gradually or abruptly.

    (2) Neurologic toxicity - early signs are paralysis of soft palate and pharyngeal muscles leading to regurgitation of fluids through the nose. More severe cases typically progress to cranial neuropathies and peripheral neuropathies. Peripheral neuritis can appear from 10 days to 3 months after pharyngeal disease and presents with proximal muscle weakness which extends to involve distal muscles with absent reflexes. Muscle weakness can be mild or severe. Glove and stocking sensory neuropathies can occur. Neurologic abnormalities resolve slowly.

3. Diagnosis

a. In most cases, diagnosis is made clinically. Diphtheria should be considered in patients presenting with mildly painful tonsillitis or pharyngitis characterized by the presence of a membrane, especially if the membrane extends beyond the tonsils and is accompanied by marked cervical adenopathy and cervical swelling or hoarsness and stridor. Nasal regurgitation of fluids strongly points to the diagnosis.

b. Differential diagnosis includes EBV mononucleosis, streptococcal pharyngitis and acute epiglottitis. The presence of membranes extending beyond the tonsils and resulting in bleeding on removal points to diphtheria as the diagnosis.

4. Treatment

a. Diphtheria anti-toxin reduces the mortality from diphtheria but must be administered early as it works only against toxin that has not been taken up into cells. The following dosages are recommended:

    (1) Pharyngeal or laryngeal disease: 20,000 - 40,000 units.

    (2) Nasopharyngeal disease: 40,000 - 60,000 units.

    (3) Extensive disease or duration > 3 days: 80,000 - 100,000 units.

b. Antitoxin may be administered IV or IM. IV therapy over 60 minutes is preferred for severe disease. Administration should always be preceded by a test dose of 1:10 antitoxin instilled into the conjunctiva or 1:100 dilution intradermally as severe hypersensitivity reactions to equine antigens can occur.

c. Antibiotics terminate toxin production, improve local disease manifestations and terminate spread to contacts. Procaine penicillin can be used until the patient can swallow oral penicillin. Erythromycin is used for penicillin-allergic patients. Both drugs are given for 14 days. Erythromycin (7 days) is the drug of choice for asymptomatic carriers. If compliance is uncertain, a single dose of benzathine penicillin IM can be used.

d. Supportive measures include bed rest, physiotherapy, attention to prevention of pressure sores, nasogastric feeding when swallowing is impaired, medical therapy for CHF. Tracheostomy is required if respiratory obstruction is imminent. Signs of laryngeal involvement should prompt early tracheostomy.

e. Strict isolation is important to prevent transmission in the hospital. Where cultures can be done, isolation is continued until three consecutive throat cultures at 24-hour intervals are negative.

f. Immunization for diphtheria should be started in the recovery phase as clinical infection does not induce immunity.

II. ENTERIC INFECTIONS

A. General

1. Enteric infections can be classified according to clinical symptoms.

Essentially all are transmitted by fecal-oral contamination as a result of food, water and close family contact. Improved hygiene, food handling and water purification are essential strategies to reduce incidence. Hospitalized patients require stool precautions. Effective treatment can reduce transmission.

2. Classification

Type of Diarrhea	Gastroenteritis (Non-inflammatory)	Dysentery (Inflammatory)
Location	Proximal small bowel	Distal small bowel, colon
Illness	Watery diarrhea, frequently with vomiting	Abdominal pain, tenesmus, small volume, mucoid, bloody stools
Stool exam	No fecal leukocytes	Fecal PMN's, frequently with rbcs
Organisms	Rotavirus, Norwalk virus Enterotoxigenic and enterohemmorhagic (O157) *E. coli* *Staphylococcus aureus* *Clostridium difficile* *Giardia lamblia* *Vibrio cholera* *Cryptosporidium* *Clostridium perfringens* *Bacillus cereus*	*Invasive E. coli* *Shigella* *Salmonella enteritidis* *Salmonella typhi* *Vibrio parahemolyticus* *Yersinia enterocolitica* *Campylobacter*

B. Evaluation
   1. History - ask about number and characteristics of stool; presence of fever, abdominal pain, tenesmus, antibiotic use, weight loss, underlying diseases.
   2. Physical exam - check for fever, toxicity, dehydration (especially common in infants).
   3. Stool examination (fresh specimen) - description of the stool (watery, mucoid, bloody), presence of fecal leukocytes, ova and parasites.
C. Gastroenteritis / Non-inflammatory diarrhea
   1. Acute Gastroenteritis in Children
      a. Acute, sporadic, watery diarrhea that occurs in young children.
      b. Can be due to rotaviruses and enterotoxigenic E. coli. It is an acute, noninflammatory diarrhea. Bile is not commonly seen in emesis. Blood and mucus are not usually seen in stool.
      c. In well-nourished infants, symptoms usually resolve in 2 - 3 days with hydration but may persist for several days. In malnourished children, diarrhea tends to persist and may be severe.
      d. Fever and vomiting may occur. With rotavirus, vomiting may precede diarrhea by 1-2 days.

    e. Treatment should be directed at restoration of fluid balance and improving nutritional status. Vomiting is not a contraindication to oral rehydration. Antibiotics are not needed.

    f. For mild dehydration (weight down 3-5%, mildly decreased urine output, eyes somewhat dry), 50 cc/kg of oral rehydration fluid either with the WHO formula or a similar "home-made" preparation should be given over 4 hours. For moderate dehydration (weight down 6-10%, decreased urine output, dry mouth and eyes), 100 cc/kg of oral rehydration fluid should be given over 4 hours. For severe dehydration (weight down 10%, altered mental status, tenting of skin, perhaps signs of shock), 20-40cc/kg of an isotonic intravenous fluid should be given rapidly and followed by ongoing intravenous, nasogastric, or oral rehydration.

    g. Once the dehydration is corrected, normal age-appropriate feedings should continue despite the diarrheal illness.

2. Traveler's diarrhea

    a. Onset of diarrhea 5-15 days after arrival in a foreign country.

    b. Symptoms include malaise, anorexia, nausea, vomiting, abdominal cramps, watery diarrhea. The diarrhea is noninflammatory, without blood or pus. Low- grade fever may be present.

    c. Usually caused by enterotoxigenic *E. coli* (50-60%).

    d. Usually self-limited and can be managed conservatively. Ciprofloxacin reduces duration of illness by 12-48hours. Antimotility agents such as imodium rapidly alleviate symptoms but must be avoided in children and in any patient with fever or bloody stool because of the risk of toxic megacolon.

    e. Prophylaxis with Pepto-Bismol 60cc qid or 2 tabs qid reduces risk. Prophylactic antibiotics (ciprofloxacin, TMP/SMX, doxycycline) are not routinely recommended.

3. *Giardia lamblia*

    a. Produces a chronic noninflammatory diarrhea. *G. lamblia* resides in the duodenum and upper small bowel.

    b. Symptoms include malaise, foul-smelling, fatty stools, abdominal bloating, belching, flatulence, weight loss.

    c. Diagnosed by finding cysts or trophozoites in the stool, but sensitivity is only 60%. Stool antigen tests are highly sensitive.

    d. Treatment is with metronidazole, tinidazole, furazolidone or paromomycin.

4. Antibiotic-associated colitis

    a. An acute colitis caused by toxins of *Clostridium difficile*. Pseudomembranes may or may not be present in the colon.

    b. Can develop after any antibiotic treatment, even short courses, by any route of administration and up to months after exposure. Most cases are related to clindamycin, ampicillin, or cephalosporins.

c. There is a wide range of clinical symptoms. The typical patient has profuse, watery diarrhea and crampy abdominal pain that develops 2 - 21days after starting antibiotics. High fever and leukocytosis are common. The stool may occasionally be bloody and often has leukocytes on stool exam.

d. Treatment
   (1) Patients with mild symptoms can be treated with discontinuation of antibiotics and supportive therapy with fluids.
   (2) Patients with fever, leukocytosis and abdominal pain should be treated with metronidazole 500-750mg tid x 7-10d. Vancomycin 125-500 mg po qid x 7-10d may be used, if available. IV metronidazole may be used if oral treatment is not possible. Cholestyramine 2 packets tid x 3-5d may decrease the frequency of diarrhea.
   (3) Patients with severe disease (toxic megacolon) may require surgery with colectomy.
   (4) Relapse occurs in 20% and requires retreatment, usually with metronidazole.

5. *Vibrio cholera*
   a. Acute noninflammatory, profuse watery diarrhea causing severe dehydration, with hypovolemic shock and death. Symptoms begin 8-24 hours after ingestion of contaminated food or water.
   b. Caused by cholera enterotoxin.
   c. Treatment is rehydration (ORF or IV). Tetracycline or doxycycline shortens the illness. Children < 8 years can be treated with TMP/SMX. Furazolidone can be used in pregnancy.

6. *Cryptosporidium parvum*
   a. Found as a primary pathogen in 3-10% of episodes of childhood diarrhea and is common in AIDS-associated diarrhea.
   b. Causes profuse watery, non-bloody diarrhea, often with recurrent episodes. Usually self-limited, but can last for several weeks in children.
   c. Treatment - none found to be effective.

7. *Isospora belli*
   a. Variable amounts of watery, non-bloody diarrhea. May be recurrent, particularly in AIDS patients.
   b. Treat with TMP/SMX 1 DS tablet bid x 10 days in normal hosts. In immunocompromised hosts use TMP/SMX 1 DS tablet qid x 10 days, then 1 DS tablet bid x 3 weeks. Children: 5 mg TMP/ 25 mg SMX per kg qid x 10 days then bid x 3 weeks. AIDS patients require long term suppression with TMP/SMX 1 DS tablet three times per week (5 mg TMP / 25 mg SMX per kg).

D. Dysentery (inflammatory diarrhea)
   1. General - Inflammatory enteritides produce acute colitis with fever and

frequent, small bowel movements accompanied by blood, mucus, and tenesmus or pain on defecation.

2. *Shigella species* (bacillary dysentery)
    a. Causes watery diarrhea and cramps initially, followed by bloody dysentery with high fever and systemic manifestations of malaise, headache and abdominal pain. Patients may develop severe rectal pain and tenesmus.
    b. Incubation period of 18 hours to 9 days (usually < 72h). Multiple cases often occur in families.
    c. Spread by direct contact or in food or water.
    d. Stool exam shows abundant WBC's and erythrocytes.
    e. Treatment will decrease duration of symptoms. TMP/SMX, ciprofloxacin or nalidixic acid for 3 days is effective but local resistance patterns vary and must be considered in choosing therapy.

3. *Salmonella enteritidis*
    a. Found in eggs and poultry.
    b. Symptoms begin 12-48h after ingestion.
    c. Produces watery diarrhea, cramps, fever and vomiting. Later stages may produce WBC's in the stool (usually less than shigellosis). Severe form can produce dysentery with bloody diarrhea and fever.
    d. May develop bacteremia (*S. choleraesuis*) especially in infants, elderly and those with sickle cell disease.
    e. Lasts 3-14 days. May develop an asymptomatic carrier state.
    f. Treat only severely ill or bacteremic patients with TMP/SMX 1 DS po bid x5d or ciprofloxacin 500mg bid x 5 days. Antibiotic therapy may prolong the carrier state.

4. *Campylobacter jejuni*
    a. Characterized by severe abdominal pain, fever, blood in stools, similar to salmonella and shigella. May also cause a watery, noninflammatory diarrhea.
    b. Associated with ingestion of contaminated water, raw milk, poorly cooked meat or poultry.
    c. Treat only if symptoms severe.
    d. Drug of choice is erythromycin for 5-7d. In adults, tetracycline or ciprofloxacin may also be used.

5. *Yersinia enterocolitica*
    a. Causes enteric fever-like picture with fever, headache, abdominal pain, diarrhea.
    b. May cause abdominal pain mimicking appendicitis.
    c. Occurs with increased frequency in patients with chronic liver disease. May have associated erythema nodosum and polyarthritis.
    d. Treatment is with chloramphenicol, TMP/SMX, tetracycline (>8 years) or ciprofloxacin (adults). It is a self-limited disease.

6. Hemorrhagic *E.coli* (O157)
  a. Occurs sporadically and with outbreaks.
  b. Severe abdominal pain, fever usually below 38.5°C, bloody diarrhea. 1-5% of patients develop hemolytic uremic syndrome.
  c. Treatment is supportive only. Antibiotics may increase risk of complications.
7. Amebic dysentery - see section IV, B, 1.
E. Typhoid Fever
  1. General
    a. Organism - *Salmonella typhi*.
    b. Typhoid fever is a serious multi-system illness marked by fever and abdominal symptoms with a prolonged clinical course. It should be suspected in patients with 1-3 weeks of persistent fever and GI complaints (especially diarrhea and abdominal pain).
    c. It is usually transmitted by ingestion of contaminated food or water via a fecal-oral route in areas of poor sanitation.
  2. Clinical presentation

Natural History of Untreated Typhoid Fever						
Time Course	Temp. Range	Pathologic Events	Disease Manifestations	Blood Cult	Stool Cult	Widal Test
0-1 wk	36.5°-38°C.	Proliferation of organisms in gut, penetration of gut mucosa	Diarrhea in 10-20% of patients	-	-	-
1-2 wk	37°-39.5°	Proliferation within gut lymphoid tissue, subsequent spread to regional lymphoid tissue and beyond, septicemia	Headache, malaise, myalgia, anorexia, nausea, cough, sore throat, constipation, possible diarrhea	+ 80%	-	+ 20%
2-4 wk	38°-39.5°	Reticuloendothelial proliferation in response to bacteremia, metastatic foci infection, focal necrosis and ulceration at sites of previous lymphoid proliferation	Toxemia, abdominal discomfort, neuropsychiatric syndromes, intestinal ulceration, genitourinary syndromes, bronchitis, relative bradycardia, hepato-splenomegaly, rose spots, anemia, leukopenia, intestinal perforation and hemorrhage	+ 80%	+ 80%	+50%
4-5 wk	36°-38°	Body defenses overcome organisms, repair and recovery of damaged tissue	Intercurrent relapse possible (3-15%)	-	+50%	+ 80%
>5 wk	---	Metastatic foci of infection possible	Cholecystitis, osteomyelitis, soft tissue abscess	-	+15%	-

3. Diagnosis

a. Blood culture is most definitive but positive in only 50-80% of cases.

b. Widal test is very problematic, frequently gives misinformation, and has marginal clinical value. The minimum positive titer must be determined in individual geographic areas and is higher in endemic regions.

c. WBC can be low or normal (leukocytosis with left shift suggests intestinal perforation).

d. In children, the diagnosis of typhoid should be considered when fever persists despite good treatment for malaria and a good search for other localized sites of infection.

4. Treatment

a. Any of the following antibiotics may be used: chloramphenicol (po as effective as IV if the patient is able to eat), TMP/SMX, quinolones, ceftriaxone. Treat relapse with additional one week of therapy.

b. Steroids - have been shown to reduce mortality in severe typhoid fever but should be reserved for toxic, delirious or obtunded patients with persistent fever and benign abdominal exam. Recommended doses are higher than those used for most other conditions. The initial recommended dose is dexamethasone 3 mg/kg IV over 30 minutes, followed by 1 mg/kg q6h x 48 hours.

c. GI hemorrhage (usually ileal) and perforation occur in about 5% of patients, and may warrant surgical intervention. Adjust antibiotic coverage to include anerobes, Gram (-) rods, and enterococci (see Sepsis: intra-abdominal, Table 1).

d. Special attention to enteric precautions is critical.

III. MENINGITIS

A. General

1. Meningitis most commonly presents as an acute infectious process with signs and symptoms developing over hours to a few days. Some meningitis pathogens typically cause a subacute or chronic course, with symptoms developing over days to weeks or months.

2. Acute encephalitis and meningitis overlap in their presentation and in some cases the disease process is best described as a meningoen-cephalitis, with features of both meningitis and encephalitis.

3. A wide variety of pathogens can cause meningitis, however the majority of cases are caused by a small number of pathogens.

4. Meningitis can also be caused by non-infectious processes; aseptic meningitis from various drugs (NSAIDS, TMP/SMX and others), and chronic meningitis from malignancy.

5. Recurrent meningitis is typically seen in patients with CSF leaks following head trauma and is caused by the usual meningitis pathogens, most commonly *S. pneumoniae*.

B. Etiologic agents

1. Three pathogens account for the majority of cases of bacterial meningitis: *Streptococcus pneumoniae*, *Hemophilus influenzae* and *Neisseria meningitidis*.
2. These pathogens commonly colonize the nasopharynx and may be carried asymptomatically, or may cause a variety of respiratory tract syndromes prior to the onset of meningitis.
3. Other pathogens must also be considered, particularly at the extremes of age, and in patients with unusual presentations or underlying immunodeficiency.
4. Empiric treatment of meningitis should take into consideration the patient's age and immune status.

Etiologic agents of Meningitis	
Condition	**Organisms**
Age: 0-8 weeks	*Strep. agalactiae* (Group B), Enteric Gram negative bacilli (*E. coli, Klebsiella pneumoniae*), *Enterococcus* (Group D Strep.), *Listeria monocytogenes, Salmonella*
Age: 8 weeks - 8 years	*H. influenzae, S. pneumoniae, N. meningitidis*
Age: 8 - 50 years	*S. pneumoniae, N. meningitidis*
Age: > 50 years	*S. pneumoniae, N. meningitidis, Listeria*, Gram negative bacilli
HIV infected	*Cryptococcus neoformans*
CSF leak / skull fracture	*S. pneumoniae, H. influenzae, a hemolytic streptococci*
Contiguous infection (otitis, sinusitis, mastoiditis)	Anaerobes, gram negative bacilli, may be polymicrobial

5. Viral meningitis
   a. A variety of viruses cause an aseptic meningitis syndrome.
   b. Characterized by (typically) a milder course with headache, neck stiffness and a lymphocytic pleocytosis with normal glucose on CSF examination.

Viral Causes of Meningitis	
Enteroviruses	Seasonal incidence (summer / fall) in temperate areas, year round in tropical and subtropical areas.
Mumps	Most common viral cause of meningitis in unimmunized population. Low CSF glucose and neutrophil predominance may suggest bacterial meningitis. Parotid enlargement may be absent.
Arboviruses	Wide variety of endemic viruses, often prominent encephalitic symptoms.
Lymphocytic Choriomeningitis virus	Acquired through contact with rodents or rodent excreta.
Herpes viruses	Aseptic meningitis (associated with primary or relapsed genital herpes or herpes zoster) Herpes simplex encephalitis
HIV	Aseptic meningitis can be seen in early HIV infection (seroconversion illness)

6. Other causes of meningitis

    a. Spirochetal meningitis - neurosyphilis, neuroborreliosis, leptospirosis.

    b. Amoebic meningoencephalitis - several species of free-living amoebas can cause meningitis / meningoencephalitis. Cases are rare, but almost universally fatal. Wet mount of CSF may demonstrate motile amoebas.

    c. Parasitic meningitis - a prominent eosinophilia of CSF should raise suspicion of parasitic meningitis due to migrating helminth larvae. *Angiostrongylus cantonensis* is an important cause of eosinophilic meningitis in SE Asia, the Pacific and the Caribbean. Other helminths such as *Schistosoma, Gnathostoma spinigerum, Taenia solium* and *Paragonimus* may cause eosinophilic meningitis. Hematologic malignancies can cause eosinophilic meningitis and must be considered in the differential.

C. Clinical

1. Symptoms of meningitis usually include fever, severe headache, and neck stiffness. Mental status changes and seizures may occur. Irritability or listlessness, poor feeding, temperature instability and vomiting are common symptoms in young infants. The onset of symptoms is usually abrupt, but occasionally may progress over several days.

2. Physical examination

    a. Older children and adults show signs of meningeal inflammation including stiff neck, Kernig's and Brudzinski's signs.

    b. Neonates and young children do not develop typical meningeal signs. In infants, a bulging fontanelle is an important finding.

    c. Confusion, delirium and coma develop later in the course of meningitis. A careful examination for associated sinusitis, otitis, and mastoiditis should be done in all cases.

    d. Focal neurologic signs occur in 10-20% of patients, most commonly cranial nerve palsies (especially III, IV, VI and VII nerves), presenting as eye movement abnormalities and facial droop. Hemiparesis suggests an associated subdural effusion.

    e. Petechial or purpuric rashes are classically associated with meningococcemia but can also be seen with overwhelming infections due to *S. pneumoniae* or *H. influenzae*.

    f. Progressive focal signs and papilledema, particularly when seen in the absence of meningismus suggest brain abscess or other space-occupying lesions.

D. Laboratory

1. Lumbar puncture should be performed immediately in patients suspected of having bacterial meningitis.

2. Antibiotic therapy should be initiated without waiting for the results of CSF analysis. If an LP can be done immediately and fluid will be sent for culture, the first dose of antibiotic can be administered as soon as CSF is obtained.

3. If any delay in obtaining CSF is anticipated, draw a blood culture and administer antibiotics immediately. Where CSF examination is limited to microscopy, cell counts and chemistry (culture not available), there is no reason to wait for the CSF to be obtained before giving the first dose of antibiotics.

4. CSF analysis should include:
   a. Tube #1: Protein and glucose
   b. Tube #2: Gram stain, culture, Acid-fast smear
   c. Tube #3: Cell count, differential
   d. Tube #4: Use for other tests such as wet mount, India Ink, cytology, syphilis serology, if indicated and initial investigations do not yield a diagnosis.

5. CSF results

CSF Findings in Meningitis					
Test	Normal	Bacterial	Tuberculosis / Fungal	Viral / Aseptic	Herpes Encephalitis
Opening pressure	< 20 cm H2O	> 20	> 20	< 20	-
WBC/mm³	Neonate ≤ 22 Others < 5 (lymphocytes)	1,000-5,000 neutrophil predominance	< 1,000 mononuclear cells (lymphs, monocytes)	< 1,000 lymphocyte predominance	< 500 lymphocytes
RBC/mm³	0 (except bloody tap)	0 - +	0 - +	0 - +	+++
Glucose	45-80 mg/dl 2/3 blood glucose	Marked decrease	Decreased	Normal (exception: mumps, LCM)	Normal
Protein mg/dl	≤ 45	100 - 500	100-5000	50 - 100	Mild increase
Special stains	No organisms seen	Gram stain: + in 60-90%	Acid fast stain is very low yield for diagnosis of TB. India ink or Gram stain may show yeast cells in Cryptococcus	No organisms seen	No organisms seen
Other tests	-	RPR	Culture for TB, fungi	-	PCR, Viral culture

6. A traumatic tap (bloody tap) will contain ~ 1 WBC for every 700 RBC present in the fluid unless the patient's WBC is markedly elevated or decreased. If only a drop of CSF is obtained, the most

helpful test to confirm bacterial meningitis is a WBC count. The presence of > 1 polymorphonuclear leukocyte / hpf on a differential stain is very suggestive of bacterial meningitis.

7. Microscopic examination of spun sediment of CSF will demonstrate the pathogen in many cases. When possible, cultures should be done to confirm the etiology and to identify a pathogen in cases where an organism is not seen on Gram stain.

Gram Stain of CSF	
Gram positive diplococcus	*S. pneumonia*
Gram negative diplococcus	*N. meningitidis*
Gram negative coccobacillus	*Haemophilus influenzae*
Gram positive bacillus	*Listeria monocytogenes*
Gram negative bacillus	*E. coli, Klebsiella* and others

E. Treatment (according to pathogen)
1. *S. pneumoniae*
a. Increasing antibiotic resistance, particularly in *S. pneumoniae* has complicated the management of bacterial meningitis. In many developing countries, optimal therapy for drug resistant *S. pneumoniae* may not be readily available. Where accurate susceptibility testing of pathogens is available, results can be used to guide therapy, particularly in *S. pneumoniae* meningitis where susceptibility is no longer predictable and unrecognized resistance may result in poor outcomes.

b. Penicillin resistance in *S. pneumoniae* is increasing around the world. Penicillin resistance is graded as intermediate (MIC 0.1 - 1.0 micrograms/ml) or high level (MIC > 1.0 micrograms/ml).

c. Non-meningeal infections due to intermediately-penicillin resistant *S. pneumoniae* can often be treated successfully with an increased dose of penicillin or ampicillin. Treatment of meningitis is complicated by poor antibiotic penetration across the blood-brain barrier and even increased doses of penicillin will not achieve adequate bactericidal levels.

d. Recommended therapy for intermediate or high-level resistant *S. pneumoniae* meningitis is a combination of ceftriaxone or cefotaxime and vancomycin (plus rifampin for high level resistant strains), drugs that are often not available in developing countries. Since penicillin resistance in *S. pneumoniae* is due to alterations in penicillin binding proteins (not beta lactamase production) use of beta-lactamase inhibitor combinations is ineffective.

e. Penicillin resistance is typically accompanied by decreased susceptibility to cephalosporins and resistance to unrelated antibiotics including erythromycin, chloramphenicol and TMP/SMX. Providing optimal therapy for drug resistant *S. pneumoniae* in resource-limited environments is very difficult and as yet there is no data on which to base treatment recommendations if third generation cephalosporins and vancomycin are not available.

   f. Use of high dose ampicillin (ie: 14 grams/day in adults) plus chloramphenicol and rifampin may be a reasonable approach if first line drugs are not available. Follow-up CSF examination to document resolution should be considered.

2. *Hemophilus influenzae* - frequently resistant to ampicillin but usually sensitive to chloramphenicol.

3. *Neisseria meningitidis* - usually sensitive to penicillin (ampicillin) but a few reports of chloramphenicol resistance have recently appeared.

F. Empiric treatment by age

Treatment of Bacterial Meningitis		
	Recommended agents and doses	**Preferred Rx (if available)**
Neonate < 7 days	Ampicillin 50mg/kg IV q12h plus Gentamicin 2.5mg/kg IV/IM q12h	Ampicillin + Cefotaxime
Neonate >7days	Ampicillin 50mg/kg IV q8h plus Gentamicin 2.5mg/kg IV/IM q12h	Ampicillin + Cefotaxime
1-2 months	Ampicillin 50-75mg/kg IV q6h plus Gentamicin 2.5mg/kg IV/IM q8h	Ampicillin + Cefotaxime
2 months to 8 years	Ampicillin 50-75mg/kg IV q6h plus Chloramphenicol 25mg/kg IV q6h	Cefotaxime or ceftriaxone
8 years to adult	Penicillin G 300,000 units/kg/d IV divided q4h or Ampicillin 75mg/kg q4h IV plus Chloramphenicol 1 gm IV q6h (100mg/kg/d). Long acting Chloroamphenicol in an oily solution has been used successfully in epidemics in West Africa.	Cefotaxime or ceftriaxone
Adults > 50 years	Ampicillin 2gm IV q4h plus Chloramphenicol 50 mg/kg/d divided q6h	Ampicillin + Cefotaxime

1. Antibiotic dosage:
   a. Cefotaxime dose - 200 mg/kg/day in 3-4 doses per day.
   b. Ceftriaxone (100 mg/kg/day divided q12h) may be used in place of cefotaxime.
   c. Cefuroxime (a second generation cephalosporin) has been associated with delayed sterilization of CSF and higher rates of relapse and complications and should not be used to treat meningitis.

2. Duration of treatment (minimum)
   a. *H. influenzae*: 7-10 days

b. *Strep. pneumoniae* - 10 days

c. *Neisseria meningitidis* - 7 days

d. Group B strep - 14-21 days

e. Gram-negative bacilli: 21 days. Treat with TMP/SMX 20/100 mg/kg/day divided q6h. Chloramphenicol is ineffective in meningitis due to enteric gram negative bacilli.

f. *Listeria monocytogenes* - 14-21 days. Ampicillin + gentamicin is usually effective. TMP/SMX may be used in patients allergic to penicillin.

3. **Rifampin prophylaxis for household contacts of meningitis cases:**

Rifampin prophylaxis (maximum dose: 600 mg)		
Neisseria meningitidis	Age < 1 month	5 mg/kg q12h x 2 days
	Age > 1 month	10 mg/kg q12h x 2 days
Hemophilus influenzae	Age < 1 month	10 mg/kg q24h x 4 days
	Age > 1 month	20 mg/kg q24h x 4 days
Strep. pneumoniae	-	Not indicated

4. **Steroids in bacterial meningitis**

a. Steroids have been demonstrated to decrease hearing deficits and other long-term neurologic sequelae in *H. influenzae* meningitis. Benefit in other bacterial meningitides is not established. The potential benefits of steroids must be balanced against the risks, and the likelihood of *H. influenzae* vs. other pathogens.

b. Steroids should only be used if they can be administered prior to any antibiotics (but administration of antibiotics should not be delayed more than a few minutes to permit steroid administration). If steroids are delayed until after antibiotics have been started, the beneficial effects are lost.

c. The recommended dose is dexamethasone 0.4 mg/kg IV q12h x 2 days.

d. In areas where cerebral malaria and meningitis overlap in occurrence and clinical presentation, use of steroids is best avoided as they have been shown to worsen the outcome of cerebral malaria. Delaying antibiotic therapy to await CSF results (to confirm meningitis vs. cerebral malaria), in order to make a decision about steroid administration is not appropriate.

5. **Pyogenic brain abscess**

a. High-dose IV penicillin plus chloramphenicol or metronidazole.

b. Surgical drainage usually is necessary.

c. Need prolonged treatment (weeks to months).

IV. PARASITIC INFECTIONS

A. Intestinal helminth infections

1. *Ancylostoma duodenale* and *Necator americanus* (hookworm)

a. Organism - adult hookworms are grayish white, 1 cm in length. Hookworms live in the upper small bowel where they are attached to the mucosa by their mouthparts. The incidence of hookworm infestation is very high in tropical and subtropical areas. Infection is acquired when larvae in soil penetrate intact skin. Larvae undergo a period of migration before reaching the gut and maturing to adult worms.

b. Clinical manifestations - larval penetration is often unrecognized but may cause local skin reactions with intense pruritus, erythema and a papular-vesicular rash. During the acute (migration) phase of infection, cough, wheezing and dyspnea may occur. When larvae reach the GI tract and begin to attach, abdominal pain, diarrhea and weight loss may occur. The major adverse effect of hookworm infection is anemia. In areas where hookworm infections are common and people harbour many adult worms, chronic iron-deficiency anemia is common. Heavily infected patients may also develop hypoalbuminemia and protein-energy malnutrition.

c. Diagnosis - eggs can be seen on direct examination of fresh stool. If the stool is not examined promptly, eggs may hatch and can be mistaken for *Strongyloides* larvae. Prompt examination or use of preservative will avoid confusion.

d. Treatment - mebendazole 100mg po bid x 3 days or albendazole 400mg po x 1 dose (same doses for children and adults). Iron supplementation (1-2 mg elemental iron per kg per day) should be given to correct any associated iron deficiency.

e. Prevention - Contact with contaminated soil for 5-10 minutes is sufficient for larval penetration. Proper waste disposal and avoidance of direct contact with soil will reduce infection rates and worm burdens.

2. *Ascaris lumbricoides* (Ascariasis, roundworm)

a. Organism - *Ascaris* is the most common helminth infecting humans. The worm is present worldwide but most prevalent in tropical areas. Adult worms are white or yellowish, 15-35cm long and live in the small intestine. Ascariasis is acquired through ingestion of eggs. Eggs hatch in the gut and larvae undergo a period of migration before returning to the gut and maturing to adults.

b. Clinical manifestations - ascariasis is frequently asymptomatic. When the worm burden is high, small bowel obstruction can be caused by large masses of worms. Adult worms sometimes migrate from their usual site and can obstruct the bile duct, pancreatic duct or appendix. Heavy worm burdens have also been associated with cognitive impairment and poor school performance. During larval migration, wheezing, cough, dyspnea and pulmonary infiltrates may occur.

c. Diagnosis - stool exam will demonstrate eggs.

    d. Treatment - use one of the following:
      (1) Mebendazole 100 mg bid x 3 days.
      (2) Albendazole 400 mg x 1 dose.
      (3) Pyrantel pamoate 11 mg/kg (max. 1 gram) daily x 3 days.
      (4) Piperazine citrate is recommended in cases of biliary or intestinal obstruction, given as 150mg/kg initially (po or NG), followed by 65mg/kg q 12h x 6 doses. Piperazine may alleviate the obstruction by narcotizing the worms.

3. *Enterobius vermicularis* (Enterobiasis, pinworm)
    a. Organism - pinworms are small, white, thread-like worms 1cm in length. Pinworm infection is prevalent around the world and is the most common helminth infection in temperate countries. Infection of one family member is usually associated with infection of most or all of the rest of the household.
    b. Clinical manifestations - infection is frequently asymptomatic. When symptomatic, infection presents with perianal and perineal pruritus. Intense itching is triggered by female worms emerging from the anus to deposit eggs on the perianal skin at night. Nocturnal restlessness and disturbed sleep can lead to daytime irritability and sleepiness in children.
    c. Diagnosis - stool examination has low sensitivity (<5%) for diagnosis of pinworms since eggs are deposited on the perianal skin, not released into the lumen of the bowel. The "scotch tape test" is the best method of diagnosis. This is most easily done by folding ~ 8 cm of clear (not "invisible") cellophane tape lengthwise over the end of a tongue depressor with the sticky side out. This should be placed along the anal verge and the buttocks closed over the tongue depressor. Remove the tongue depressor and place the tape, sticky side down on a microscope slide. Eggs will be seen under low power. The scotch tape test should be done in the early morning. A single scotch tape test will detect ~50% of infections, 3 tests on separate days will detect 90%.
    d. Treatment - use one of the following:
      (1) Mebendazole 100 mg x 1 dose, repeat in two weeks.
      (2) Albendazole 400 mg x 1 dose, repeat in two weeks.
      (3) Pyrantel pamoate 11 mg/kg (max. 1 gram) q 2 weeks x 3 doses.
      (4) Treat all members of the household at the same time.

4. *Trichuris trichiura* (Trichuriasis, whipworm)
    a. Organism - adult worms are pinkish gray with an average length of 40mm. The anterior end of the worm is elongated and very thin (whip-like), this part of the worm embeds in the mucosa of the cecum and ascending colon where enzymes secreted by the worm break down local tissues.
    b. Clinical manifestations - low-grade infections are usually

asymptomatic. Heavily infected patients may present with iron deficiency anemia and bloody diarrhea caused by damage to the intestinal mucosa. Irritation caused by embedded worms causes repetitive straining, which may lead to rectal prolapse in children.

c. Diagnosis - stool examination will demonstrate eggs.

d. Treatment - mebendazole 100mg po bid x 3 days or albendazole 400mg po x 1 dose. Heavily infected patients may require re-treatment.

5. *Strongyloides stercoralis* (Strongyloidiasis)

a. Organism - adult worms are colorless, semi-transparent, 0.7mm - 2.2 mm in length. Strongyloidiasis is most prevalent in tropical and subtropical areas. Infection is initiated when larvae in soil penetrate intact skin. Larvae undergo a period of migration before maturing to adults and reaching the upper small intestine where they burrow into the mucosa. *Strongyloides* is capable of auto-infection (larvae re-infect the host by penetrating the intestinal mucosa or peri-anal skin, without having to pass through a period of development in soil). Untreated infections can therefore persist for decades. Immuno-compromised hosts may develop very high parasite burdens due to repeated cycles of auto-infection.

b. Clinical manifestations (symptoms correlate with the stage of infection)

(1) Larval penetration of skin causes a pruritic papular erythematous rash similar to that seen with hookworm infection.

(2) Migration of larvae through the lungs causes cough, wheezing and dyspnea with pulmonary infiltrates and eosinophilia (Loeffler-like syndrome).

(3) Penetration of the intestinal mucosa by adults produces an acute gastroenteritis-like syndrome with nausea, vomiting, burning or colicky abdominal pain, diarrhea and the passage of mucus.

(4) With chronic infection, malabsorption and weight loss can occur. Eosinophilia is common and may be persistent because of ongoing migration of auto-infecting larvae.

(5) Hyperinfection syndrome - in immunocompromised hosts, an overwhelming infection can occur with massive invasion of tissues with larvae. Larvae may carry bacteria from the gut as they migrate resulting in infections of various tissues (usually gram-negative). Clinical manifestations seen in hyperinfection syndrome include dyspnea and pulmonary infiltrates, abdominal pain and peritonitis, meningitis and generalized sepsis. Patients with hematologic malignancies, steroid therapy, lepromatous leprosy, HIV infection and severe malnutrition are susceptible to hyperinfection syndrome. Eosinophilia may be absent in overwhelming infection with *Strongyloides*.

      c. Diagnosis - stool examination will demonstrate larvae (not eggs!) in feces. Larvae must be distinguished from hookworm larvae in stools that have not been examined promptly. Since the number of larvae in stool may be small, a concentration technique or repeated stool exams may be necessary. In hyperinfection syndrome, larvae may be identified in sputum, CSF or tissues.

      d. Treatment - use one of the following:

          (1) Thiabendazole 25 mg/kg po bid x 2 days (max. 3 g/day).

          (2) Albendazole 400 mg po once daily x 3 days.

          (3) Ivermectin 200 micrograms/kg/day po x 2 days.

          (4) Hyperinfection syndrome requires treatment for 2-3 weeks.

6. Cestodes (tapeworm)

      a. Organism - cestodes (or tapeworms) are segmented worms. Human disease can be due to adult worms living in the GI tract, or larval stages in tissues.

      b. Clinical manifestations

          (1) Intestinal infections - tapeworm infections usually come to the patient's attention when worm segments (which are actively motile) are passed in stool or emerge from the anus. Other symptoms (abdominal discomfort, nausea, anorexia and weight loss) are usually mild. Infections with the fish tapeworm can present with features of vitamin B12 deficiency.

          (2) Extraintestinal infections - larval tapeworm infections cause symptoms when larval cysts enlarge causing a space-occupying lesion or when encysted larvae die, causing local inflammation.

             (a) Cysticercosis - larval tapeworm infection due to *Taenia solium* (pork tapeworm). Encysted larvae (cysticerci) can be found in any organ of the body but symptoms usually result from cysticerci in the brain. Inflammation caused by dying larvae causes seizures and focal neurologic signs. In some areas of the world, neurocysticercosis is the most common cause of adult onset seizures. Symptoms and signs of increased intracranial pressure (headache, nausea, vomiting, ataxia and confusion) and chronic meningitis can also occur. Multiple small subcutaneous nodules may provide a clue to the diagnosis in heavily infected patients.

             (b) Hydatid disease - larval infection due to *Echinococcus* species are most prevalent in sheep-rearing areas where sheep serve as the main intermediate host. Outside sheep-rearing areas, a wide range of other species can be intermediate hosts. Hydatid cysts most commonly develop in the liver, followed by spleen, lung and other tissues. Clinical symptoms arise from pressure on adjacent tissues from the enlarging cyst (RUQ pain / mass), allergic reactions to leaking cyst fluid (urticaria, eosinophilia, anaphylaxis), and cyst rupture (anaphylaxis, cough, chest pain, hemoptysis, dissemination of larvae to other organs).

(3) Diagnosis
   (a) Intestinal tapeworm infections are diagnosed by stool examination (eggs or worm segments).
   (b) Plain radiographs of soft tissues may demonstrate typical calcified "puffed rice" lesions in muscles in patients with cysticercosis.
   (c) CSF in neurocysticercosis typically shows decreased glucose, increased protein and mononuclear cell pleocytosis.
   (d) Abdominal ultrasound is helpful in the diagnosis of hydatid disease. Occasionally hydatid cysts calcify and can be seen on plain radiographs. Total calcification of the cyst implies that the parasite is non-viable and no treatment is required but lesser degrees of calcification do not guarantee non-viability.

(4) Treatment

Treatment of Cestode Infections	
Diphyllobothium latum (Fish)	Praziquantel 10mg/kg x 1 dose for children and adults
Dipylidium caninum (Dog)	
Taenia saginata (Beef)	
Taenia solium (Pork)	
Hymenolepis nana (Humans)	Praziquantel 25 mg/kg x 1 dose for children and adults
Hymenolepis diminuta (Rat)	
Neurocysticercosis (*T. solium*)	Praziquantel 50 mg/kg/day in 3 doses x 15 days Albendazole 15 mg/kg/day in 2 doses x 8-30 days (max 400 mg bid) Dexamethasone +/- anticonvulsants should be given to reduce risk of seizures.
Hydatid disease (*Echinococcus*)	Complete surgical excision of the cyst is the preferred treatment but requires expert surgical skill. Injection of scolicidal agents (95% ethanol, 30% saline) into the cyst prior to resection is recommended to decrease the risk of seeding tissues with viable larvae if cyst leakage occurs during resection.Fine needle aspiration with instillation of scolicidal agents and reaspiration is an alternative to surgery. Antihelminthic chemotherapy can be used for patients where operative management is not possible or pre-operatively to decrease the risk of dissemination with cyst rupture. Albendazole 15 mg/kg/day in 2 doses (max 400 mg bid) x 28 days. Stop drug for two weeks then repeat albendazole course x 2 (total of 3 cycles) Mebendazole 50-70 mg/kg/day for several months (not as effective as albendazole).

B. Intestinal protozoan infections

    1. *Entamoeba histolytica* (Amoebiasis)

        a. Organism - *E. histolytica* is an amoeba that principally causes intestinal disease but can become invasive and cause disease outside the GI tract, primarily in the liver. *E. dispar*, a closely related amoeba, is indistinguishable from *E. histolytica* on stool exam but is non-pathogenic. In the developing world 10-50% of individuals carry either *E. histolytica* or *E. dispar.* Carriers of *E. histolytica* excrete cysts, which survive in the environment and transmit the disease to others when ingested. Contamination of water supplies can result in large outbreaks of amoebiasis. Improved sanitation is the primary preventative strategy.

        b. Intestinal amoebiasis

            (1) Asymptomatic cyst passers - cysts are found in the stool in the absence of clinical symptoms. Some asymptomatic cyst passers will subsequently develop invasive disease. Those who are carrying pathogenic strains are an important source of infection for others. Treatment is recommended both to reduce the risk of progression to invasive disease and the risk of transmission.

            (2) Symptomatic intestinal disease can present as:

                (a) Mild intermittent colitis - non-bloody diarrhea, mucus, abdominal pain, flatulence and weight loss.

                (b) Acute dysenteric colitis - bloody diarrhea, abdominal pain and tenderness, tenesmus, and dehydration. Fever is uncommon.

                (c) Fulminant colitis - severe bloody diarrhea with progression to bowel wall necrosis, perforation, or toxic megacolon.

                (d) Amoeboma - localized chronic granulomatous lesion in the bowel, presents with obstructive symptoms. May be mistaken for bowel carcinoma.

                (e) Perianal ulceration can develop in patients with active diarrhea due to *E. histolytica* from direct invasion of the peri-anal skin by trophozoites.

            (3) Diagnosis

                (a) Stool exam - cysts or trophozoites identified in the stool must be distinguished from non-pathogenic species. Trophozoites with ingested RBC are characteristic (but not invariable) in invasive disease due to *E. histolytica*. Patients with acute diarrhea usually excrete only trophozoites, which disintegrate quickly after being passed in the stool. When *E. histolytica* is suspected, stool must be examined immediately or placed in preservative to prevent deterioration of the trophozoites. For patients with asymptomatic infection or intermittent diarrhea, cysts are often excreted only intermittently and multiple stool examinations may be required to prove the diagnosis. A single

stool exam will identify only 1/3 of infected patients.
- (b) Proctoscopy may show colitis with punctate hemorrhagic areas or small ulcers, but can be normal in early disease.
- (4) Treatment is recommended for all persons with documented infection with *E. histolytica*, even in the absence of symptoms. See table below.

c. Amoebic liver abscess
- (1) Liver abscess is the most common extra-intestinal manifestation of *E. histolytica* infection. There may or may not be evidence of a previous or concurrent intestinal infection with *E. histolytica*.
- (2) Clinical
  - (a) Clinical presentation is extremely variable. Diarrhea occurs in 30-40% of patients. Few patients have detectable cysts or trophozoites in the stool, however very sensitive laboratory techniques will demonstrate intestinal colonization in most. Failure to eradicate intestinal colonization has been associated with recurrences of liver abscesses.
  - (b) Acute form - spiking fever, leukocytosis, right upper quadrant pain and exquisite tenderness over the liver. Pain may be referred to the right shoulder. Hepatomegaly is often absent. 10-15% of cases present as "fever of unknown origin".
  - (c) Subacute form - fatigue, weight loss, and hepatomegaly. Less than one half of patients have fever or abdominal pain. Must differentiate from hepatoma.
- (3) Complications
  - (a) Pleuropulmonary involvement is the most common complication of amoebic liver abscess, usually due to rupture or erosion through the diaphragm. Patients present with cough, pleuritic chest pain, dyspnea and dullness and crackles at the right lung base. Extension of infection into the pericardium will result in a pericardial friction rub and effusion.
  - (b) Intraperitoneal rupture occurs most commonly in abscesses of the left lobe. Sudden perforation presents with a rigid, distended abdomen that suggests a perforated viscus. The mortality rate is very high.
  - (c) Cerebral amoebiasis - *E. histolytica* is a rare cause of brain abscess. This complication should be considered in patients with known amoebiasis who suddenly develop altered mental status or focal neurologic signs. Onset is very abrupt with rapid progression to death in 12-72 hours without adequate therapy.
- (4) Laboratory
  - (a) Leukocytosis with a left shift, without eosinophilia.
  - (b) Mild anemia occurs in ~ 50%.
  - (c) Hyperbilirubinemia is unusual and suggests severe disease or

peritonitis.
- (d) Elevated alkaline phosphatase is present in 80%. Transaminases are often normal, may be elevated in severe disease.
- (e) Stool exam is usually negative for *E. histolytica* cysts or trophozoites.

(5) Chest x-ray
- (a) Elevation of the right hemidiaphragm. Atelectasis or infiltrates in the right lower lobe.
- (b) Pleural effusions are often present and may be serous or purulent (from rupture of an abscess through the diaphragm).

(6) Abdominal ultrasound
- (a) Hepatic lesions are typically single, hypodense, round or oval in shape, located peripherally near the capsule and in the right lobe in 3/4 of the cases.
- (b) Early lesions may appear solid or heterogeneous.
- (c) If the abscess is centrally located, intrahepatic bile ducts may be dilated.
- (d) Even in experienced hands, ultrasound cannot always differentiate amoebic abscess from hepatoma.

(7) Treatment

Therapy for Amoebiasis	
Disease	**Drug**
Cyst passers	Iodoquinol 650 mg tid x 20 days (10 mg/kg tid)
	Paromomycin 10 mg/kg tid x 7 days
	Diloxanide furoate 500 mg tid x 10 days (10 mg /kg tid)
Colitis (Dysentery)	Metronidazole 750 mg tid x 10 day (15 mg/kg tid)* **followed by** iodoquinol, diloxanide or paromomycin
	Tinidazole 1 gram q12h (25 mg/kg q12h) x 3 days **followed by** iodoquinol, diloxanide or paromomycin
	Tetracycline 250 mg qid x 15 days **plus** chloroquine base 600 mg stat, 300 in 6 hours then 150 mg TID x 14 days
Liver abscess	Metronidazole 750 mg tid x 5-10 days (15 mg/kg tid) **followed by** iodoquinol, diloxanide or paromomycin. Clinical response should be evident within 3 days.
	Chloroquine base, 600 mg stat, 300 mg in 6 hours, then 300 mg daily x 14-28 days (10 mg base / kg daily). Can be used in pregnancy or added to metronidazole in patients who do not respond promptly to treatment.
	Tinidazole 600 mg bid - 800 mg tid (20 mg/kg tid) x 5 days **followed by** iodoquinol, diloxanide or paromomycin
	Aspiration (using ultrasound guidance) is indicated in patients who fail to respond to metronidazole, or in very large cysts (>10cm) with an increased risk of rupture. In seriously ill patients, aspiration of the abscess may shorten the recovery time. Open drainage is usually best avoided because of the risk of secondary bacterial infection. Occasionally laparotomy with needle aspiration may be required for drainage of deep abscesses, especially in the left lobe.

*Alternative dosing regimens for metronidazole: 2.4 grams once daily for 2-3 days, 50 mg/kg stat (single dose).

Do not use iodoquinol, diloxanide or tetracycline in pregnancy. Recommendations regarding use of metronidazole in pregnancy are conflicting. Avoid in 1st trimester, use with caution in 2nd and 3rd. Paromomycin and chloroquine may be used in pregnancy.

2. *Giardia lamblia* (Giardiasis)
   a. Organism - *Giardia* is a flagellated protozoan that inhabits the upper small intestine of many species. Infection is acquired through ingestion of contaminated food or water.
   b. Clinical manifestations
      (1) 50% of infected individuals are asymptomatic.
      (2) Symptomatic infections may be manifested by mild, intermittent diarrhea, often with prominent bloating and flatulence, recurrent episodes of diarrhea, or severe diarrhea with malabsorption and steatorrhea.
      (3) Giardiasis is more severe and prolonged in patients with immunoglobulin deficiencies or AIDS. In AIDS patients, giardiasis may fail to respond to treatment or recur each time treatment is stopped.
   c. Diagnosis can be difficult due to intermittent cyst excretion and repeated stool examinations may be required. Both cysts and trophozoites may be seen in the stool. Where available, stool antigen tests for *Giardia* are useful and have higher sensitivity than stool microscopy.
   d. Treatment is with metronidazole 250mg (5mg/kg) po tid x 5 days or albendazole 400mg po once daily x 5 days.
3. *Isospora belli*
   a. Organism - *Isospora belli* is a coccidian parasite that inhabits the upper small bowel. Humans are the only known hosts. It is found mainly in tropical and subtropical areas.
   b. Clinical manifestations
      (1) In immunocompetent hosts, *Isospora* causes a self-limited diarrheal illness, indistinguishable from other non-inflammatory diarrheas.
      (2) In immunocompromised hosts, especially HIV-infected hosts, prolonged diarrhea is the rule and infection may be complicated by malabsorption, hemorrhagic colitis and dehydration.
   c. Diagnosis - oocysts are shed intermittently and in small numbers, thus, concentration methods or repeat stool exam may be necessary. Oocysts can be detected by wet mounts or modified acid fast stains. Eosinophilia is sometimes present.
   d. Treatment

    (1) TMP/SMX 160/800 mg bid x 10 days (10/50 mg/kg/day).

    (2) In AIDS patients, give 160/800 mg qid x 10 days then bid x 3 weeks. For children with HIV infection, give 20/100 mg/kg/day in 4 doses x 10 days then 10/50 mg/kg/day in 2 doses x 3 weeks.

    (3) Chronic suppressive therapy is required after initial treatment for immunocompromised hosts. TMP/SMX 80/400 (5/25 mg/kg) once daily or 160/800 (10/50 mg/kg) three times weekly is effective. Pyrimethamine 75 mg/day with folinic acid 10mg/day can be used in sulfa-allergic patients.

4. *Cryptosporidium parvum*

    a. Organism - *Cryptosporidium* is primarily a parasite of cattle, transmissible to humans through contaminated food and water.

    b. Clinical manifestations

        (1) In immunocompetent hosts, *Cryptosporidium* causes an acute, self-limited watery diarrhea. In children, diarrhea can persist for several weeks.

        (2) Immunocompromised hosts may develop high volume, watery diarrhea resulting in severe dehydration and electrolyte disturbances.

    c. Diagnosis - modified acid-fast staining of stool is required to demonstrate oocysts. Oocyts are differentiated from *Cyclospora* oocysts based on size.

    d. Treatment - to date, no effective treatment has been identified for *Cryptosporidium*. In normal hosts, the symptoms will subside within 10 days but shedding of oocysts may persist for months. In immunocompromised hosts, careful attention must be given to maintaining hydration and electrolyte balance.

5. *Cyclospora cayetanensis*

    a. Organism - *Cyclospora* is an important cause of traveler's diarrhea and pediatric diarrhea in developing countries. It has recently been recognized as an important cause of foodborne diarrhea in North America, primarily from fresh fruits and herbs imported from developing countries. The organism will not be detected on routine stool exams and it is likely that it is an under-recognized cause of foodborne diarrhea.

    b. Clinical manifestations - *Cyclospora* causes prolonged watery diarrhea with prominent fatigue, anorexia and weight loss.

    c. Diagnosis - modified acid-fast staining of stool will demonstrate oocysts.

    d. Treatment is with TMP/SMX 160/800 mg bid x 10 days (5/25 mg per kg bid) in both normal and immunocompromised hosts. Immunocompromised hosts may require long-term suppression with TMP/SMX to prevent recurrences.

C. Tissue helminth infections (extraintestinal helminth infections)

1. **Cutaneous larva migrans** (creeping worm)
   a. Organism - creeping worm is caused by a variety of worms that wander through skin and subcutaneous tissues, most commonly non-human hookworms, such as dog and cat hookworm. Larvae are unable to complete the normal migration cycle in humans and wander through skin until they die. Creeping worm can also be caused by *Strongyloides* or *Gnathostoma spinigerum.*
   b. Clinical manifestations - symptoms start within hours of larval penetration of skin. An itchy papule develops at the site of penetration and evolves into a vesicle. As the larvae wander through the skin, they leave a serpiginous, elevated, intensely puritic red track.
   c. Diagnosis - usually apparent on examination. When secondary infection is present it may be more difficult to detect the track. Hookworm larvae can be differentiated from *Strongyloides* based on the speed of migration of the track. Hookworm larvae move slowly (< 1 cm / day) and persist for months. *Strongyloides* larvae move rapidly (up to 10 cm / hour) and are very transient, lasting only hours. *Strongyloides* CLM typically occurs on the buttocks.
   d. Treatment
      (1) Thiabendazole 50 mg/kg/day for 2-4 days or once weekly x 4 weeks.
      (2) Albendazole 400 mg po x 1.
      (3) Topical application of 10% thiabendazole ointment 2-3 times daily for 5 days is also very effective. (To make 10% thiabendazole ointment, crush one 500 mg tablet of thiabendazole and mix in a small amount of sterile water. Mix in 3.3 grams of any water soluble ointment base such as hydrous emulsifying ointment or glaxal base).

2. *Trichinella spiralis* (Trichinosis)
   a. Organism - *Trichinella spiralis* is a roundworm of carnivorous animals and birds. Humans are infected when they eat undercooked meat (especially pork) contaminated with infective larvae. Infection can occur worldwide but is most common in temperate climates.
   b. Clinical manifestations
      (1) The severity of symptoms depends on the number of ingested larvae. Light infections are asymptomatic.
      (2) Moderate infections present with fever, muscle pain, abdominal pain and diarrhea. Characteristic signs of trichinosis include periorbital edema and multiple splinter hemorrhages beneath finger and toenails.
      (3) In heavy infections, migration of larvae may cause myocarditis, pneumonitis and meningoencephalitis with seizures. As larvae cease migration and encyst in tissues, acute symptoms resolve but muscle pain may persist.

   c. Diagnosis - periorbital edema and splinter hemorrhages with marked eosinophilia should raise suspicion of trichinosis. If the diagnosis is in doubt, a muscle biopsy done in the 3rd to 4th week of illness will demonstrate encysted larvae.

   d. Treatment

     (1) Trichinosis is self-limited - mild infections resolve in 2-3 weeks. More severe infections will resolve in several months.

     (2) Bedrest, antipyretics and analgesics are useful for patients with significant symptoms.

     (3) In patients with severe myositis or myocarditis a short course of prednisone (1 mg/kg daily x 5 days) may be helpful.

     (4) Anti-helminths are ineffective against encysted or migrating larvae and do not change the outcome but may decrease the duration of symptoms (mebendazole 15mg/kg bid x 10-14 days or albendazole 400mg bid x 14 days).

3. Visceral Larva Migrans

   a. Organism - visceral larva migrans (VLM) is a syndrome of tissue damage caused by migration of larval roundworms through visceral tissues. Most cases in temperate areas are caused by infection with dog or cat roundworms (*Toxocara* spp.); in other areas *Gnathostoma* spp. and *Spirometra* spp. are important causes of VLM.

   b. Clinical manifestations

     (1) Toxocariasis is most common in young children who ingest soil containing roundworm eggs. Migrating worms cause hemorrhage, granulomatous inflammation and tissue necrosis. Mild infections are asymptomatic.

     (2) More significant infections present with fever, anorexia, failure to thrive, weight loss, cough and wheeze.

     (3) Heavy infections cause myocarditis, pneumonitis, meningoencephalitis and hepatosplenomegaly. Ocular involvement may be mistaken for retinoblastoma. Eosinophilia is usually present.

   c. Diagnosis - biopsy of involved tissue will demonstrate larvae. Stool exam is not helpful since the larvae causing VLM are unable to complete their migration cycle in the human host.

   d. Treatment

     (1) Symptoms are self-limited but when severe, steroid therapy may be indicated to reduce the inflammatory response and resultant tissue damage.

     (2) Antihelminthic therapy does not affect the outcome but may decrease the duration of symptoms (mebendazole 100-200mg bid x 5 days, albendazole 400mg bid x 5 days or diethylcarbamazine 2mg/kg tid x10 days).

4. Filariasis

a. Lymphatic filarial disease

(1) Organism - tissue roundworm infections caused by *Wuchereria bancrofti* (most widespread), *Brugia malayi, Brugia timori*. Adult worms are found in lymph channels and lymph nodes especially in the lower extremity. Symptoms result from the host response to adult worms. Chronic inflammation of the vessel wall produces thickening, stasis of lymph flow, and, with time, complete obstruction of the vessel. Large numbers of microfilaria produced by adult worms circulate through the blood stream but cause relatively few symptoms. Microfilaria are transmitted from person to person through the bite of infected mosquitoes.

(2) Clinical manifestations

   (a) Periodic acute episodes of lymphangitis or lymphadenitis with high fever, headache, local pain, backache and tenderness. Edema and erythema occur in skin overlying affected lymphatic channels.

   (b) Acute orchitis or epididymitis may occur, most commonly with *W. bancrofti*. Chyluria results from rupture of lymph channels into the urinary tract.

   (c) Chronic lymphadenopathy may be the only feature of infection in some patients. Recurrent episodes of acute and chronic inflammation leads to lymphedema and elephantiasis (non-pitting edema of the extremities with thickening and fissuring of the skin). With very advanced disease the skin takes on a warty appearance. Ulceration and secondary infections are common in severely affected extremities. Hydroceles are very common and may be massive, interfering with ambulation.

(3) Diagnosis

   (a) Definitive diagnosis of lymphatic filariasis requires demonstration of microfilaria in blood films. If specimens taken during the day are negative, films should be obtained between 2300 and 0100 hours as some species of microfilaria circulate primarily at night. In both early and late disease, blood films may be negative for microfilaria.

   (b) In endemic areas, episodes of relapsing acute lymphangitis and typical features of lymphedema are strongly suggestive of filarial disease. Eosinophilia supports the diagnosis. The differential diagnosis includes chronic venous disease, congenital lymphatic abnormalities (Milroy's disease), and lymphatic damage secondary to skin absorption of inorganic compounds from the soil. The lower extremities are typically involved but other sites such as the arms and breasts can also be affected.

    (4) Treatment
- (a) Diethylcarbamazine (DEC) is given after meals according to the following schedule:

                Day 1: 50mg po (1mg/kg)
                Day 2: 50mg po tid (1mg/kg tid)
                Day 3: 100mg po tid (2mg/kg tid)
                Days 4 - 21: 2 mg/kg tid

- (b) Ivermectin in a single dose of 200-400 micrograms/kg may be given. It is more effective when given with albendazole 400mg x 1.
- (c) All drugs clear microfilaria but are less effective against adult worms. Ivermectin has less effect on adult worms than DEC and microfilaria reappear in the blood more rapidly than after DEC treatment. Mass treatment of the community at 6-12 month intervals may reduce transmission.
- (d) Repeat blood films at least one month after treatment, and if microfilaria are found, repeat the treatment course.
- (e) Reactions to treatment (fever, arthralgia, myalgia, and GI symptoms) may occur and are usually mild. Treat with antihistamines or in severe cases, corticosteroids.

b. Onchocerciasis
- (1) Organism - *Onchocerca* volvulus, transmitted by the *Simulium* blackfly, which lives near rapid flowing streams and rivers. Adult worms live in subcutaneous tissues for up to 12 years and produce large numbers of microfilaria. Microfilaria circulate through the skin and subcutaneous tissue. Immune reactions to dead or injured microfilaria are responsible for most of the symptoms of the disease.
- (2) Clinical manifestations - the cardinal features are subcutaneous nodules (containing the adults worms), dermatitis (itching and depigmentation) and eye lesions.
  - (a) Symptoms - itching is the most common and troubling symptom. The severity of symptoms depends upon the patient's sensitivity to the microfilaria, not the number of microfilaria. Some individuals have minimal symptoms with heavy microfilarial loads, while others have intense symptoms with only a few microfilaria.
  - (b) Signs - the skin becomes thickened with papular eruptions, hyperpigmentation and a leathery texture, especially over the buttocks and lower extremities. Subcutaneous nodules containing adult worms develop over bony prominences. With long-standing disease, depigmentation, premature aging and atrophy of the skin occurs, especially on the legs. With advanced disease, pendulous folds of skin in the inguinal area

(hanging groin), scrotal enlargement and hydrocele are common. **Sowda** is a condition in which the host has a very strong immune response to microfilaria resulting in extreme pruritus, scaly papules, swelling of the skin, and regional lymphadenopathy, often limited to one extremity.

(c) Ocular microfilaria cause inflammatory damage to the cornea, iridocyclitis, glaucoma, choroiditis and optic atrophy. Inflammatory damage leads to night blindness, visual field loss and blindness. In endemic areas onchocerciasis is an important cause of blindness and shortened life expectancy.

(3) Diagnosis

(a) Skin snips demonstrate the presence of microfilaria.

(b) Mazzotti test - Diethylcarbamazine (DEC) 50 mg as a single challenge dose causes intense itching 1-24 hours after administration. The Mazzotti test can induce vision-threatening complications when microfilaria are present in the eye and should not be used routinely. Patients with heavy infections may develop severe systemic symptoms with fever, malaise, swollen lymph nodes, facial and peri-orbital edema and potentially serious complications. Do not use the Mazzotti test in debilitated patients or in any patient in whom the diagnosis can be established by skin snip examination.

(4) Treatment

(a) Indications for treatment - severe skin lesions and itching, Sowda, early eye changes, night blindness or visual field loss.

(b) Ivermectin (Mectizam) is the drug of choice. It eliminates microfilaria for 6-12 months, and has fewer adverse effects than DEC. It should not be used in pregnant or lactating women and children under five years. Give 150 micrograms/kg as a single dose, with water, on an empty stomach. Annual retreatment is required to control microfilaremia as the adult worms are not affected. The life span of adult worms is 12-15 years.

(c) Ivermectin is also used in mass treatment of populations in areas where onchocerciasis is an important health problem. Annual retreatment is required.

(d) Moxidectin is a macrofilaricide (kills adult worms), which has shown promising results in clinical trials, but has not yet been licensed for human use.

(e) Surgical removal of filaria nodules will remove some of the adult worms, and lessen the microfilaria burden. This has proven to be more useful in Central and South America than in Africa.

c. Loiasis

    (1) Organism - *Loa loa*, endemic to areas of West and Central Africa, transmitted by biting tabanid flies. Adult worms live in subcutaneous tissues, microfilaria circulate through the blood with a daytime periodicity.

    (2) Clinical manifestations

      (a) Calabar swellings are the most common manifestation of loiasis. Painless swellings 5-20 cm in diameter appear at irregular intervals, most often at the wrists and ankles and last for hours to days.

      (b) Migration of the adult worm through the conjunctiva or under the skin typically does not cause a significant local reaction and is very transient, lasting a few minutes.

      (c) Intermittent episodes of urticaria may occur.

      (d) Complications include endomyocardial fibrosis, peripheral neuropathy, nephropathy, pleural effusions, arthritis.

    (3) Diagnosis - in endemic areas, the diagnosis is usually made on clinical grounds. Microfilaria may be seen in blood smears obtained at midday, but smears are frequently negative.

    (4) Treatment

      (a) DEC will kill microfilaria but does not kill adult worms. In patients with a high microfilarial load, DEC treatment may precipitate encephalopathy. Diethylcarbamazine is given in a similar protocol to Bancroftian filariasis but the dose for Day 4 - 21 is increased. (Day 1: 50 mg x1, Day 2: 50 mg tid, Day 3: 100 mg tid, Day 4-21: 3 mg/kg tid).

      (b) Albendazole 200 mg bid for 3 weeks or ivermectin 200 micrograms/kg may also be used.

      (c) Mass treatment of communities with ivermectin q3 months or DEC 5mg/kg x 3 consecutive days each month can decrease transmission.

      (d) Persons temporarily resident in endemic areas can use DEC 300 mg weekly as prophylaxis.

5. Schistosomiasis (bilharziasis)

  a. Organism - humans are the definitive hosts for 5 species of schistosomes. Adult worms live in small veins of the mesenteric system or the vesicular plexus (around the bladder). Eggs are expelled into the bloodstream and make their way across the vessel wall into urine or stool. If eggs contact water, they hatch, releasing larvae, which undergo further development in intermediate snail hosts before transmission back to humans. Humans are infected during fresh water contact by free-swimming larvae (cercaria) that penetrate intact skin.

Schistosoma species infecting humans		
Species	Disease	Endemic areas
S. hematobium	Urinary	Middle East, Africa
S. mansoni	Intestinal	Arabia, Africa, S. America, Caribbean
S. japonicum	Intestinal	China, Philippines
S. mekongi	Intestinal	Southeast Asia
S. intercalatum	Intestinal	West and Central Africa

b. Presentation

(1) A pruritic papular rash (swimmer's itch) may occur at the site of cercarial penetration. Resolution occurs in 7-10 days without treatment.

(2) Katayama syndrome occurs 4-8 weeks after infection, as adult worms begin egg-laying. Symptoms include acute onset of fever, headache, and cough; lymphadenopathy, hepatosplenomegaly and eosinophilia are found on physical examination. Resolution occurs within several weeks.

(3) Chronic diseaseis due to the host inflammatory response to eggs trapped in tissues. Early chronic intestinal schistosomiasis presents with bloody diarrhea and colicky abdominal pain. With prolonged infection, hepatosplenomegaly and portal hypertension develop. In advanced disease ascites, esophageal varices and cachexia occur. Early urinary schistosomiasis presents with terminal hematuria and dysuria. Granulomatous masses in the bladder wall and ureters result in obstructive uropathy. Involvement of the female genital tract results in ulcerating, polypoid or nodular lesions.

(4) Recurrent *Salmonella* urinary tract infections or bacteremias result from infection of the adult worms with *Salmonella*. Antimicrobial therapy is ineffective in eradicating *Salmonella* from the worms. Treatment of the schistosomiasis is necessary to prevent further recurrences.

(5) Eggs can be carried away by the bloodstream and deposited in ectopic sites resulting in a variety of unusual disease manifestations such as transverse myelitis and cor pulmonale. *S. japonicum* is an important cause of focal seizures and meningoencephalitis in the Far East.

c. Diagnosis is established by identifying schistosome eggs in stool or urine. Snip biopsies of the rectal mucosa may demonstrate eggs in cases where no eggs are seen in the stool.

d. Treatment - all species of schistosomes are treated with praziquantel as follows:

Praziquantel Treatment for Schistosomiasis	
S. hematobium	40 mg/kg x 1 dose or 20 mg/kg bid x 1 day
S. mansoni	40-60 mg/kg x 1dose or 20 mg bid/tid x 1 day
S. japonicum	20 mg/kg tid x 1 day
S. mekongi	
S. intercalatum	

6. Other Trematodes
  a. Liver flukes
   (1) *Clonorchis sinensis, Opisthorchis viverrini* and *O. felineus* are important human liver flukes. Adult worms live in intrahepatic bile ducts and excrete eggs into bile. Infection is acquired through consumption of raw or inadequately cooked fish containing encysted larval stages. Larvae released from cysts migrate up the extrahepatic biliary system to small intrahepatic bile ducts where they mature and begin laying eggs.
   (2) Many infected individuals are asymptomatic or have mild non-specific symptoms of fatigue, anorexia and indigestion. Suggestive symptoms include right upper quadrant pain, hepatic and/or gallbladder enlargement, gallstones and impaired gallbladder function.
   (3) Complications such as cholangitis, cholecystitis, obstructive jaundice and ascites may occur. Infection with liver flukes is strongly associated with the development of cholangiocarcinoma.
  b. Fascioliasis
   (1) *Fasciola hepatica* (sheep liver fluke) and *Fasciola gigantica* (cattle liver fluke) infect humans through ingestion of larvae encysted on aquatic plants grown in water contaminated by feces of the host animal. Like the human liver flukes, adult stages live in the bile ducts. Larvae are released from cysts in the upper GI tract, migrate across the intestinal wall and peritoneum, penetrate the liver capsule and migrate through liver tissue to bile ducts.
   (2) Clinical symptoms result from damage to liver tissue as larvae migrate, and from proliferation of bile duct endothelium in response to the presence of adult worms. Acute manifestations during the migration phase include RUQ pain, diarrhea, weight loss, cough, fever, hepatosplenomegaly, anemia and marked eosinophilia. Chronic manifestations include RUQ pain, cholestatic jaundice, pruritus, hepatomegaly, ascites and fatty food intolerance. Intermittent episodes of cholangitis or cholecystitis may occur.
  c. Intestinal flukes
   (1) Multiple species of intestinal flukes infect humans either through consumption of encysted larvae on water plants or in tissues of

fish, snails, crabs, clams or shrimp. Larvae released from cysts in the upper GI tract attach to the intestinal mucosa causing local inflammation and ulceration.

(2) Clinical manifestations include diarrhea, abdominal discomfort, anorexia, anemia and eosinophila. *Fasciolopsis buski* is a large fluke and has been found to cause intestinal obstruction and vitamin B12 deficiency.

d. Lung flukes

(1) *Paragonimus* species are widely distributed through Asia, Africa, Latin America and South America. Humans are infected through consumption of encysted larvae in crabs, shrimp or crayfish. Larvae excyst in the upper GI tract and migrate across the intestinal wall, through the peritoneal cavity, penetrate the diaphragm and migrate through the lung. Larvae develop into adults in the lung and begin egg laying. Eggs are coughed up and either expectorated in sputum or swallowed and excreted in feces.

(2) Clinical manifestations include cough with blood-tinged or rusty sputum, chest pain and night sweats. Pleural effusion and pneumothorax may occur. In endemic areas, paragonimiasis should also be considered in patients presenting with bronchiectasis, "tuberculosis" unresponsive to anti-tuberculous treatment, and bronchopneumonia unresponsive to antibiotic therapy, particularly when eosinophilia is present. Ectopic parasites reaching the brain or spinal cord cause eosinophilic meningitis or spastic paraplegia.

e. Diagnosis of all species of liver, intestinal and lung fluke infections is made by examining eggs that are excreted in stool. Each species has characteristic egg morphology that allows specific identification. Eggs may also be found in sputum and gastric washings in paragonimiasis.

f. Treatment is as follows:

Treatment of Trematode Infections		
	Species	**Treatment**
Liver Flukes	*Opisthorchis*	Praziquantel 25 mg/kg tid x 1 day
	Clonorchis	Praziquantel 25 mg/kg tid x 1 day Albendazole 10 mg/kg/d x 7 days
	Fasciola	Bithionol 30-40 mg/kg every other day x 10-15 doses (max 2 grams/day) Praziquantel 15 mg/kg stat
Intestinal Flukes	*Fasciolopsis*	Praziquantel 25 mg/kg tid x 1 day
	Heterophyes	
	Echinostoma	
	Metagonimus	
Lung Flukes	*Paragonimus*	Praziquantel 25 mg/kg tid x 2 days

D. Tissue protozoan infections (excluding malaria)
  1. American Trypansosomiasis (Chaga's disease)
    a. Organism - *Trypanosoma cruzi*, transmitted by the Reduviid bug, is endemic in Central and South America. The Reduviid bug deposits organisms on the skin while feeding. Organisms are inoculated through the skin by scratching induced by the bite, or inoculated into the conjunctiva when bites occur near the eye. Transmission can also occur through blood transfusion or transplacentally. Neurotoxins produced by *T. cruzi*, and the host immune response damage autonomic nerves leading to the clinical manifestations of chronic disease.
    b. Clinical manifestations
      (1) Early symptoms include local swelling and inflammation at the site of inoculation (Chagoma). When infection occurs through the conjunctiva, unilateral peri-orbital edema results (Romaña's sign). Fever, generalized lymphadenopathy and hepato-splenomegaly may be present.
      (2) Chronic disease
        (a) Asymptomatic infection is common.
        (b) Megaesophagus causes difficulty swallowing, esophagitis, aspiration, recurrent aspiration pneumonia, parotid hypertrophy, wasting and inanition.
        (c) Megacolon causes severe constipation and fecal impaction, as well as volvulus.
        (d) Cardiac disease causes abnormal conduction (heart block, RBBB), dysrhythmias, dilated cardiomyopathy, thromboembolic disease.
    c. Diagnosis - in acute disease, parasites may be detected in blood smears. Thick films and buffy-coat smears and centrifugation techniques will improve sensitivity. Organisms are more readily found in children than in adult patients.
    d. Treatment should be provided to all patients in the acute stages of infection. Treatment is less likely to be beneficial in chronic infections where extensive tissue damage has already occurred. Treatment is recommended for children and for adults within 2 years of infection.
      (1) Nifurtimox - adults 8-10 mg/kg tid, children 15 mg/kg tid x 90 days with close observation for peripheral neuropathy and hemolysis. Polyneuropathy is an indication to terminate therapy.
      (2) Benznidazole - adults 2.5 mg/kg bid, children 2.5-5 mg/kg bid x 60 days with close observation for photosensitivity, peripheral neuritis, neutropenia, thrombocytopenia.
  2. African Trypanosomiasis (sleeping sickness)
    a. Organism - two different subspecies of *Trypanosoma brucei* cause

sleeping sickness, *T.b. rhodesiense* and *T. b. gambiense*. The subspecies differ in areas of endemicity with overlap in a few areas. The parasites are transmitted by the bite of the tsetse fly. Humans are the preferred host of *T .b. gambiense* and clinical disease is milder with asymptomatic carriers playing an important role in sustaining the disease in the community. *T. b. rhodesiense* primarily infects ungulates (both domestic and wild), which are the main reservoirs of the parasite. Clinical disease in humans is severe and progresses rapidly to neurologic involvement.

b. Clinical manifestations

    (1) Following infection, a painful, indurated papule (chancre) develops at the site of the bite in some patients. This lesion resolves spontaneously over several weeks.

    (2) Early symptoms - an initial febrile episode lasting 1-7 days develops in some patients. Following the initial febrile episode, intermittent attacks of fever with malaise, headache, myalgias, weight loss, and generalized pruritus occur. Irritability, personality change and insomnia may be seen in some patients. Painful edema of hands and feet and an evanescent rash may occur. Generalized lymphadenopathy (+/- hepatosplenomegaly) develops as the disease progresses. In *T. b. gambiense*, prominent enlargement of the posterior cervical nodes is characteristic (Winterbottom's sign).

    (3) Late symptoms - the onset of CNS disease is usually insidious, and occurs in weeks in *T. b. rhodesiense* and in months to years in *T.b. gambiense*. Affected patients exhibit personality changes, lethargy, daytime somnolence and nocturnal insomnia. Movement disorders and extrapyramidal signs, hypertonicity and cerebellar ataxia are common features but cranial nerve palsies and long tract signs are unusual. The disease may mimic Parkinson's disease (slurred speech, shuffling gait, tremors and muscular rigidity). With advanced disease, severe pruritus, wasting and immobility ensue with progression to coma in the preterminal stage.

c. Diagnosis is made by demonstration of the organisms in fluid aspirated from a chancre or lymph node, peripheral blood or CSF. Buffy-coat smears and thick smears stained with Geimsa are more sensitive than routine thin films. Multiple smears should be examined as the parasites tend to appear in the blood in waves. Concentration techniques should be used, if available. Serum and CSF levels of IgM are markedly elevated. CSF exam shows increased protein and a mononuclear pleocytosis. Anemia, thrombocytopenia, coagulation abnormalities and liver function abnormalities are commonly present but non-specific.

    d. Treatment

      (1) Early disease - suramin is the drug of choice for both subspecies if the CSF exam is normal. Suramin must be administered by slow IV infusion and carries substantial risk of severe adverse effects. Pentamidine (4 mg/kg/d IM x 10 days) may be used in early disease due to *T. b. gambiense.*

      (2) Late disease (CNS involvement) - Melarsoprol is the drug of choice for patients with CNS involvement or for patients failing suramin treatment in early disease. Pretreatment with 2 to 4 doses of suramin is recommended for patients with advanced CNS disease. Toxic reactions to melarsoprol may be severe and include toxic encephalopathy, exfoliative dermatitis and renal dysfunction.

3. Leishmaniasis

    a. Organism - a variety of Leishmania species, transmitted by sandflies. Disease manifestations depend on the species of parasite. Different species of Leishmania grow best at different temperatures. Species preferring cooler temperatures cause skin (*L. tropica, L. mexicana. L. braziliensis*) or mucocutaneous disease (*L. braziliensis*). Visceral disease (Kala-azar) is caused by *L. donovani* which grows at higher temperatures. Immunocompromised patients such as AIDS patients are at increased risk of progressive disease and relapse following treatment.

    b. Clinical manifestations

      (1) Visceral leishmaniasis - causes fever, hepatosplenomegaly, lymphadenopathy, weight loss, anemia, thrombocytopenia, leukopenia, hypergammaglobulinemia, increased susceptibility to infections. Mucosal and skin lesions may occur with visceral disease.

      (2) Cutaneous leishmaniasis - a variety of skin lesions occur (chronic ulcers, nodular lesions, plaques and papules), usually on exposed areas of skin. When multiple lesions are present they tend to appear, progress and resolve in synchrony. They spread along lymphatics with subcutaneous nodules appearing in a linear pattern. Lesions may last for months to years before healing, leaving a depressed scar.

      (3) Mucocutaneous disease - individuals with infections due to *L. braziliensis* may develop metastatic mucosal lesions. Mucosal lesions may appear in the nasal, buccal or pharyngeal mucosa and may appear years after healing of the cutaneous lesions. Mucosal lesions can be extensive, resulting in destruction of the nasal septum, palate, lips and larynx.

    c. Diagnosis - demonstration of the organism in affected tissues is the main method of diagnosis. Splenic aspiration is the most sensitive method of confirming the diagnosis in Kala-azar but this procedure requires an experienced physician and surgical support as it may be complicated by splenic laceration and hemorrhage. Organisms may also be detected in bone marrow, lymph node aspirates, buffy-coat and liver. Thus, in most cases, splenic aspiration should be reserved for patients with suspected disease in whom the diagnosis is not established after sampling these other sites. Aspiration or biopsy of the indurated margin of cutaneous or mucocutaneous lesions can yield diagnostic material.

  d. Treatment

    (1) Pentavalent antimonials such as sodium stibogluconate and meglumine antimoniate are still widely used for treatment of visceral and cutaneous disease.

    (2) Amphotericin B and pentamidine have also been used, particularly in patients who fail treatment with pentavalent antimonials.

    (3) Ketoconazole has been used for treatment of cutaneous disease due to *L. panamensis* but is ineffective in *L. brasiliensis*.

4. Toxoplasmosis

  a. Organism: *Toxoplasma gondii*, an endemic pathogen worldwide. Risk of infection is highest in areas where hygiene is poor (fecal-oral contamination of food/water with cat feces) and where raw meat is consumed. Infection occurs through ingestion of oocysts contaminating food, or tissues cysts in meat. Transmission can also occur through blood transfusion or transplacental transmission.

  b. Clinical manifestations

    (1) Acute disease in the normal host

      (a) Acute mononucleosis-like syndrome and cervical lymphadenopathy.

      (b) Rarely, acute severe visceral disease affecting liver, lung, heart, and muscle occurs.

      (c) Chorioretinitis can occur but is unusual (<1% of acute infections).

    (2) Toxoplasmosis in AIDS patients

      (a) Encephalitis is a common presentation in AIDS patients with CD4 counts < 100. Symptoms include fever, headache, altered mental status and focal neurologic signs.

      (b) Pneumonitis

      (c) Chorioretinitis

    (3) Congenital toxoplasmosis

      (a) Severe disease presents as hydrocephalus, cerebral calcifications, mental retardation and chorioretinitis. Anemia, jaundice, thrombocytopenia, rash and deafness may be associated.

    (b) Chorioretinitis - retinal lesions may be apparent at birth or may not be detectable until the second or third decades of life. Severe congenital disease results in cataracts, strabismus and microphthalmia.

  c. Diagnosis - usually made by serologic testing demonstrating seroconversion or a positive IgM. In areas where serologic testing is not available, empiric treatment of AIDS patients with suspected toxoplasmosis is appropriate as improvement will be apparent within 2 weeks. Failure to improve in this time period makes toxoplasmosis unlikely and other diagnoses should be considered.

  d. Treatment

    (1) No treatment is required for normal hosts except in unusually severe cases.

    (2) Treatment of infection during pregnancy can reduce the risk of transmission to the fetus. Congenitally infected infants should be treated for the first year of life. Spiramycin is used for treatment during pregnancy. Post delivery infants are treated with 3 week cycles of spiramycin (100 mg/kg/day) alternating with sulfadiazine (50-100 mg/kg/day)/pyrimethamine (0.5-1.0 mg/kg/day)/folinic acid.

    (3) Chorioretinitis is treated with sulfadiazine 500 mg qid + pyrimethamine 25 mg. Steroids should be given along with antiparasitic therapy. Treatment is continued for 10 days after resolution of inflammation. Folinic acid supplementation should be given.

    (4) Toxoplasmosis in AIDS patients is treated with sulfadiazine 1-2 g qid + pyrimethamine 50-75 mg/day with folinic acid x 6 weeks. After completing the initial course of therapy, AIDS patients should continue suppressive therapy for life with dapsone or TMP/SMX.

    (5) Clindamycin can be substituted for sulfadiazine in patients with significant adverse reactions to sulfa compounds.

V. MALARIA

A. General

  1. In many areas of the developing world malaria is the most important cause of morbidity and mortality, particularly in young children. Drug susceptibility patterns vary widely in different regions and knowledge of local patterns is essential to appropriate management.

  2. Immunity

    a. The immune status of the patient is an important variable in management. True immunity that completely prevents malaria episodes does not occur in malaria, instead individuals are considered semi-immune or non-immune.

   b. Semi-immune patients are those who have grown up in highly
   endemic areas (and have not left these areas for more than 6 months)
   and, through continuous exposure, have acquired a degree of
   resistance to symptomatic malaria. Even semi-immune individuals
   can still develop severe and life threatening episodes of malaria,
   although less frequently than non-immune subjects.

   c. Non-immune patients remain vulnerable to severe and frequent
   malaria attacks. Expatriates from non-endemic areas should be
   managed as non-immune, regardless of their duration of exposure and
   history of malaria attacks. Local residents who leave endemic areas
   for more than 6 months lose immunity and are vulnerable to severe
   attacks upon return to the endemic area.

3. Etiology

   a. Malaria is caused by the protozoan parasite *Plasmodium*.

   b. *P. falciparum* causes the most serious disease, and is the most
   prevalent species around the world. *P. falciparum* is predominant
   throughout Africa, Papua New Guinea and Haiti.

   c. *P. vivax* is less common in Africa with the exception of North Africa
   but is common in other endemic areas.

   d. *P. ovale* is found in West Africa. *P. vivax* and *P. ovale* are
   characterized by persistent liver stage parasites which can cause late
   relapses of malaria even years after leaving an endemic area.

   e. *P. malariae* is relatively uncommon outside of Africa and is
   characterized by the ability to sustain prolonged (years), low grade,
   asymptomatic parasitemias. *P. malariae* is an important cause of
   nephrotic syndrome in children in sub-Saharan Africa due to the
   persistence of malarial antigens in the circulation.

B. Clinical

   1. Symptoms

   a. Fever, chills, headache, myalgias, arthralgias, anorexia, nausea,
   vomiting, abdominal pain, diarrhea are common symptoms. The fever
   pattern often lacks periodicity until the infection has been established
   for a number of days. Malaria must not be ruled out on the basis of
   absence of periodic fever.

   b. Symptoms of malaria often mimic other common diseases such as
   gastroenteritis, pneumonia, pyelonephritis and meningitis.

   2. Signs

   a. There are no specific features of malaria and most cases have minimal
   physical findings other than fever, tachycardia and tachypnea.

   b. Severe malaria in young children may cause lactic acidosis and
   present with deep, "driven" respirations (Kussmaul breathing).

   c. Cerebral malaria and/or hypoglycemia present with decreased level of
   consciousness, seizures or focal neurologic signs.

   d. Pregnant women with unrecognized malaria may present abruptly with
   severe respiratory distress in the immediate post partum period.

    e. Jaundice is unusual but may be present in patients with severe disease. With longstanding or frequently recurrent infection, anemia, splenomegaly, and hepatomegaly may be present.

3. Laboratory

    a. Thrombocytopenia is very common and will be present in most cases. Anemia is seen in prolonged, severe or frequently recurrent disease. The white blood count is typically normal or reduced and when significantly elevated, a careful search should be made for an associated bacterial infection.

    b. Albuminuria, hemoglobinuria, and, occasionally, increased urobilinogen may be seen. Total and unconjugated bilirubin may be increased and liver enzymes (AST, ALT) are often elevated.

    c. Metabolic abnormalities include mild hyponatremia, reduced serum bicarbonate and raised serum lactate. Systemic acidosis is common in small children with severe disease. Hypoglycemia is most likely to occur in young children, pregnant women, patients with severe disease and those treated with quinine.

4. Diagnosis

    a. Wherever possible, a clinically suspected case of malaria should be confirmed by a positive malaria smear. Clinical diagnosis is frequently inaccurate and can lead to inappropriate use of antimalarial agents, which contributes to the evolution of resistance. In some cases, multiple smears taken over several days may be required to identify the organism, particularly in non-immune individuals with low-grade parasitemias.

    b. New diagnostic tests using rapid dipstick technology to detect malarial antigens in the blood are becoming more widely available (i.e. *Para* Sight™-F, ICT Malaria Pf™, OptiMAL tests). These tests may be useful in areas where blood smear microscopy cannot be done, but accuracy is limited when tests are performed by untrained individuals and they should not be used as a substitute for blood smear examination where microscopy is available. *Para* Sight™-F and ICT Malaria Pf™ detect only *Plasmodium falciparum,* OptiMAL differentiates all four species of malaria. These tests may be positive in asymptomatic parasitemia in semi-immune individuals and must be used with caution to avoid over-diagnosis and unnecessary use of antimalarials in these patients. They may also detect residual antigens present in the blood following successful treatment and are therefore not useful for following response to therapy.

C. Severity of disease

    1. Mild disease is frequent in semi-immune individuals. Disease is typically manifested by fever, myalgias, headache and mild GI symptoms.

    2. Severe disease

a. Defining criteria of severe disease include cerebral malaria (unarousable coma, altered level of consciousness), severe anemia, renal failure, pulmonary edema, hypoglycemia, circulatory collapse/shock, spontaneous bleeding/DIC, repeated generalized convulsions, acidemia/acidosis, malarial hemoglobinuria.

b. Other manifestations include impaired level of consciousness, rousable coma, prostration/extreme weakness, hyperparasitemia, jaundice, hyperpyrexia.

c. Severe malaria is associated with a much higher rate of an adverse outcome, including death. Treatment must be initiated immediately with the most effective and reliable agent available. Close monitoring for complications is essential.

d. Individuals most at risk for severe malaria include young children, pregnant women (especially first and second pregnancies) and non-immune individuals.

e. In children, hypoglycemia and systemic acidosis are common in severe malaria. The presence of systemic acidosis should be suspected when deep, rapid respirations are present. Rapid improvement of tissue perfusion and oxygenation by intravenous rehydration, blood transfusion and treatment of hypoglycemia is critical to a successful outcome.

D. Management

1. **Dosing of antimalarial agents** - may be expressed in terms of **base** or **salt**. Always confirm whether dose recommendations refer to base or salt.

Base/Salt Equivalents of Selected Antimalarial Agents		
Drug	Base (mg)	Salt (mg)
Chloroquine phosphate	150	250
Chloroquine sulfate	100	136
Clindamycin phosphate	150	225
Mefloquine	250 228	274 250
Quinine dihydrochloride	16.7	20
Quinine sulfate	250	300

2. **Simple malaria**

a. Chloroquine

(1) Effective in most cases of mild to moderate disease caused by chloroquine-sensitive organisms. The presence and degree of resistance varies by region and accurate knowledge of local patterns are essential in making appropriate treatment decisions.

(2) Definition of resistance

(a) R1 - clearance of parasites by day 7 with recurrence of parasitemia by day 28.

(b) R2 - reduction of parasitemia by greater than 75% at 48 hours but failure to clear parasitemia by day 7. Parasitemia may clear by day 9 without further treatment in some patients.

(c) R3 - parasitemia fails to decrease by 75% by 48 hours or increases.

(3) It is important to differentiate true resistance from failures of drug compliance, administration, absorption or prescribing. Clinical response to treatment should be followed carefully and, where chloroquine is used in the presence of resistance, follow-up blood films should be done to document an appropriately decreasing parasitemia. Watch for late relapses (2-4 weeks), particularly in vulnerable children.

(4) The total recommended dose of chloroquine is 25mg/kg of base, given as either 10mg/kg base stat, 5mg/kg in six hours, then 5mg/kg daily x 2 days or 10mg/kg base stat, 10mg/kg on day 2 and 5mg/kg on day 3.

b. Sulfadoxine/pyrimethamine (Fansidar)

(1) Use in suspected chloroquine resistance or in patients who develop chloroquine-induced itching. Avoid in 1st trimester and in the last 2 weeks of pregnancy. Resistant disease occurs in SE Asia, is increasing in Africa and is uncommon in South America.

(2) Dosage is 20mg sulfadoxine/1mg pyrimethamine per kg. One tablet contains 500mg sulfadoxine/25mg pyrimethamine.

(a) Infant 6 weeks - 1 year: ¼ tablet

(b) Child 1 year-3 years: ½ tablet

(c) Child 4 years-8 years: 1 tablet

(d) Child >8 years to adult: 3 tablets

3. Resistant malaria

a. Quinine

(1) Dosage - 30mg/kg/day po divided tid for 7 days. Quinine has a short half-life and shorter courses of quinine monotherapy should be avoided to reduce the risk of treatment failure and promotion of resistance.

(2) Quinine should be combined with a second agent such as tetracycline 250mg po qid x 7 days, doxycycline 100mg po bid x 7 days, clindamycin 10mg/kg qid x 7 days (safe in children) or fansidar given at the end of the quinine course (where fansidar is reliably effective).

(3) Side effects of quinine include cinchonism (tinnitus, hearing loss, nausea, vomiting), and, less commonly, cardiac arrhythmias and hypoglycemia. Mild side effects such as tinnitus and decreased hearing are expected at therapeutic blood levels of quinine and are not an indication to discontinue or shorten the quinine course. The hearing loss resolves once the quinine course is completed. When quinine is given to patients who have been treated with

mefloquine or halofantrine in the preceding two weeks, the risk of cardiac arrhythmias is increased.

b. Mefloquine

(1) Side effects include nausea, vomiting, diarrhea, and neuropsychiatric problems (anxiety, depression, sleep disturbances, psychosis). Contraindications to mefloquine must be respected to minimize serious adverse reactions. Mefloquine is contraindicated in patients with a history of seizures, psychosis or significant depression, previous hypersensitivity reactions to mefloquine and cardiac conduction defects. Mefloquine should be used with caution in the first trimester of pregnancy but may be used in pregnancy when other agents may not provide optimal coverage. Mefloquine levels in breastmilk are inadequate to protect a breastfeeding infant.

(2) Mefloquine dosage is 1 tablet (250mg) per 10kg, 25mg/kg as a single dose or 15mg/kg stat followed by 10mg/kg in 8 hours. In partially immune individuals, the total dose may be reduced to 10mg/kg (full doses should be used in Thailand even in semi-immune subjects).

c. Halofantrine - narrow therapeutic index with toxic effects occurring at levels close to those required for effective treatment. WHO no longer recommends use of halofantrine.

d. Malarone - 250mg atovaquone + 100mg proguanil per tablet has excellent safety and tolerability but has not been approved for use in pregnancy. The adult dose is 4 tablets once daily for 3 days. Children are treated with 20mg/kg/day atovaquone + 8mg/kg/day proguanil for 3 days.

4. Severe malaria

a. General measures

(1) Check CBC, malaria smear, glucose. Follow the hematocrit and glucose closely. Transfuse as necessary.

(2) Monitor urine output closely and watch for appearance of "black" urine. Overhydration may cause pulmonary edema.

(3) Children with Kussmaul respirations require rapid intravenous resuscitation with IV fluid or blood to correct hypoperfusion, anemia and hypoglycemia (if present).

b. Quinine

(1) Give IV quinine hydrochloride 20mg/kg (salt) in 10ml/kg isotonic fluid over 4 hours as a loading dose, then 10mg/kg (salt) over 4 hours every 8 hours starting 8 hours after the beginning of the loading dose infusion. Switch to oral administration as soon as the patient can take oral drugs and add tetracycline, doxycycline or Fansidar.

    (2) If more than 3 days of parenteral therapy are required, decrease the dose of IV quinine by 1/3 to 1/2.

    (3) Quinine induces insulin release and increases the risk of hypoglycemia, especially in infants and pregnant women. Blood sugar levels should be monitored.

    (4) IM quinine is not recommended due to muscle necrosis and sterile abscess formation, but may be useful if IV is not possible (in equivalent doses). If intramuscular quinine is used, the following precautions must be observed: dilute the quinine to a concentration of 60mg/ml before injection. Then, inject deeply into the anterior thigh (not buttocks).

c. Artemesinin derivatives (artemether, artesunate)

    (1) These drugs are at least as effective as quinine in treatment of severe malaria. Although fever and parasite clearance times are decreased compared to quinine, reduction in mortality or the incidence of residual neurologic deficit has not been established. In one study, coma time was prolonged in children receiving artemether compared to quinine. Use of artemesinin derivatives is best reserved for treatment of severe or resistant malaria.

    (2) Recrudescence rates are high if courses of less than 5 days are used as monotherapy. Combination with mefloquine is highly effective.

    (3) Artemesinin derivatives are available in oral, parenteral and rectal form preparations. Rectal preparations are particularly useful for initial treatment of severe malaria in primary health clinics while the patient is en route to a referral centre.

    (4) Dosage is as follows:

Dosing regimens for artemesinin derivatives		
Drug	**Loading dose**	**Subsequent doses**
Artemesinin suppositories	40 mg/kg	20 mg/kg at 4, 24, 48 and 72 hours
Artesunate suppositories	200 mg (adult dose)	200 mg at 4, 8, 12, 24, 36, 48 and 60 hours
Intramuscular Artesunate	2.4 mg/kg	1.2 mg/kg at 12 and 24 hours then daily x 6 days
Intramuscular Artemether	3.2 mg/kg	1.6 mg/kg daily x 3 days until oral therapy is possible

d. Chloroquine

    (1) May be used for treatment of severe malaria only in areas where there is no resistance.

    (2) Parenteral chloroquine should be reserved for severe malaria, since there is a risk of severe adverse reactions. High blood concentrations of chloroquine (rapid IV infusion, large IM doses) cause hypotension. Intravenous infusions must be given very

slowly and are difficult to administer in the absence of a controlled rate infusion pump (back to back infusions of 5 mg base/kg over 6 hours, repeated 5 times to achieve a total dose of 25 mg/kg in 30 hours).

(3) Intramuscular doses should not exceed 3.5 mg base/kg every 6 hours. As soon as oral dosing is possible, discontinue parenteral administration and complete the required dose orally to a total of 25mg/kg.

e. Management of respiratory distress in children with severe malaria

(1) In the past, respiratory distress in children with malaria has often been attributed to heart failure from anemia. This has resulted in a reluctance to transfuse, use of inappropriately slow infusion rates or use of diuretics to minimize volume overload.

(2) It is now recognized that respiratory distress in these children is much more likely to be due to hypoperfusion, lactic acidosis and impaired oxygen delivery due to both hypoperfusion and anemia. In these children, rapid correction of hypovolemia and anemia is lifesaving. Delay in transfusion and overuse of diuretics is dangerous.

f. Management of hypoglycemia in malaria

(1) High risk patients (very young children, pregnant women, those with high grade parasitemias and those treated with quinine, especially parenteral quinine) should be monitored prospectively for development of hypoglycemia.

(2) Hypoglycemia should be suspected when the patient exhibits any of the following: decreased level of consciousness, unusual behaviour, irritability, abnormal posturing (decerebrate or decorticate rigidity), decreased tone/floppiness, convulsions, twitching, stertorous breathing, or unexplained clinical deterioration.

(3) Hypoglycemia should be treated with 25% or 50% dextrose in a dose of 0.5g/kg by infusion over several minutes followed by a continuous infusion of dextrose or dextrose/saline. In children, dilution of high concentration dextrose solutions (25%, 50%) to a 10% solution will reduce the osmotic gradient and minimize the risk of precipitating rapid fluid shifts in the CNS.

(4) When giving IV quinine, administer in 10% dextrose to reduce the risk of hypoglycemia. Close monitoring of blood sugars is recommended as hypoglycemia can occur despite infusion of 10% dextrose.

g. Unproven treatments for severe malaria which should not be used

(1) Steroids have no proven benefit in severe malaria and should not be used. Some studies have shown increased mortality, prolonged duration of unconsciousness and increased rates of steroid-induced complications.

(2) Sodium bicarbonate to treat acidosis is not recommended as it does not address the underlying reason for acidosis and may worsen central nervous system acidosis. Dichloroacetate has been used to lower serum lactate levels but has no proven effect on survival and is not recommended.

(3) Desferrioxamine - initial studies suggested a decreased duration of coma in children with cerebral malaria, which has not been substantiated in further studies. Increased mortality has been observed in later studies and, therefore, desferrioxamine should not be used.

(4) Adrenaline - some older sources recommend use of adrenaline prior to quinine therapy, however, no benefit has been demonstrated and there are many potential risks (increased risk of arrhythmias, exacerbation of lactic acidosis, splenic rupture).

(5) Other therapies that are not recommended include dextran, heparin, osmotic agents to reduce cerebral edema (urea, mannitol, invert sugar), pentoxifylline (Trental).

E. Complications

1. Cerebral malaria

a. Presents with fever and altered mental status, including coma, without other signs of meningitis. Seizures are common.

b. Since it can be difficult to clinically differentiate between meningitis and cerebral malaria, and meningitis can be accompanied by acute malaria, all children with suspected cerebral malaria should be investigated with a lumbar puncture. CSF shows normal opening pressure, WBC <5 cells/mm3 and elevated protein. With antimalarial treatment, symptoms may rapidly clear, however cerebral malaria is a serious complication and is associated with significant mortality.

2. Anemia

a. Anemia in malaria is multifactorial, due to immune-mediated hemolysis, rupture of infected red cells, marrow suppression and splenic sequestration. Significant anemia may develop acutely during a severe episode of malaria but can also develop as a result of frequent episodes of malaria in children, particularly those with poor iron stores due to inadequate intake or intestinal iron loss from helminth infestations.

b. Decisions about when to transfuse must balance the risks of transmission of blood-borne pathogens, and risks of severe anemia. Arbitrary transfusions at specific hemoglobin levels should be avoided, although some experts recommend transfusion for all children with acute malaria and hemoglobin < 4 g/dl (hematocrit < 12 %). When the hemoglobin is less than 5 g/dl (50 g/l), a careful clinical assessment for signs of altered mental status, respiratory distress or heart failure should be done to determine the need for transfusion.

c. For children who are clinically stable, rapid initiation of anti-malarial therapy with the most effective agent available and close observation will usually avert the need for transfusion. Children with hyperparasitemia can be expected to sustain a rapid and significant fall in hemoglobin and will require transfusion at higher hemoglobin levels than those with low-grade parasitemias. The major indication for transfusion in a child with severe anemia is respiratory distress. Children with impaired consciousness should be transfused more liberally than those who are fully alert. A transfusion threshold of 5 g/dl is recommended in these children even in the absence of respiratory distress. When a child with severe anemia is deemed not to require transfusion, it may be appropriate to identify a suitable donor or unit that can be available in case of unexpected deterioration. Where prompt transfusion cannot be guaranteed, a higher transfusion threshold will be necessary.

d. Children with frequent episodes of malaria should be monitored closely for progressive anemia. Use of insecticide-impregnated nets and chemoprophylaxis may avert the need for transfusion. Iron supplementation should be provided for iron deficient children and should be expected to raise the hemoglobin by 1.5-2.0 g over 2 weeks. The timing of iron therapy is debated. Theoretical concerns that iron therapy in the acute stages may exacerbate malaria must be balanced against the advantages of prompt initiation of therapy. A reasonable approach is to delay iron therapy only until there is demonstrated response to anti-malarial therapy and the child is eating. A recent study found that 28 days of iron replacement started in hospital yielded a better hemoglobin after one month compared to transfusion. The benefits of folate supplementation are uncertain. Folate may decrease the efficacy of treatment with fansidar and should be avoided when this agent is used for treatment.

3. Acute renal failure

a. Acute renal failure is seen with high levels of parasitemia and hemolysis, or with hypoperfusion. It is more common in adults. In some patients, oliguric renal failure is present early with hepatic dysfunction, jaundice and metabolic acidosis. Death is usually due to pulmonary edema. A more slowly developing form of acute oliguric or non-oliguric renal failure occurs during recovery from acute malaria and carries a better prognosis.

b. In all patients with oliguria, careful assessment of intravascular volume should be made and volume depletion rapidly corrected. If this does not restore urine output, furosemide 40 mg IV may be tried to restore urine output. If this fails to reestablish urine flow, the dose can be doubled to a maximum of 400 mg. If there is no response to 400 mg, further diuretic therapy should be abandoned. Where feasible, a brief period of peritoneal dialysis may be required to control hyperkalemia or uremic symptoms.

c. Blackwater fever (passage of black or dark red-brown urine) refers to sudden, massive hemolysis resulting in precipitation of free hemoglobin in the renal tubules. When massive hemolysis is recognized early, forced alkaline diuresis may reduce the risk of renal failure by improving the solubility of hemoglobin and preventing formation of casts. Alkalinization of the urine can be achieved by an isotonic infusion of 0.45 % saline with 50 mls of 8.4% sodium bicarbonate added to each litre. Loop diuretics (furosemide) should be avoided as they acidify the urine. In patients presenting with established oliguric renal failure from hemolysis, attempts to induce diuresis by infusion of large fluid volumes may precipitate volume overload.

4. Splenomegaly

a. Common in patients with recurrent episodes of malaria.

b. Massive splenomegaly due to an abnormal immune response to malaria results in Hyperreactive Malarial Splenomegaly Syndrome (previously called Tropical Splenomegaly). This is commonly seen in areas where there is intense, chronic exposure to malaria. The massive splenomegaly results in pancytopenia, often with symptomatic anemia (even in the absence of acute malarial episodes) and increased susceptibility to infection. Although thrombocytopenia is present, overt bleeding is unusual. The blood slide is negative except when an acute attack of malaria intervenes. These patients may present with sudden onset of acute left upper quadrant pain representing an acute splenic infarction. During pregnancy, the massive splenomegaly may interfere with uterine enlargement.

c. Treatment - the goal of treatment is to eliminate further exposure to malaria. Complete avoidance of exposure is guaranteed only for those who can remove themselves from endemic areas. Use of insecticide-impregnated mosquito nets and chemoprophylaxis is indicated for those who cannot leave the endemic area. Chemoprophylaxis needs to be consistent and sustained for the duration of exposure in order for regression of splenomegaly to occur. Splenectomy should be avoided as it does not deal with the underlying cause of the disease and is typically followed by enlargement of the liver.

F. Malaria in Pregnancy

1. In low transmission areas, the maternal case fatality rate is increased significantly in severe malaria. Pregnant women are especially prone to hypoglycemia, particularly when treated with quinine. Hypoglycemia may contribute to fetal distress and bradycardia. Pregnant women in low transmission areas are also prone to acute pulmonary edema, which can develop abruptly in the immediate post-partum period.

2. In areas of high malaria transmission, the risk and intensity of parasitemia is increased in pregnancy, especially in the first and second pregnancy. Parasitemia is most frequent during the second trimester. Placental parasitemia with adverse fetal effects may occur in the absence of peripheral parasitemia or maternal symptoms. Maternal malaria and placental parasitemia may cause, or contribute to, spontaneous abortion, intrauterine death, premature labour, stillbirth and low birth weight. Typical manifestations of malaria in pregnancy in high transmission areas are maternal anemia and low birth weight.

3. Placental malaria may impair delivery of maternal antibodies to the fetus and promote transmission of HIV from infected mothers to their infants.

4. Pregnant women, especially in first and second pregnancies, should be targeted for malaria prophylaxis.

G. Prevention

1. Non-immune individuals at risk for malaria should use the most effective chemoprophylactic agent possible. Even individuals with extensive prior exposure to malaria remain at high risk of severe disease and should continue regular prophylaxis. In endemic areas, where it is not feasible to provide continuous prophylaxis for all young children, use of bednets should be encouraged and chemoprophlaxis targeted to high risk children (see below).

2. Prophylaxis for semi-immune individuals should be targeted to high-risk groups:
   a. Pregnancy - especially primigravida and secundigravida.
   b. Children with sickle cell anemia.
   c. Children and adults with hypertrophic malarial splenomegaly.
   d. Malnourished children.
   e. Children with progressive anemia or growth faltering due to repeated malaria episodes.

3. Use of measures to prevent or minimize mosquito contact is important as an adjuct to chemoprophylaxis. Insecticide-impregnated bed nets are effective in decreasing malaria morbidity and mortality. Permethrin, deltamethrin and lambdacyhalothrin are safe and effective insecticides for use on fabrics and may be safely used even for infants. Permethrin requires re-impregnation every 6 months; deltamethrin and lambdacyhalothrin require re-impregnation every 12 months. Permethrin can also be applied to clothing - a 13.3% solution will provide residual activity for about 4 weeks. Application of DEET to exposed skin can help provide additional protection. Children should use products containing 10% DEET (reapplication every 3-4 hours is required), adults can use 30-35% DEET which has a longer duration of action. Sustained release formulations of DEET are now available and provide more prolonged protection with a single application. When using DEET follow application instructions found on the product carefully as these are tailored to the specific concentration and formulation.

4. Chemoprophylaxis:

a. Chloroquine is no longer an effective agent in most endemic areas and should not be used for prophylaxis in non-immune individuals except in areas where the parasites remain fully susceptible. Prophylactic chloroquine dosage is 5mg/kg (max 300mg base) po weekly. Chloroquine prophylaxis should be limited to 5 years duration.

b. Proguanil (Paludrine) 3mg/kg daily. Proguanil monotherapy has limited efficacy and is not recommended for non-immune individuals. Proguanil may be useful with or without chloroquine for semi-immune individuals with hypertrophic malarial splenomegaly.

c. Chloroquine and proguanil in combination provides improved chemotherapeutic efficacy, but, in many areas, this combination is still inadequate to protect non-immune hosts.

d. Doxycycline 100 mg daily for adults, 1.5 mg /kg once daily for children over 8 years and > 25 kg. Doxycycline should not be used in children under 8 years of age, in pregnancy or breastfeeding. Doxycycline is the first-line choice for malaria prevention in non-immune individuals in chloroquine and mefloquine resistant areas and for individuals with contraindications to mefloquine.

e. Mefloquine (250mg base once weekly, 5mg/kg once weekly) is the first-line choice for malaria prevention in non-immune individuals in chloroquine-resistant areas. Side effects associated with prophylactic doses are usually mild and self-limiting; <5% individuals need to discontinue prophylaxis because of adverse effects. Severe neuropsychiatric side effects are infrequent at prophylactic doses (1:10,000 users) but are more frequent when used inappropriately in individuals with clear contraindications to mefloquine. Contraindications to mefloquine include seizure disorder, a history of psychosis or severe depression and a previous severe reaction to mefloquine. Mefloquine should be used with caution in the presence of underlying cardiac conduction abnormalities.

f. Malarone (250mg atovaquone + 100mg proguanil) has been shown to be an effective prophylactic agent for semi-immune individuals.

g. Primaquine is effective in preventing infection with *P. falciparum* as well as preventing relapses of *P. vivax* and *P. ovale*. G6PD deficiency must be excluded before prescribing primaquine to avoid risk of severe hemolytic reactions. This agent should be reserved for individuals in whom other agents are inappropriate.

h. Drugs unsuitable for chemoprophylaxis: quinine, halofantrine, artemisinin derivatives, pyrimethamine/sulfadoxine, amodiaquine and clindamycin. Azithromycin has weak antimalarial activity and should only be considered for prophylaxis when no other choices are suitable.

5. Malaria prophylaxis in pregnancy

a. Non-immune women and their infants are at high risk of serious complications from malaria during pregnancy. Careful attention should be paid to minimizing mosquito contact through use of appropriate clothing (covers exposed skin, light coloured), and insecticide-impregnated bed nets and avoidance of outdoor activities after dusk. Information regarding the safety of DEET in pregnancy is limited, but in high risk areas the benefits of avoiding malaria may outweigh potential risks of DEET. In pregnancy, limit DEET concentrations to 10%. Chemoprophylaxis should employ the most effective agent suitable for use in pregnancy.

(1) In areas where there is no chloroquine resistance, chloroquine is a safe and effective agent throughout pregnancy.

(2) Mefloquine is the most effective chemoprophylactic agent available for chloroquine-resistant areas. It is known to be safe for use in pregnancy from the beginning of the second trimester. The safety of mefloquine in first trimester is not as well established - limited data suggest a possible association with increased risk of spontaneous abortion. For non-immune women, the increased risk of severe malaria (for both mother and fetus) must be weighed against the potential for an adverse fetal outcome.

(3) Chloroquine + proguanil may be used for prophylaxis in areas where there is minimal chloroquine resistance and an additional degree of protection is desirable. For areas where higher degrees and frequency of chloroquine resistance is well established, this combination provides sub-optimal protection. If used as an alternative to mefloquine during the first trimester, melfloquine should be substituted at the onset of the second trimester.

(4) Doxycycline is contraindicated throughout pregnancy.

(5) Primaquine is contraindicated throughout pregnancy as the fetus' G6PD status cannot be established.

(6) Fansidar is contraindicated in the first trimester and during the last 2 weeks of gestation.

b. Semi-immune women and their infants will also benefit from chemoprophylaxis during pregnancy. Where chemoprophylaxis cannot be offered to all women, a chemoprophylactic program should target primigravidae and secundigravidae and all HIV-infected women, regardless of number of prior pregnancies.

(1) Weekly chloroquine may be used in areas without resistance.

(2) Fansidar has been shown to be effective in reducing placental malaria and the incidence of low birth weight infants when given as two full (treatment) doses during pregnancy (once in second trimester and once in third trimester). In HIV-infected women, monthly treatment with fansidar was more effective than the two dose regimen.

(3) Folic acid supplementation should be provided with all of the above regimens.

Antimalarial agents				
	Adult dose		**Pediatric dose**	
Agent	**Treatment**	**Prophylaxis**	**Treatment**	**Prophylaxis**
Chloroquine 150 mg base	4 tablets stat 4 tablets on day 2 2 tablets on day 3	300 mg base weekly	10 mg/kg base stat 10 mg/kg day 25 mg/kg day 3	5 mg /kg base weekly
Fansidar (500 mg Sulfadiazine/ 25 mg Pyrimethamine)	3 tablets stat	-	20 mg Sulfadoxine/ 1 mg Pyrimethamine per kg	-
Mefloquine 250 mg base	< **60 kg**: 3 tablets stat, 2 in 8 hours > **60 kg**: 3 tablets stat, 2 tablets in 8 hours,1 tab. in a further 8 hr.	250 mg once weekly	25 mg/kg or 15 mg/kg stat, 10 mg/kg in 8 hrs	5 mg base / kg weekly
Proguanil 100 mg	-	200 mg daily	-	3 mg/kg daily
Doxycycline 100 mg[a]	100 mg BID	100 mg daily	1.5 mg/kg bid (>8 years)	1.5 mg/kg daily (>8 years)
Clindamycin 150 mg[a]	600 mg q8h	-	10 mg/kg stat then 5 mg/kg q8h	-
Malarone (250 mg Atovaquone/100 mg Proguanil)	4 tablets daily x 3 days	1 tablet daily	20 mg atovaquone 8 mg proguanil per kg daily x 3 days	11-20 kg: ¼ tab/day 21-30 kg: ½ tab/day 31-40 kg: ¾ tab/day
Primaquine 15 mg base[b]	Radical cure: P. vivax15 mg base / day x 14	Primary prevention 30 mg base daily	Radical cure: P. vivax 0.3 mg base / day x 14	Primary prevention: 0.5 mg/kg base daily
Quinine sulfate 300 mg salt (250 mg base) per tablet	10 mg / kg salt tid x 7 days	-	10 mg/kg base tid x 7 days	-
Quinine dihydrochloride	20 mg / kg salt stat then 10 mg / kg q8h	-	20 mg/kg salt stat then 10 mg/kg q8h	-
Maloprim (100 mg dapsone/ 12.5 mg pyrimethamine)	-	1 tablet weekly	-	6-11 yrs: ½ tab weekly > 12 yrs: 1 tab weekly
Artesunate (oral)	4 mg / kg daily x 5-7 days	-	4 mg/kg daily x 5-7 days	-

Antimalarial agents (continued)				
	Adult dose		Pediatric dose	
Agent	Treatment	Prophylaxis	Treatment	Prophylaxis
Artesunate (IV)	2 mg/kg stat, 1 mg/kg at 12 hours, 1 mg/kg daily until oral Rx possible	-	2 mg/kg stat, 1 mg/kg at 12 hours, 1 mg/kg daily until oral Rx possible	-
Artemether (IM)	3.2 mg/kg stat, 1.6 mg/kg q24h until able to take oral meds	-	3.2 mg/kg stat, 1.6 mg/kg q24h until able to take oral meds	-
Artemesinin (suppository)	10 mg/kg stat, repeat in 4 hours then 7 mg/kg at 24, 36, 48 & 60 hours	-	10 mg/kg stat, repeat in 4 hours then 7 mg/kg at 24, 36, 48 & 60 hours	-

a. For use with quinine (Quinine x 7 days with 7 days of doxycycline or clindamycin)

b. Primaquine may be used for primary prevention of P. falciparum or for radical cure after infection with P. vivax or P. ovale. Rule out G6PD deficiency before use.

Halofantrine is no longer recommended for routine use. Rule out prolonged QT syndromes and avoid use with drugs that prolong QT intervals. Avoid use after mefloquine.

VI. SEXUALLY TRANSMITTED DISEASES

A. Gonorrhea

1. **Organism** - *Neisseria gonorrhea* (Gram negative diplococci).
2. **Clinical**
   a. Males - dysuria and urethritis with purulent urethral exudate. Incubation period usually 3-4 days (range 2-12 days).
   b. Females - vaginal discharge, lower abdominal pain, urethritis, dysuria, acute pelvic inflammatory disease (PID). May frequently have minimal or no symptoms.
   c. Complications
      (1) Males - epididymitis, prostatitis, urethral strictures (late).
      (2) Females - sterility after PID, tubo-ovarian abscess, Bartholin's gland abscess.
      (3) Either - disseminated disease (arthritis-dermatitis syndrome). Initially febrile and variably toxic due to bacteremia. Characteristic scattered skin lesions develop in 2/3 of cases (5-15 mm tender, erythematous papules, that develop a pustular, hemorrhagic, necrotic center). Patients also develop polyarticular arthralgias, and tenosynovitis. After one week, the skin lesions resolve. A monarticular or oligoarticular purulent arthritis may then develop (WBC in joint fluid > 25,000).

3. Diagnosis

a. Gram stain of urethral smear in males - sensitivity greater than 90%.

b. Gram stain of cervical (not vaginal) smear in females - sensitivity greater than 65%.

c. Culture for definitive diagnosis, if possible.

4. Treatment (always treat for chlamydial co-infection)

a. Uncomplicated infection (single dose)

   (1) Ciprofloxacin or another quinolone as a single dose (resistance is occurring in Asia).

   (2) Cefixime as a single 400 mg oral dose (no resistance reported) or cefuroxime acetil 1 gm orally.

   (3) Amoxicillin/clavulanate as a single 3 gm oral dose.

b. Alternative regimens (single dose)

   (1) Ceftriaxone 125 mg IM.

   (2) Spectinomycin 2 gm IM if penicillin allergic.

c. Pelvic inflammatory disease - usually due to gonorrhea or chlamydia but also consider Gm (-) rods and anerobes.

   (1) Remove intrauterine device (IUD), if present.

   (2) Sexual partners of all patients with PID need to be treated for both GC and chlamydia infection.

   (3) Outpatient treatment (low grade temp, WBC near-normal, no signs of peritonitis or pelvic abscess) - use one of the following regimens:

     (a) Amoxicillin/clavulanic acid 3 gm single dose followed by doxycycline 100 mg bid for 7 days.

     (b) Ceftriaxone 125 mg IM (single dose) + doxycycline 100 mg po bid for 7 days.

     (c) Ofloxacin 400 mg po bid + metronidazole 500 mg po bid for 7 days.

   (4) Inpatient treatment (temp > 38°C., peritonitis or pelvic abscess, pregnancy, failure to improve with outpatient treatment, unlikely to comply with treatment as outpatient) - use one of the following regimens:

     (a) Ampicillin 1gm IV q6h + gentamicin 1.5 mg/kg IV q8h + metronidazole 500 mg po or IV q6h or chloramphenicol 500 mg po or IV q6h.

     (b) Cefoxitin 2 gm IV q6h or cefotetan 2 gm IV q8-12h until improved + doxycycline 100mg po bid.

     (c) Clindamycin 600 mg IV q8h + gentamicin 1.5 mg/kg IV q8h (or 4mg/kg as a single daily dose).

     (d) Ofloxacin or other newer quinolones for 7-10 days.

     (e) Continue IV treatment until at least 48h after the patient is clinically improved, then doxycycline 100 mg po bid to complete a total of 14 days of therapy.

(f) If tubo-ovarian abscess is present, try conservative treatment with antibiotics, as above. If the patient deteriorates or does not improve (remains febrile, pain persists, WBC remains elevated), perform surgical drainage.

d. Disseminated gonococcal infection
   (1) Ceftriaxone one gm IV/ IM followed by cefixime for 5 days.
   (2) Amoxicillin/clavulanic acid 3 gm as a stat dose orally followed by 500 mg tid for 7 days.
   (3) Ciprofloxacin 500 mg bid x 7-10d.
   (4) Continue IV treatment for at least 24 hrs after the patient is clinically improved, then complete 7-10 days of treatment with oral anti-gonococcal drug.

B. Nongonococcal urethritis

1. **Organisms** - *Chlamydia trachomatis* (50%), *Ureaplasma urealyticum*, *Mycoplasma genitalium*.

2. **Clinical**
   a. Males - scanty, watery, mucoid urethral discharge. Commonly seen after treatment for gonococcal urethritis.
   b. Females - acute urethritis with pyuria, cervicitis, or salpingitis due to *C. trachomatis*.

3. **Diagnosis** - based on clinical features, and failure to respond to treatment for gonorrhea.

4. **Treatment** - choose one of the following:
   a. Tetracycline 500 mg po qid, or doxycycline 100 mg po bid x 7d.
   b. Erythromycin 500 mg po qid x 7d.
   c. Azithromycin 1 gm po as single dose.
   d. Ofloxacin 300 mg po q12h x 7d.
   e. Pregnant women - erythromycin 500 mg po qid x 7d, amoxicillin 500 mg po tid x 10d or azithromycin 1gm po x 1 dose.

C. Syphilis

1. **Organism** - *Treponema pallidum*.
2. **Incubation period** - 1-12 weeks.
3. **Stages**
   a. Primary
      (1) Characterized classically by the development of a single, firm, indurated, painless ulcer (chancre) at site of contact, usually genital. However, only 50% of primary syphilitic ulcers are typical.
      (2) Chancre spontaneously disappears in 4-6 weeks.
      (3) Painless inguinal lymphadenopathy may be present.
   b. Secondary
      (1) Occurs 2 weeks to 6 months (average 6 weeks) after the appearance of the chancre.
      (2) Characterized by the development of anorexia, nausea, malaise, headache, and myalgias.

(3) A rash is frequently present. It may be of any type, but frequently is papulosquamous (has a scale). It is usually non-pruritic. The distribution is bilateral, symmetric, and involves the hands and soles. Hyperpigmented, circular lesions are common.

(4) Mucocutaneous lesions are commonly present. Condylomata lata are broad, moist, gray-white, exudative lesions that are found on the genitals; they are highly infective.

   c. Latent - normal examination, with positive VDRL (or RPR).

   d. Tertiary - appears years after the original infection. Cardiovascular form causes aortic root dilatation and aortic regurgitation. Neurosyphilis is usually asymptomatic, but, if left untreated, may cause progressive neurologic symptoms, including dementia and posterior column disease characterized by loss of position sense in the feet and an ataxic, slapping gait.

4. Diagnosis - must rely on physical signs and the VDRL.

   a. The VDRL becomes reliably positive by 4 weeks after infection in most patients. It remains positive for years in untreated disease. False positive VDRL tests have been reported in a variety of diseases, especially infections (malaria), in pregnancy, and immune complex disease. These are usually weakly positive. Confirm the positive VDRL with a specific treponemal test if available (FTA-ABS or MHA-TP).

   b. Neurosyphilis - CSF exam is indicated in all patients with signs and symptoms of neurosyphilis and those with syphilis > 1 year duration. Typical CSF findings are 10-100 lymphocytes, increased protein, and a positive CSF VDRL. Some far advanced cases may have normal CSF. Follow the patient after treatment to insure improvement in VDRL titers and CSF abnormalities.

5. Treatment

   a. Penicillin is the drug of choice for all stages of syphilis. Document penicillin allergy before using alternative drugs. In pregnant women with penicillin allergy, desensitization to penicillin should be considered, as alternative agents are less effective in preventing congenital disease.

   b. Primary, secondary, and early latent (< 1 yr) stages - benzathine penicillin 2.4 million units IM once, doxycycline 100 mg po bid x 14 days, or erythromycin 500 mg po qid x15 days (higher risk of relapse).

   c. Late latent (> 1 yr) stage - benzathine penicillin 2.4 million units IM weekly x 3 doses, or doxycycline 100 mg po bid x 30d, tetracycline 500 mg po qid x 30d, or erythromycin 500 mg po qid x 30d.

   d. Neurosyphilis - any of the following are acceptable:

(1) Aqueous PCN G 2-4 million units IV q4h x 10-14d.

(2) Procaine PCN G 2.4 million units IM qd + probenecid 500 mg po qid x 10-14d.

    (3) Doxycycline 200 mg po bid x 21 days.

    (4) Ceftriaxone 1 gm IM qd x 14 days.

    (5) Amoxicillin 3 gm po bid + probenecid 500 mg po bid x 15 days.

    (6) Chloramphenicol 2 gm IV or 500 mg po q6h x 30 days.

6. Follow up - defining cure

  a. VDRL - repeat the test at 3, 6, and 12 months (and 24 months in late syphilis). In successfully treated primary and secondary stage disease the VDRL slowly reverts to negative over one to two years in most patients. It remains positive longer after treatment of late or repeated episodes of disease. A fourfold decrease in the VDRL titer at 6 months, or eight-fold decrease at 12 months indicates successful treatment in primary and secondary disease. In late disease, a fourfold decrease in VDRL titer at 12 months indicates successful treatment. The FTA remains positive for life and cannot be used to monitor therapy.

  b. Neurosyphilis - CSF abnormalities return to normal following treatment. The CSF VDRL may be reactive for greater than one year.

7. HIV infection and syphilis

  a. The presentation, serologic response, and response to treatment may be atypical in HIV-positive patients with syphilis.

  b. Some authorities recommend CSF examination for all patients co-infected with syphilis and HIV regardless of clinical stage. CSF examination is especially important in:

    (1) All patients with infection of greater than 1 yr duration (or latent syphilis of unknown duration).

    (2) Syphilis of any stage with neurologic signs or symptoms.

    (3) Treatment failure in syphilis at any stage.

  c. Treatment

    (1) Patients who have a normal CSF may be treated with standard regimens, but follow-up to assure cure is important.

    (2) Higher drug doses and longer duration of treatment may be necessary for cure.

    (3) Even high dose IV therapy may fail in neurosyphilis.

D. Anogenital warts (Condylomata accuminata)

  1. Etiology - Human papilloma virus.

  2. Description - moist, papular lesions that are usually located in the perineal or genital area. Larger lesions may become cauliflower-like. Differentiate from syphilis (condylomata lata).

  3. Treatment - no form of treatment has been shown to eradicate the virus. No treatment is uniformly effective in treating or preventing recurrence. The following may be helpful:

    a. Podophyllin 25% in tincture of benzoin

      (1) Use on lesions < 2 cm.

      (2) Protect the surrounding tissue with petroleum jelly.

      (3) Apply to warts, remove after 4 hours.

      (4) Repeat the treatment weekly x 4wk. If no regression after 4 weeks, consider alternative treatment.

      (5) Contraindicated in pregnancy.

    b. Bi - or tri-chloroacetic acid in a 30-50% solution

      (1) Apply 2x per month.

      (2) Can treat larger lesions.

      (3) Can be used in pregnancy.

    c. For large or resistant lesions use surgical excision, cryotherapy, or imiquimod cream (apply 3 times a week for 12 weeks).

E. Chancroid

  1. Organism - *Haemophilus ducreyi.*

  2. Signs and symptoms

    a. Incubation period is about one week.

    b. Produces one or more small papules that rapidly progress to painful, ragged, undermined genital ulcers. Later, tender adenopathy develops which may ulcerate if left untreated.

  3. Diagnosis

    a. Identification based on clinical appearance is difficult. Must also consider syphilis, HSV II, and lymphogranuloma venereum.

    b. Perform Gram stain looking for gm (-) coccobacillus. Aspirate from inguinal nodes may be positive. Culture is unreliable.

    c. Consider a therapeutic treatment trial.

  4. Treatment - use any of the following:

    a. Erythromycin 500 mg po qid x 7 days or until ulcers heal.

    b. Ceftriaxone 250 mg IM as single dose.

    c. Azithromycin 1 gm po as single dose (failures reported in HIV patients).

    d. Ciprofloxacin 500 mg po bid x 3 days.

F. Granuloma inguinale

  1. Organism - *Calymmatobacterium granulomatis.* Common in various parts of the world.

  2. Signs and symptoms

    a. Lesions begin as painless papules, progress to beefy-red, granulomatous, friable ulcers with elevated margins. The usual location is the genital area.

    b. Multiple ulcerative lesions may be present, spread locally and coalesce forming large ulcerative masses. These typically remain painless unless secondarily infected.

    c. Healing occurs with scar formation.

  3. Diagnosis

    a. Based on the characteristic appearance of the lesions.

    b. Demonstration of Donovan bodies (intracellular bacilli found in macrophages taken from scrapings or biopsies of the margins of lesions).

4. Treatment

    a. Doxycycline 100 mg po bid, TMP/SMX 1 DS tab po bid, or erythromycin 500 mg po qid.

    b. Healing usually begins within one week, but treatment is continued until healing is complete.

G. Lymphogranuloma venereum

1. Organism - *Chlamydia trachomatis.*

2. Signs and symptoms - initial genital lesion is a papule or ulcer that rapidly heals, followed by rapid enlargement of inguinal nodes over 2-6 weeks. The nodes frequently ulcerate, forming multiple sinuses with purulent drainage.

3. Diagnosis - suspected by appearance and clinical course.

4. Treatment - doxycycline 100 mg po bid or erythromycin 500 mg po qid x 21days.

H. Herpes genitalis

1. Organism - Herpes simplex type II.

2. Signs and symptoms - the initial lesions are vesicular, located in the perineal area, and associated with pain, fever, and malaise. They rapidly ulcerate, leaving multiple shallow, painful ulcers. The lesions heal in 5-7 days. Recurrent episodes occur which are usually milder than the initial episode.

3. Diagnosis

    a. Based on the clinical appearance and history (especially if recurrent).

    b. Tzanck smear - Wright-Giemsa stain of smear taken from ulcer shows multinucleated giant cells.

    c. Viral culture is diagnostic, if available.

4. Treatment

    a. Analgesics and local treatment.

    b. Anti-viral therapy (begin within 24 hours of onset)

       (1) Acyclovir 400 mg po tid x 5 days (initial episode - treat for 10 days).

       (2) Famciclovir 125 mg po bid x 5 days (initial episode - 250 mg tid x 5 days).

    c. For severe recurrent disease, acyclovir 400 mg po bid or famciclovir 250 mg po daily reduces the frequency and severity of recurrences.

VII. Soft Tissue and Bone Infections
A. Lymphadenopathy
1. General
a. Common patterns of superficial lymph node drainage

Patterns of lymph node drainage	
Submental Submandibular	Mouth Salivary glands
Jugular Supraclavicular Suboccipital	Head and neck
Supraclavicular	Intrathoracic and intra-abdominal
Pre-auricular Post-auricular	Eyes, ears, scalp
Central and lateral axillary	Upper extremities Chest wall Breast Intrathoracic structures
Epitrochlear	Forearm and hand
Inguinal	Lower extremities Genitalia
External iliac and femoral	Lower extremities Genitalia Pelvic structures

b. Deep node enlargement
  (1) Thoracic (hilar or mediastinal) lymph node enlargement may cause secondary effects from compression of the following structures:
     (a) Trachea or mainstem bronchi - cough, dyspnea, wheezing, stridor.
     (b) Esophagus - dysphagia.
     (c) Superior vena cava or subclavian vein - venous congestion in the face, neck, arm.
     (d) Phrenic nerve - paralysis of the diaphragm.
     (e) Recurrent laryngeal nerve - hoarseness.
  (2) Internal iliac or pelvic lymph node enlargement may cause venous or lymphatic congestion in the legs or external genitalia.
  (3) Abdominal and pelvic lymph node enlargement may occasionally be palpable on exam.

2. Significance of lymph node enlargement
a. Certain lymph nodes are palpable under normal circumstances. Submandibular nodes <1 cm are common in children and young adults. Inguinal nodes 0.5 - 2 cm are common in adults. The factors below help determine the significance of lymphadenopathy.

    b. Clinical setting
- (1) Age of the patient - lymphadenopathy in patients <30 years old is usually benign or infectious.
- (2) Associated symptoms - fever, night sweats, weight loss suggests tuberculosis or malignancy. Erythema and warmth of the surrounding tissue suggests pyogenic infection. Generalized symptoms may be associated with HIV disease.

    c. Physical characteristics (firmness, mobility, tenderness)
- (1) Tender and fluctuant with inflamed overlying skin - infectious.
- (2) Suppurative - tuberculosis or staphylococcal infection.
- (3) Firm, fixed, non-tender - tumor.
- (4) Large, firm, mobile, symmetric - lymphomatous process.

    d. Location - certain locations suggest malignancy (supraclavicular, abdominal or retroperitoneal).

3. Generalized lymphadenopathy

    a. Definition: lymphadenopathy affecting more than 2 separate anatomic areas.

    b. Significance - generalized lymphadenopathy has a different differential than localized or regional lymphadenopathy and should always be considered significant.

    c. Important diagnostic possibilities in generalized lymphadenopathy
- (1) Infectious - rheumatic fever, brucellosis, secondary syphilis, rubella, infectious mononucleosis, toxoplasmosis, tuberculosis, kala-azar, HIV infection, tularemia, sleeping sickness, Chaga's disease.
- (2) Neoplastic - lymphoma, lymphatic leukemia.
- (3) Collagen vascular diseases - Still's disease, rheumatoid arthritis, lupus, dermatomyositis.
- (4) Other - serum sickness, scabies infestation, phenytoin, sarcoidosis, amyloidosis, hyperthyroidism, storage diseases.

4. Diagnostic approach

    a. If an infectious cause is suspected, treat for 10 - 14 days with antibiotic to cover strep and staph (ie: cephalexin, cefuroxime, amoxicillin/clavulanic acid, clarithromycin). Suppurating nodes should be aspirated and cultured, if possible. Re-evaluate after 2 weeks. It is important to accurately measure and record lymph node location and size on each visit.

    b. If nodes are fixed and firm or the patient shows other signs of malignancy, the nodes should be biopsied as soon as possible.

c. If huge suppurating nodes are present and haven't responded to antibiotics a biopsy is strongly recommended. AFB stains and culture for TB should be performed as well as routine pathology. Where such resources are unavailable, the presence of gross caseation on bisection of the node is strong evidence for TB and warrants TB treatment. Impression smears can be done for Gram stain and AFB should be done but are less sensitive than culture. Where diagnostic facilities are extremely limited, empiric TB treatment (for scrofula) may need to be considered.

d. If no response, consider other etiologies - Burkitt's lymphoma, sarcoidosis, amyloidosis, mucocutaneous lymph node syndrome, histiocytic disorders.

B. Osteomyelitis
1. Types
a. Hematogenous

(1) Primary hematogenous osteomyelitis is most common in children and typically involves the metaphysis of a long bone. Minor trauma (often unrecognized) causes thrombosis in capillary loops in the metaphysis, increasing local vulnerability to infection. Infection is initiated when a transient bacteremia seeds the site. Secondary hematogenous osteomyelitis refers to a relapse of osteomyelitis in older children and adults with a history of remote primary osteomyelitis.

(2) Organism - common organisms in hematogenous osteomyelitis reflect the most common age-related causes of bacteremia.

Organisms in Hematogenous Osteomyelitis	
Infants < 1 month	*Staph. aureus* Group B Streptococci *E. coli*
Infants > 1 month Children	*Staph. aureus,* *Hemophilus influenzae* Group A Streptococci
Adults	Primary hematogenous: *Staph. aureus* Secondary hematogenous: original organism

Salmonella is an important pathogen in individuals with sickle cell anemia and HIV infection, but may also be seen in the absence of these underlying conditions, especially in areas where *Salmonella* infections are highly prevalent.

b. Secondary to a contiguous focus of infection

(1) Most patients will have a history of previous surgery, trauma or soft-tissue infection, which introduces organisms into bone.

(2) Organisms - *Staph. aureus* is the single most common isolate. In posttraumatic cases with extensive contamination with environmental flora, polymicrobial infections may occur.

c. Associated with vascular insufficiency or neuropathy

(1) Vascular insufficiency due to diabetes or peripheral vascular disease leads to loss of skin integrity and damage to local soft tissues. Peripheral neuropathy from diabetes or leprosy can result in damage to soft tissues of the feet from repetitive trauma. Infection of underlying bone is commonly associated with chronic ulcerations.

(2) This form of osteomyelitis usually involves the small bones of the feet and is typically chronic. Osteomyelitis associated with vascular insufficiency may be recalcitrant to treatment in the absence of revascularization.

(3) Organisms - usually polymicrobial, including *Staphylococcus aureus*, Streptococci (including *Enterococcus*), gram-negative bacilli and anerobes.

2. Diagnosis
   a. Clinical signs

(1) Acute osteomyelitis typically presents with fever, local tenderness, swelling and limitation of motion. Children often present with vague symptoms, lacking fever or other signs suggestive of an acute infection. Pseudoparalysis (refusal to use the limb) or limping are important signs in children.

(2) In chronic infections, draining sinuses are usually present.

(3) Osteomyelitis related to vascular insufficiency often presents with minimal or no pain due to associated peripheral neuropathy. Ulcerations are usually present. Osteomyelitis should be suspected if exposed bone is present in the ulcer bed, or if probing the ulcers encounters bone.

   b. X-ray findings

(1) Acute - signs of osteomyelitis (periosteal thickening or elevation and focal osteopenia) do not appear until after the second week of infection. Lytic changes appear even later. Local soft tissue swelling is usually present before bony changes are evident.

(2) Chronic - look for mottling of the bone with areas of lucency from bone destruction and radiopaque areas representing sequestra and involucra formation.

   c. Cultures

(1) Blood cultures are helpful in identifying the organism in some cases of acute hematogenous osteomyelitis (~60% positive).

(2) Sinus tract cultures are unreliable in predicting organisms present in bone with both false positives (isolation of organisms that are not present in bone) and false negatives (failure to isolate true pathogens). An exception to this is when *Staph. aureus* is recovered from a sinus tract culture, it can be assumed to be present in bone also, but may not be the only pathogen.

(3) Culture of aspirated fluid or biopsy material should be attempted, if possible.

3. Treatment
a. Acute
(1) Perform immediate needle aspiration of the site. In children, subperiosteal needle aspirations can be done if point tenderness is present. When large amounts of subperiosteal pus are present, surgical drainage is required. Drilling of bone to decompress intramedullary pus may be required.

(2) Choice of antibiotics depends on Gram stain or culture, if available. Treatment should include parenteral antibiotics at high dose until a good clinical response is obtained (resolution of fever and leukocytosis, local signs of infection improved), then oral antibiotics for a total of 4-6 weeks of therapy. If cultures cannot be done, treatment should be based on the organisms expected based on the patient's age and mechanism of osteomyelitis (hematogenous, contiguous, vascular).

(3) Treatment of diabetic foot infections should provide coverage for *Staphylococcus aureus*, gram negatives and anaerobes. Cultures of bone are useful to exclude *Pseudomonas*. If *Pseudomonas* is present, treatment should include an anti-pseudomonal agent. Anaerobes should always be assumed to be present in diabetic foot infections, as these are not easily recovered in culture.

(4) The erythrocyte sedimentation rate should start to improve within 1-2 weeks and should consistently decline to normal throughout treatment.

b. Chronic
(1) Antibiotic therapy alone is unlikely to cure chronic osteomyelitis.

(2) Surgical debridement to remove all dead bone (sequestrectomy) is essential. Packing the wound open and allowing granulation tissue to fill in the defect over several weeks may be successful.

(3) Antibiotics targeted to the causative organism should be provided. If an attempt to cure is made, then several weeks of high dose intravenous therapy throughout the surgical and post-op period, while the wound granulates in, is appropriate. A prolonged course of oral antibiotics following healing may improve the chance for cure.

c. Antibiotics

Empiric Antibiotic Treatment of Osteomyelitis		
Hematogenous osteomyelitis	Infant < 1 month	Ampicillin + Gentamicin
		Ampicillin + Ccfotaxime
	Child > 1 month	Cloxacillin + Chloramphenicol
		Cefuroxime
		Cloxacillin + TMP/SWX
	Adult	Cloxacillin or Cefazolin
Contiguous osteomyelitis	Child	Cloxacillin + TMP/SWX
		Cloxacillin + Chloramphenicol
	Adult	Cloxacillin + Ciprofloxacin
Diabetic foot	**No** *Pseudomonas*	Cloxacillin + Chloramphenicol
		Cefazolin (cephalexin) + Metronidazole
		Amoxicillin / clavulanic acid
		Clindamycin + TMP/SWX
	Pseudomonas	Ciprofloxacin + Metronidazole
		Add Cloxacillin if *Staph. aureus* present

(1) In *Staph aureus* osteomyelitis, addition of rifampin (20 mg/kg/d, max 600 mg) may be helpful.

(2) If third generation cephalosporins are available, cefotaxime or ceftriaxone can be used in place of chloramphenicol or TMP/SWX for children and adults with hematogenous or contiguous osteomyelitis. Cefuroxime (a second generation cephalosporin) is useful in children as it provides coverage for *S. aureus*, Group A streptococci and *H. influenzae* (but not *Salmonella*).

(3) Surgical intervention is advisable if the patient has not responded to appropriate antibiotics within 48 hours.

(4) Patients with longstanding chronic osteomyelitis or frequent recurrences may require chronic suppressive antimicrobial therapy with low dose oral antibiotics. An initial period of parenteral therapy to settle acute systemic signs of infection may be necessary. Cultures to identify the organism and antibiotic susceptibility are important to guide antibiotic selection, when they are available.

C. Necrotizing soft tissue infections

1. **General** - necrotizing soft tissue infections are rapidly progressive infections in which bacterial toxins or synergistic combinations of bacterial species promote tissue breakdown and rapid bacterial replication.

2. **Microbiology**

   a. Necrotizing fasciitis may be due to Group A streptococcus (GAS) or a polymicrobial infection with anaerobes and facultative gram negative bacilli. Necrotizing fasciitis due to Group A strep may be associated with toxic shock syndrome.

81

b. Clostridia can cause a variety of soft tissue infections.

3. **Clinical presentation**

    a. Rapidly progressive infection of skin, subcutaneous tissue, underlying fascia and/or muscle. Rapid expansion of the involved area and pain out of keeping with visible changes of inflammation should raise the suspicion of necrotizing fasciitis.

    b. Other danger signs include: prominent edema extending beyond areas of erythema, multi-coloured skin lesions, bullae, especially if filled with hemorrhagic fluid, presence of anaesthetic areas or crepitus and foul smelling "dishwater" pus.

    c. In suspicious cases of necrotizing fasciitis, make a small incision and insert a metal probe to the level of the fascia. Unhindered movement of the probe through the fascial layer indicates necrosis.

4. **Type 1 necrotizing fasciitis** (mixed anaerobes and facultative Gram-negative bacilli)

    a. Risk factors include diabetes, obesity, peripheral vascular disease, general debility and breaches in the GI or GU mucosa due to surgery, trauma or malignancy.

    b. Typically involves the perineum, lower extremities and abdomen.

    c. A portal of entry is evident in most cases.

    d. Systemic toxicity is pronounced, with fever, leukocytosis and shock.

    e. Scattered areas of skin necrosis and ulceration with intervening areas of normal skin. Crepitus is present in about 25% of cases. Cutaneous anaesthesia is not found.

5. **Type 2 necrotizing fasciitis** (Group A streptococci - occasionally other ß-hemolytic streptococci)

    a. GAS necrotizing fasciitis typically occurs in young healthy individuals without underlying disease.

    b. Portal of entry is present in about 50% of individuals (minor soft tissue lesions such as burns, abrasions etc. In children varicella is a common precipitant.)

    c. Systemic toxicity is marked.

    d. Early skin findings may be very subtle. Pain often precedes other findings. Early on there may be only mild erythema with local tenderness and pronounced pain. As the infection progresses, the extent of visibly involved skin extends rapidly. Erythema becomes more prominent and may be replaced by multi-coloured, blue-gray areas of necrosis. Patchy cutaneous anaesthesia is a late sign. Crepitus does not occur.

6. **Clostridial infections**

    a. Simple contamination of traumatic wounds is common. Most contaminated wounds do not progress to infection unless there is necrotic or devitalized tissue present. Good wound management with cleansing and debridement of devitalized tissue is important to prevent serious clostridial infections.

b. Clostridial cellulitis - necrotizing infection of subcutaneous tissues, sparing muscle and fascia.
    (1) Onset is gradual but spread is rapid once disease is established.
    (2) Pain and systemic toxicity are mild.
    (3) Crepitus is very prominent.

c. Clostridial myoncrosis / gas gangrene
    (1) Severe pain and marked systemic toxicity.
    (2) Abrupt onset and rapid progression.
    (3) Crepitus is present but less prominent than in clostridial cellulitis. Extensive gas is evident on x-ray.

7. Treatment

a. Early and aggressive surgical debridement is essential in the management of necrotizing infections. Repeated re-exploration of the wounds should be undertaken at regular intervals (q8-12 hours) until no further necrosis is demonstrated.
    (1) Gram stain of tissue obtained at the initial debridement can be used to guide antimicrobial therapy. Several different sites should be sampled.
    (2) Gram-positive cocci suggest Group A streptococci, large Gram-positive bacilli suggests Clostridia. The presence of mixed organisms suggests Type 1 necrotizing fasciitis due to anaerobes and facultative Gram- negative bacilli.

b. Antimicrobial therapy
    (1) GAS necrotizing fasciitis - clindamycin + penicillin.
    (2) Type I necrotizing fasciitis - metronidazole + 3rd generation cephalosporin or metronidazole + ciprofloxacin. Where these agents are unavailable, chloramphenicol may be used.
    (3) Clostridial cellulitis/myonecrosis - the combination of penicillin + clindamycin has synergistic activity. Penicillin should not be combined with metronidazole in clostridial infection as this combination is antagonistic. Penicillin or clindamycin monotherapy should be avoided due to the possibility of resistance. Chloramphenicol may be used in penicillin-allergic patients.

8. Group A streptococcal toxic shock syndrome (TSS)

a. Diagnostic criteria
    (1) Isolation of Group A streptococci
        (a) From a sterile body site.
        (b) From a non-sterile body site.
    (2) Clinical signs of severity
        (a) Systolic BP < 90mmHg
        (b) Two or more of the following:
            i. Renal impairment (creatinine >2x normal).
            ii. Coagulopathy (platelet count <100,000 or DIC).

        iii. Liver impairment (AST, ALT, bilirubin >2x normal).

        iv. Adult respiratory distress syndrome.

        v. Rash (erythroderma) with subsequent desquammation.

        vi. Necrotizing soft tissue infection.

  (3) Definite case: 1a + 2a + 2b

  (4) Probable case: 1b + 2a +2b.

b. Treatment

  (1) Supportive care - fluid rescuscitation, inotropes, ventilatory support, transfusion.

  (2) Antibiotics - clindamycin 900mg IV q8h + penicillin 24 million units IV per day in divided doses. If IV clindamycin is unavailable, oral clindamycin is well absorbed and can be used in patients able to take oral medications.

  (3) Where available, intravenous immune globulin 150mg/kg/day x 5 days will improve survival.

  (4) Surgical intervention is necessary where TSS accompanies necrotizing fasciitis.

D. Pyomyositis

1. General

a. Pyomyositis - primary muscle abscess, a bacterial infection of muscle that develops in the absence of a predisposing infection or penetrating trauma. Pyomyositis is common in the tropics.

b. Organism: 75-95% of cases are caused by *Staphyloccocus aureus*. Group A Streptococcus is the second most common organism. Less common pathogens include other streptococci, Gram-negative bacilli and anaerobes.

c. Epidemiology

  (1) Pre-disposing conditions include diabetes, alcoholic liver disease, steroid therapy, hematologic malignancies, sickle cell disease and HIV infection. In the tropics, most patients lack underlying conditions, however, HIV infection should be considered.

  (2) Pyomyositis occurs in all age groups, but is more frequent in children in the tropics.

d. Etiology

  (1) In most cases, organisms likely reach muscle through a transient bacteremia. In up to 50% of cases a history of recent blunt trauma or vigorous exercise is present and may produce minor trauma to the muscle that provides an environment conducive to initial bacterial replication.

  (2) Eosinophilia is often present in patients with tropical pyomyositis suggesting that migrating helminths may be the source of bacterial inoculation in some cases.

2. Clinical presentation

a. The early stage of pyomyositis is characterized by subacute onset of fever, with local swelling of the involved area but no erythema and only mild pain and tenderness. At this stage, the muscle feels woody or indurated rather than fluctuant, and aspiration does not yield pus. The early stage typically lasts 10-12 days.

   b. As infection progresses, localized muscle swelling and pain become more prominent and the overlying skin develops characteristic signs of inflammation. (With very deep muscle infections, skin changes may remain minimal or appear only late). Aspiration at this stage will yield pus.

   c. If the infection is not treated promptly, it can progress to systemic sepsis and metastatic infection in other muscles and tissues. Some patients will present with abrupt onset of high fever and/or signs of toxic shock syndrome.

   d. Large muscle groups of the lower extremities are most commonly affected.

3. Diagnosis

   a. Suspect this diagnosis in patients with localized pain and swelling, usually in an extremity. Pyomyositis at unusual sites may be mistaken for other disorders. For example, iliopsoas pyomyositis mimics appendicitis, iliacus pyomyositis mimics septic hip, psoas involvement may suggest spinal disease. Fever and leukocytosis are usually present.

   b. Fluctuance may not be detectable in deep abscesses. Ultrasound may be helpful in localizing the abscess. Needle aspiration of pus is diagnostic.

4. Treatment

   a. Antibiotic therapy should be initiated as soon as the diagnosis is suspected. Empiric antibiotics should cover *S. aureus* (cloxacillin, cefazolin, cephalexin, clindamycin). Parenteral antibiotics are preferred until systemic signs of infection resolve.

   b. Surgical drainage - once an abscess has formed, surgical drainage is essential. If ultrasound is not available, blind needle aspiration can be helpful in confirming the presence of a collection of pus, particularly when the collection is deep in muscle and fluctuance is difficult to detect. Pus should be sent for Gram stain (and culture, if possible). If the Gram stain demonstrates an organism other than Gram-positive cocci in clusters (presumptive *S. aureus*) modification of antimicrobial therapy will be indicated.

   c. Duration of treatment - drainage of the abscess will result in prompt clinical improvement with normalization of temperature and leukocytosis. With adequate drainage, fever usually resolves promptly. A 10 day course antibiotic therapy is recommended. In patients presenting with evidence of systemic sepsis, or where a positive blood culture for *S. aureus* has been obtained, 2 weeks of anti-staphylococcal therapy should be given to reduce the risk of late metastatic infection with *Staph. aureus*. Continued fever after drainage suggests incomplete evacuation of pus or metastatic sites of infection.

  d. Complications include compartment syndrome and metastatic infections (bone, heart, other organs).

E. Buruli ulcer
  ### 1. General
    a. Buruli ulcer is a chronic, progressive ulceration of soft tissues prevalent in rural areas of many tropical and subtropical countries. Buruli ulcer is especially prevalent in West Africa and appears to be increasing in incidence. The disease is particularly prevalent in marshy areas.

    b. The mechanism of infection is unknown but frequent contact with stagnant or slow-running water is noted in areas where the disease is prevalent.

    c. 70% of cases occur in children under 15 years of age.

  ### 2. Organism - *Mycobacterium ulcerans*. *M. ulcerans* produces a lipid toxin which triggers cell death and suppresses the normal host immune response.

  ### 3. Clinical presentation
    a. The disease typically starts with a painless subcutaneous nodule or nodules attached to the skin. Over a period of several months the lesions evolve to ulcers. Ulcers may remain small or progressively enlarge to involve extensive areas of skin and underlying soft tissue with extensive undermining of the edges. Discomfort is minimal and may result in delay in seeking medical attention.

    b. Bone involvement can occur. With severe disease, extensive deformities can result. Constitutional symptoms and lymphadenopathy are uncommon.

  ### 4. Treatment
    a. Surgical excision of lesions is recommended. Skin grafting and reconstruction may be required.

    b. Antimicrobial therapy is of limited success. The combination of an aminoglycoside (amikacin or streptomycin) plus rifampin is effective in animal models.

  ### 5. Differential diagnosis includes tropical phagedenic ulcers, cutaneous leishmaniasis, lupus vulgaris (*Mycobacterium tuberculosis*), sickle cell disease-related ulcers, venous stasis ulcers, yaws, cutaneous diphtheria, and malignant ulcers.

F. Tropical ulcer
  ### 1. General
    a. Tropical ulcers are chronic ulcerations usually involving the lower extremities.

b. They are prevalent in hot, humid, tropical and subtropical environments, especially Central and East Africa.

2. Pathogenesis

   a. Lesions are usually initiated by trauma, however, the inciting event can be trivial and may not be recognized. Undernutrition and micronutrient deficiencies, while unproven, have traditionally been considered important as contributing factors.

   b. The infection is polymicrobial and fusobacteria and spirochetes appear to play a key role. Following recovery from a tropical ulcer, some patients develop multiple recurrences.

3. Clinical presentation

   a. Tropical ulcers typically begin with a small papule or bullous lesion, usually over the anterior surface of the tibia. The papule rapidly breaks down to form an ulcer, which can persist for many years in the absence of treatment. The ulcer border has a well-defined edge with a purulent base.

   b. Tropical ulcers are typically very painful (in contrast to Buruli ulcers). Ulcers can penetrate deeply and damage underlying bone and tendons.

   c. Squamous cell carcinoma may complicate long-standing ulcers.

4. Treatment

   a. Antibiotics - penicillin +/- metronidazole or amoxicillin/clavulanic acid.

   b. Rest and elevation of the extremity helps promote healing in severe cases.

   c. Topical therapy

   (1) In the early stages of treatment, while the wound is very dirty, use of a debriding agent is indicated. Where available, commercial debriding agents such as Debrisan, Granuflex and Varidase are useful. Where these agents are not available, a 1:3 dilution of 6% w/v hydrogen peroxide can be used. Since peroxide will damage healthy cells, it should be replaced with simple saline cleansing as soon as the wound is adequately debrided.

   (2) Sugar/povidone-iodine dressings can also be used until the wound is clean and granulation tissue is developing. At that point, a simple non-stick dressing such as Vaseline gauze can be used.

   (3) Once healthy granulation tissue covers the ulcer base, skin grafting should be considered.

   d. Supplement vitamins A, B and C, and zinc in areas where micronutrient deficiencies are common.

   e. Protect the healed ulcer site. Healing results in very fragile, thin skin in the area of the ulcer that is especially prone to reulceration with minimal trauma.

5. Differential diagnosis - see Buruli ulcer.

G. Cancrum oris (Noma)
1. General
a. Cancrum oris is a severe, tissue-destructive infection of the facial soft tissues affecting debilitated children aged 2-6 years.

b. An acute illness such as measles or malaria triggers an acute ulcerative gingivitis, which progresses rapidly to gangrene and loss of the tissues of the cheek.

2. Treatment
a. Improvement of nutrition is an essential aspect of treatment. Protein and micronutrient deficiencies should be corrected.

b. Antimicrobial therapy with penicillin.

c. Local wound care.

d. Extensive reconstructive surgery is often required.

VIII. TUBERCULOSIS
A. Organism
1. Tuberculosis is caused by *Mycobacterium tuberculosis*. *M.bovis* and *M. africanum* cause some cases of TB.

2. Tuberculosis is usually transmitted from person to person when organisms in the lung are aerosolized during coughing, sneezing and speaking. The aerosolized bacteria remain suspended in the air for several hours and can be inhaled into terminal air passages where initial bacterial replication occurs.

3. Pulmonary tuberculosis is the most common form of disease due to *M. tuberculosis*. Extra-pulmonary tuberculosis occurs in < 20% of cases and can occur in any organ or tissue of the body.

4. *M. bovis* is a pathogen of cattle and is transmitted to humans through ingestion of unpasteurized milk. *M. bovis* typically causes cervical lymphadenitis or gastrointestinal TB.

B. Clinical syndromes
1. Primary tuberculosis
a. Initially, inhalation of Mycobacteria is followed by local bacterial replication in the alveoli. At this stage of infection, before an immune response develops, organisms are disseminated widely throughout the body. The outcome of infection is determined by the efficacy of the host's immune response in controlling bacterial replication. In most individuals, the immune system is able to exert control over bacterial replication, although organisms are not killed. The chest x-ray may show evidence of primary infection: a small peripheral lesion (usually in the lower lobes) with associated hilar adenopathy (Ghon complex).

b. Inadequate immune control over bacterial replication results in "progressive primary disease". This is most common in children less than 4 years of age or in patients with immune deficiency (HIV infection, malnutrition, etc.). Rapid bacterial replication results in enlargement of the primary lesion and further enlargement of hilar nodes. Compression of bronchi from enlarged nodes can cause segmental or lobar collapse (typically right middle lobe collapse). Cavitation and empyema can occur. Patients with progressive primary disease are acutely ill with fever, night sweats, cough and weight loss. Some patients will go on to develop extra-pulmonary disease, particularly meningitis or miliary disease.

2. Post primary tuberculosis

a. Post primary disease is caused by re-activation of dormant organisms in the lung, usually in the apical-posterior segments of the upper lobes or the superior segments of the lower lobes, where high oxygen tension provides optimal conditions for mycobacterial growth. Patients presenting with cough of > 3 weeks duration should be investigated for TB. Fever, night sweats, and weight loss may be present.

b. Chest x-ray will show infiltrates in the apical posterior portion of the lung. Cavities may be seen. With prolonged disease, loss of volume in the upper lobes pulls the hilum superiorly. Pleural thickening over the apex may be present.

3. Extrapulmonary tuberculosis

a. General

(1) Early after infection, organisms are widely disseminated to all organs and tissues of the body. In most infected individuals, host defenses gain control over bacterial replication leaving viable but "inactive" organisms in the tissues.

(2) Failure of host defenses triggered by aging or immunocompromising conditions (HIV, steroid therapy, malnutrition, measles, etc.) will allow these organisms to replicate unchecked and cause disease. The most common sites of extra-pulmonary disease are: lymph nodes, pleura, genitourinary, bone and joint, meninges and peritoneum. Extra- pulmonary disease is common in HIV infected individuals.

b. Miliary TB

(1) Widely disseminated disease with involvement of many organs.

(2) Clinical manifestations are non-specific (fever, night sweats, anorexia, weight loss and hepatosplenomegaly).

(3) Chest x-ray shows diffuse "millet seed" infiltrates.

c. Lymphatic TB

(1) Most commonly involves the cervical nodes (>90%) but can involve other areas. Node enlargement is slow and painless, without local signs of inflammation. Typically, several smaller nodes surround a single large node. Over time the nodes become matted together and the skin may become fixed.

      (2) Sinus formation occurs when caseous nodes rupture through the skin. Constitutional symptoms are frequently absent. Examination of the cut surface of an excised node may show caseation but organisms are difficult to find on AFB smears.

d. Genitourinary TB

      (1) Renal TB is common because of the high blood flow and high oxygen tension in the kidney, conditions that favour mycobacterial replication. Renal involvement presents with symptoms of bladder irritation (dysuria, frequency, hematuria) and, occasionally, renal colic. Sterile pyuria (with or without proteinuria) is the hallmark of renal TB. Acid-fast smears of urine have poor sensitivity and can be misleading due to the presence of non-pathogenic AFB contaminating urine.

      (2) Genital TB in males presents with epididymitis or prostatitis, often with a palpable mass. Infertility is common.

      (3) Genital TB in females most commonly affects the fallopian tubes and results in scarring and distortion of the tubes. Infertility, amenorrhea, irregular menstruation and pelvic pain may occur.

e. Bone and joint TB

      (1) Skeletal TB most commonly affects the spine (50%), hip (15%) and knee (15%) but can affect any site.

      (2) Spinal TB usually involves the lower thoracic spine with T10 most commonly affected. Pain and reluctance to bend over are common early features. Later in the disease, as bone damage progresses, collapse of vertebral bodies produces visible angulation in the spine (gibbus).

      (3) Infection begins at the superior or inferior edge of the anterior portion of the vertebral body and spreads across the disc space to involve the adjacent vertebral body. Neurologic compromise can occur from instability of the spine or from soft tissue masses compressing the spinal cord.

f. Abdominal TB

      (1) Any part of the GI tract can be affected by TB, most commonly the terminal ileum. Abdominal pain, masses and bowel obstruction are most common.

      (2) Anal fistula should prompt consideration of rectal TB.

g. Peritoneal TB

      (1) Results from hematogenous dissemination of TB bacilli to the peritoneum, from rupture of a caseous mesenteric node or intestinal focus into the peritoneum or from spread of genitourinary TB through the fallopian tubes.

      (2) Peritoneal TB typically presents with progressive ascites and constitutional symptoms. In many endemic areas, it must be distinguished from ascites secondary to cirrhosis from hepatic schistosomiasis or hepatocellular carcinoma.

(3) Peritoneal fluid analysis will show a high protein content (exudative) and lymphocytosis. AFB are rarely found on smear. Nodules studding the peritoneum will be seen at laparotomy or laparoscopy.

(4) Some patients with peritoneal TB do not develop ascites. In these patients, disease is manifested by matting of the abdominal organs with tender abdominal masses and the classic "doughy" abdomen on examination.

h. Meningeal TB

(1) TB meningitis typically has an insidious onset with low-grade fever, malaise, headache, irritability or listlessness and neck stiffness. Cranial nerve palsies (especially cranial nerves III, IV, VI and VIII), hemiplegia and involuntary movements may be seen. Hydrocephalus with nausea, vomiting and decreased consciousness is common. Without treatment, TB meningitis is typically fatal in 3-6 weeks.

(2) CSF examination will show elevated WBC with lymphocyte predominance, high protein and low glucose. Since the CSF findings may be atypical early in disease (neutrophil predominance, normal glucose), CSF exam should be repeated after several days, if in doubt. AFB are rarely seen in the CSF. The yield of CSF examination for AFB can be increased by examining the sediment obtained by prolonged centrifugation of several milliliters of CSF or allowing CSF to stand overnight.

i. TB of the brain

(1) Tuberculomas in the brain present as space-occupying lesions with focal neurologic signs or signs of increased intracranial pressure.

(2) Rupture of a tuberculoma into the CSF spills large numbers of mycobacteria into the subarachnoid space and results in fulminant TB meningitis.

j. Pericardial TB

(1) TB bacilli reach the pericardium either through hematogenous dissemination or through direct extension from lungs or mediastinal nodes. Fever, chest pain and a pericardial friction rub are typical manifestations.

(2) Some patients develop large pericardial effusions, with progression to pericardial tamponade, while others develop a calcified, thickened pericardium leading to constrictive pericarditis.

k. Laryngeal TB

(1) Infection of the larynx (inoculated with organisms when the patient expectorates organisms from the lung) results in a highly contagious form of TB.

(2) Patients present with pain (often severe) and hoarseness.

4. TB in HIV-infected patients

a. HIV-infected patients are at increased risk of progressive disease after primary infection with TB. Those with latent TB are at increased risk of reactivation (~10% per year compared to 10% lifetime risk for non-HIV infected). The increased risk for TB occurs early in HIV disease, often before the patient has been actually diagnosed with HIV. HIV infection should, therefore, be considered in all new diagnoses of TB.

b. Pulmonary TB in HIV-infected patients is atypical, more frequently involving the middle and lower lung fields. Cavitation and AFB smear positivity are less common than in non-HIV infected patients.

c. Extrapulmonary disease is more common in HIV infected patients that in uninfected patients.

d. Common features of TB in HIV-infected patients include fever with no apparent source, night sweats, weight loss, and cough. These are also common manifestations of other opportunistic infections and neoplasms (particularly lymphoma).

C. Diagnosis

1. Clinical clues

a. A diagnosis of TB should be suspected in patients with the following symptoms:
(1) Persistent cough for > 3 weeks.
(2) Fever, night sweats and weight loss.
(3) Malnutrition unresponsive to 4 weeks of intensive nutritional therapy.

b. A history of contact with a patient with smear positive sputum is an important diagnostic clue but is typically absent in adults with reactivated disease. In infants and young children (who must have primary disease), there should be an identifiable close contact with smear positive pulmonary TB. When no such contact can be identified, a presumptive of TB in the child should be questioned.

2. Acid fast stains (AFB)

a. The sensitivity of acid-fast stains is poor, especially in extra-pulmonary TB. TB should never be ruled out on the basis of a negative acid-fast stain.

b. Patients with smear positive sputum are highly infectious and close contacts should be screened for infection.

c. Sputum or urine for AFB smears should be collected in the early morning. At least three specimens should be examined.

3. Mantoux (PPD) testing detects delayed type hypersensitivity responses that develop in response to infection with mycobacteria.

a. In areas where BCG is used routinely and infection is highly prevalent, PPD testing is often considered of limited value. However the mantoux reaction post-BCG is usually small. A significant reaction even post BCG is suggestive of infection.

b. If BCG has not been administered, PPD positivity reflects infection with TB bacilli but does not necessarily indicate active disease. A negative PPD test does not rule out disease, particularly in patients with impaired delayed type hypersensitivity (HIV/AIDS, malnutrition etc.).

c. Interpretation of results - the standard dose of PPD is 5 units (0.1 ml). Care must be taken to ensure that the PPD is administered intradermally - (a 6-10 mm wheal should be produced). Only a properly administered dose should be used for interpretation. The result should be read at 48-72 hours after administration. The area of induration is measured transversely to the long axis of the forearm and recorded in mm. Erythema is not significant and should not be recorded. A reaction of > 10 mm is considered a positive result except in situations where the likelihood of TB is high. A reaction of > 5 mm is considered positive in the following situations:

(1) Close contacts of smear- positive cases.
(2) Chest x-ray changes consistent with TB.
(3) Immunocompromised hosts (HIV, prolonged use of steroid therapy).
(4) Other high risk patients (diabetes mellitus, severe renal insufficiency, malnutrition, leukemia, lymphoma).

4. Radiographs

a. Chest x-rays are helpful in the diagnosis of TB but specificity is poor. Post primary disease is typically located in the apical-posterior segments of the upper lobes or the superior segments of the lower lobes.

b. Cavitations are highly suspicious for TB but can be due to tumors, fungal or parasitic infections or bacterial abscesses.

c. Miliary TB is characterized by tiny "millet seed" infiltrates throughout the lungs.

d. Spinal TB is suggested by collapse of vertebral bodies. In most cases, several adjacent vertebral bodies are affected.

5. Trials of therapy are often suggested when the clinical setting suggests TB but the diagnosis is not clear. A TB trial implies that the patient is given TB drugs on a time-limited basis to see if a response occurs. If there is no response to treatment, the TB drugs are discontinued. Such "TB trials" should generally be discouraged because they promote inappropriate use of TB drugs and increase the risk of emergence of resistance to TB drugs. However there are occasional patients for whom a TB trial may be appropriate. The following conditions should be met before considering a TB trial.

a. An objective and easily measured indicator of response must be available. This indicator must change rapidly in response to treatment so that a response can be detected within one to two weeks. Almost the only parameter which fulfills these criteria is persistent fever, documented in the hospital.

    b. Consider common "TB mimics", investigate as intensively as possible and provide empiric treatment for alternative diagnoses where reasonable before considering a TB trial. For most patients, one or two courses of empiric broad-spectrum antibiotic therapy should be given before undertaking a TB trial. Some TB drugs have broad antibacterial effects and an apparent response may simply be due to the antibacterial activity of the drug.

    c. In patients with "fever of unknown origin", a naprosyn test should be considered before embarking on a TB trial. The patient should be monitored for a sufficient period of time to establish a clear fever pattern, then initiated on naprosyn 250mg q12h (not PRN) x 2-3 days. A complete, rapid response to naprosyn suggests a neoplastic cause for fever. Failure of a complete response is suggestive of an infectious cause of fever. This test can be particularly helpful in HIV-infected patients where lymphoma is an important differential diagnosis.

    d. When undertaking a trial, use the usual protocols for treatment of TB (not a single drug). Trials should be no more than 2 weeks duration. If there is a response to treatment, the full course of TB treatment should be given. If there is no response, all TB drugs should be discontinued and the patient monitored carefully.

D. Treatment

1. Principles of treatment

    a. TB bacilli exist in different environments that influence their response to anti-tuberculous drugs. There are actively growing extracellular organisms, dormant extracellular organisms and slowly growing intracellular organisms. Combination chemotherapy is required to provide adequate activity against these different populations of organisms, as each of the anti-TB drugs preferentially works against a selected population.

    b. TB bacilli are naturally resistant to TB drugs at low frequencies (approximately 1 in 10^3 to 10^8 organisms, depending on the drug). Simultaneous resistance to 2 drugs occurs in about 1 in 10^{12} organisms. In patients with very high bacterial loads (such as those with cavities), the presence of these naturally resistant organisms constitutes a risk for the development of acquired resistance if too few drugs are used for treatment, or if the patient has already has a strain of TB that is fully resistant to one or more drugs. Natural resistance is one reason why drug regimens for TB must include several different drugs. A combination of at least three effective drugs will reduce the risk of inducing acquired resistance by selecting out naturally resistant mutants.

    c. "Persisters" are viable but very slowly or intermittently growing organisms that are relatively resistant to TB therapy because of their extremely low metabolic activity. These organisms can persist throughout therapy and give rise to relapse. Rifampin and pyrazinamide are the most effective agents against these organisms and, when included in a treatment regimen, will give a high rate of success with "short course" therapy (6-9 months). When these drugs cannot be used due to resistance, 18-24 months may be required for adequate treatment of these organisms.

   d. Never add a single drug to a failing regimen. A minimum of two (and preferably more) agents should be added in order to minimize the chance of promoting further resistance.

2. First line anti-TB agents

   a. Isoniazid (H)

      (1) Bactericidal but active only against actively growing organisms.

      (2) Side-effects include peripheral neuropathy, hypersensitivity (rash, fever), hepatic toxicity including hepatitis (presents as anorexia, nausea, jaundice and dark urine). Monitor LFTs if possible. Discontinue if LFTs increase to 3x baseline.

      (3) Try to give with pyridoxine 50mg/day to prevent peripheral neuropathy particularly in poorly nourished children and adults. If pyridoxine supplies are limited, reserve for patients at higher risk of toxicity (pregnant, malnourished, pre-existing neuropathy).

      (4) Supplied as 100mg 300 mg tablets. Safe in pregnancy.

   b. Rifampin (R)

      (1) Bactericidal, active against all bacterial populations.

      (2) Side-effects include orange coloration of urine and secretions, nausea, vomiting, hepatitis, hypersensitivity reactions (rash, eosinophilia, fever). With intermittent dosing, some patients will develop a flu-like syndrome that can progress to hemolytic anemia, thrombocytopenia and renal failure.

      (3) Supplied as 300mg. tablets. Safe in pregnancy.

   c. Pyrazinamide (Z)

      (1) Bactericidal only against intracellular organisms. Active against "persisters".

      (2) Side effects include hepatic toxicity, hyperuricemia, hypersensitivity (fever, arthralgias, rash).

      (3) Supplied as 500mg tablets. Not tested for safety in pregnancy but has been widely used in pregnancy. IUATLD (International Union Against TB and Lung Disease) does not recommend withholding PZA in pregnancy.

   d. Ethambutol (E)

      (1) Bacteriostatic, helps promote bactericidal activity of isoniazid.

      (2) Side-effects include hypersensitivity, optic neuritis (loss of color vision), hyperuricemia, peripheral neuropathy. Not recommended in children under 5 years due to inability to monitor visual changes (use streptomycin).

      (3) Supplied as 400mg tablets. Safe in pregnancy.

e. Streptomycin
- (1) Bactericidal but active only against extracellular organisms.
- (2) Side-effects include nephrotoxicity, ototoxicity, vestibular toxicity. Check for complaints of dizziness, vertigo or poor balance before each injection. Transient dizziness and peri-oral tingling immediately after injection does not require termination of therapy. Persistent dizziness or tinnitus requires discontinuation of therapy.
- (3) Supplied as 1gm. vials. Avoid in pregnancy.

3. Second line anti-TB agents

a. Kanamycin
- (1) An aminoglycoside closely related to streptomycin. Can be used in place of streptomycin if streptomycin is unavailable.
- (2) Side-effects are similar to streptomycin.
- (3) Do not use in pregnancy.

b. Cycloserine
- (1) Bacteriostatic against both intracellular and extracellular organisms.
- (2) Side-effects include seizures, peripheral neuropathy, mental changes.
- (3) Give 50-100mg pyridoxine daily to decrease CNS toxicity. Do not use in pregnancy.

c. Ethionamide
- (1) Bacteriostatic, only active against extracellular organisms.
- (2) Do not use in pregnancy.

d. Para-amino salycilic acid (PAS)
- (1) Bacteriostatic.
- (2) GI side effects are often dose limiting. Compliance is often difficult.
- (3) Can be used in pregnancy.

e. Ciprofloxacin / Ofloxacin
- (1) Quinolone antibiotics that have anti-tuberculous activity.
- (2) Avoid in pregnancy and in children.

f. Thiacetazone
- (1) Bacteriostatic, but a very weak anti-tuberculous agent.
- (2) Side-effects include GI and skin (rash which may progress to severe Stevens-Johnson syndrome). Rash may occur in up to 20% of HIV patients, with up to a 3% mortality. Use with caution in areas of high HIV prevalence.
- (3) Avoid in pregnancy.

g. Clofazimine
- (1) Primarily used in treatment of leprosy.
- (2) Reserve for use in multi-drug resistant TB, where options are limited.

Drug Doses for TB Treatment

	Daily	Two Times Weekly
Isoniazid 100 mg, 300 mg	Adult: 5-10 mg/kg (300 mg) Child: 10-15 mg/kg (300 mg)	Adult: 15 mg/kg (900 mg) Child: 20-40 mg/kg (900 mg)
Rifampicin 300 mg	10 mg/kg >50 kg: 600 mg <50 kg: 450 mg Child: 10-20 mg/kg (600 mg)	10 mg/kg (600 mg) Child: 10-20 mg/kg (600 mg)
Pyrazinamide 500 mg	15-30 mg/kg >50 kg: (2 gm) <50 kg: (1.5 gm) Child: 15-30 mg/kg (2 gm)	50-70 mg/kg (4 gm) Child: 50-70 mg/kg (4 gm)
Ethambutol 400 mg	15-25 mg/kg (2.5 gm) Child above age 5 yrs: 15-25 mg/kg (2.5 gm)	50 mg/kg Child: 50 mg/kg
Streptomycin 1 Gm Inj	10-15 mg/kg 500-1000 mg 5 times/wk Child: 20-30 mg/kg (1 gm)	20-25 mg/kg (1.5 gm) Child: 25-30 mg/kg (1.5 gm)

4. Treatment protocols:
a. Drug protocols for daily administered regimens.

Daily Treatment Regimens for Tuberculosis

Regimen	Phase	Drugs	Duration
Pulmonary & extra-pulmonary disease in children and adults	Intensive	H, R, Z and E or S	8 wks
	Continuation	H and R	16 weeks*
Where PZA cannot be used	Intensive	H, R and E or S	8 weeks
	Continuation	H and R	24 weeks
Suspected drug resistant TB	Intensive	H, R, Z, E and S**	8-12 weeks
	Continuation	H, R, Z	21 months

* In miliary disease, bone and joint TB and TB meningitis, prolong treatment to 12 months.

** Include at least 2 drugs that the patient has never had before. This may require use of second line agents in addition to those indicated.

b. The following table is a summary of protocols for intermittent dosing of anti-TB agents. These intermittent dosing regimens are intended for use as part of a directly observed program of drug administration. The initial phase often includes a more intensive phase of daily drug administration.

Intermittent Treatment Regimens for Tuberculosis			
Regimen	**Frequency**	**Drugs**	**Duration**
Pulmonary & extra-pulmonary disease in children and adults	Daily	H, R, Z and E or S then →	8 wks
	Twice weekly	H and R	16 weeks
Where PZA cannot be used	Daily	H, R, Z and E or S then →	2 weeks
	Twice weekly	H and R	16 weeks
Suspected drug resistant TB	Thrice weekly	H, R, Z and E or S	24 weeks

E - ethambutol, H - isoniazid, R - rifampicin, S - streptomycin, Z - pyrazinamide.
In areas where the incidence of drug resistance is very low (<4%) and where the patient has never had any TB treatment in the past, the fourth drug can be omitted from the initiation phase of each protocol.

    c. Directly observed therapy (DOT) implies that the patient is observed to take each dose of medication by a health care worker or designated responsible layperson who understands the importance of good compliance. The advantage of intermittent dosing is that it can permit cost effective implementation of DOT. Intermittent treatment regimens should always be used in conjunction with directly observed therapy, never as self-administered treatment.

  5. Duration of therapy

    a. Patients with previously untreated pulmonary TB can be treated with 6 or 9 month regimens. Regimens that are ≤ 9 months in duration must contain both INH and rifampin. Six-month regimens must contain both INH and rifampin, with PZA during the initial phase.

    b. Many countries have national guidelines for the management of TB. These regimens should be adhered to for routine cases.

    c. A 6-month regimen consisting of isoniazid, rifampin, and pyrazinamide given for 2 months followed by isoniazid and rifampin for 4 months should be considered standard therapy. Include ethambutol or streptomycin in the initial phase when isoniazid resistance is suspected, where the prevalence of resistance to one or more TB drug is ≥ 4%, or in patients with extensive or cavitary disease where a high bacterial load is present.

    d. Children should be treated in essentially the same way as adults using appropriately adjusted doses of drugs. Quinolone antibiotics (second line agents) are not approved for use in children.

    e. Miliary, bone and joint, and meningeal TB should be treated for a total of one year.

    f. HIV patients respond to standard regimens. In early HIV disease, standard duration of treatment is acceptable. Follow the patient closely for evidence of relapse. In severely immunocompromised patients, lifelong suppression with INH after treatment may be indicated. Avoid use of thiacetazone, if possible, due to frequent occurrence of severe Stevens-Johnson syndrome.

6. Drug resistance
  a. Suspect resistance in the following situations:
  (1) Sputum remains smear positive after 3 months of treatment.
  (2) History of previous TB therapy, especially if sporadic or interrupted dosing.
  (3) The source for the patient's infection was a case of known or suspected drug-resistant TB or had a history of erratic therapy.
  (4) HIV infection in some countries is associated with a higher risk of resistance.
  b. When drug resistance is suspected:
  (1) Never add a single drug to a failing regimen.
  (2) Consult with someone experienced in managing drug-resistant TB.
  (3) If at all possible, try to get susceptibility testing done to guide therapy.
  (4) Commit to fully supervised therapy.
  (5) Before starting new drugs, set aside all drugs that will be required in order for that patient to complete the course of therapy so that there is no risk of running out of drugs midway through treatment.
  (6) Treatment is individualized and will be based in part on the patient's history of prior TB drug exposures.
  (7) Plan on a long course of therapy - for smear positive patients, at least 12 months after sputum has converted to negative, often 24 months.

IX. VIRAL INFECTIONS
A. Dengue
1. General
  a. Organism - Dengue virus is an Arbovirus with four serotypes.
  b. Vector - *Aedes aegypti* mosquito
  (1) Feeds during the day (early morning, late afternoon).
  (2) Adapted to human habitat, often bites indoors.
  (3) Breeds in small quantities of water in peri-domestic environment.
  (4) *Aedes albopticus* is a secondary vector - widespread distribution, including non-tropical areas.
  c. Distribution
  (1) World wide throughout the tropics, expanding distribution into previously dengue-free areas.
  (2) Can occur as sporadic cases or as large epidemics.
  (3) Increasing disease activity is noted in Africa, Asia and the Americas.

2. Three clinical syndromes
  a. Dengue fever (classic or breakbone fever)
  b. Dengue hemorrhagic fever
  c. Dengue shock syndrome
3. Dengue fever syndrome (breakbone fever)
  a. General
    (1) Disease severity is influenced by patient's age and immune status from prior infections with other dengue serotypes.
    (2) Many cases are asymptomatic, especially in younger patients (up to 80% of pediatric cases are asymptomatic).
    (3) In symptomatic young children, a first episode of dengue commonly presents as undifferentiated febrile illness, indistinguishable from other febrile illnesses. Symptoms are usually mild and resolve in 1-3 days. Upper respiratory symptoms are often present.
    (4) Incubation period is 4-7 days (range 2-14 days).
  b. Clinical (initial presentation is indistinguishable from other viral infections)
    (1) Symptoms
      (a) Abrupt onset of fever and chills occurs in the majority of patients. A transient maculopapular rash may be present early in the febrile period.
      (b) Severe frontal headache, retro-orbital pain, pain on eye movement, musculoskeletal and lumbar pain are present in 2/3 of patients.
      (c) Anorexia, nausea, vomiting occur in half of patients.
      (d) Abdominal pain, respiratory distress, and mental status changes occur less frequently and may represent more severe disease.
      (e) The illness often follows a biphasic course with the initial fever (+/- rash) lasting 2-7 days, remitting for 24-48 hours followed by recurrence of both fever and rash (maculopapular).
    (2) Signs
      (a) Initial examination is usually nonspecific. Look for scleral injection, tender, generalized lymphadenopathy, relative bradycardia (slower heart rate than expected for degree of fever).
      (b) Rash - several different types of rash may be seen. In the first phase of illness a diffuse flushing or transient pinpoint erythematous lesions may be seen. After several days of illness, with the onset of the second phase, maculopapular or scarlatiniform rashes appear in approximately 50% of patients. This rash begins on the trunk, spreads to extremities. Although the palms and soles are spared by the rash, desquamation of the palms and soles is common in the recovery phase of the illness.

Towards the end of the febrile period some patients will develop clusters of petechiae on the extremities.

(c) Easy brusing, petechiae or positive tourniquet test is usually found. The tourniquet test is performed by inflating a blood pressure cuff to midway between the diastolic and systolic blood pressure for five minutes. Greater than 3 petechiae/cm2 (20 petechiae per square inch) is considered positive.

c. Laboratory

(1) CBC: neutropenia (< 5000 with granulocytopenia), lymphopenia and atypical lymphocytosis, thrombocytopenia (< 100,000), rising hematocrit.

(2) UA: proteinuria, microscopic hematuria.

(3) Elevated liver enzymes usually present.

d. Differential diagnosis is broad. Especially consider influenza, malaria, leptospirosis, typhoid fever, EBV mononucleosis syndrome and viral hemorrhagic fevers.

4. Dengue hemorrhagic fever and dengue shock syndrome (DHF/DSS)

a. General

(1) Usually seen in patients who have previously been sensitized by prior infection with a different viral serotype. Pre-existing antibodies are unable to neutralize different viral serotypes but are believed to play a role in enhanced disease severity, perhaps by promoting increased release of cytokines and inflammatory mediators.

(2) The key features of DHF/DSS are:

(a) Abnormal vascular permeability with marked fluid shifts which lead to hemoconcentration.

(b) Abnormal hemostasis resulting in bleeding (thrombocytopenia, vascular fragility and clotting factor abnormalities all contribute to the increased risk of bleeding).

(c) Hypovolemia leads to impaired tissue perfusion and oxygenation.

b. Clinical

(1) Initial clinical presentation is indistinguishable from uncomplicated dengue fever.

(2) With defervescence, rapid deterioration occurs, characterized by hemorrhagic manifestations and hypovolemic shock.

(3) Hepatomegaly is common in DHF/DSS (> 90% of children).

(4) Pleural, peritoneal and retroperitoneal effusions are common.

c. Diagnosis (the following must be present):

(1) Fever or history of recent fever.

(2) Hemorrhagic manifestations (epistaxis, spontaneous bruising, bleeding from venipuncture sites, gum bleeding, etc.).

(3) Platelet count ≤ 100,000/mm3.

(4) Capillary leak manifested by elevated hematocrit (20% or more over baseline), low serum albumin, pleural or other effusions.

5. WHO criteria for categorizing DHF/DSS

 a. Grade 1 - fever, non specific constitutional signs, positive tourniquet test.

 b. Grade 2 - Grade 1 features plus spontaneous hemorrhagic manifestations.

 c. Grade 3 - circulatory failure (tachycardia, pulse pressure < 20 mmHg, hypotension).

 d. Grade 4 - profound shock with undetectable pulse and blood pressure.

 e. Grades 3 and 4 represent dengue shock syndrome.

6. Treatment

 a. No specific treatment is available. Aspirin must be avoided due to the risk of Reye's syndrome and the frequent occurrence of gastrointestinal tract bleeding. NSAIDs should also be avoided.

 b. Vitamin K supplementation may be helpful since vitamin K dependent clotting factors may be depleted.

 c. Symptomatic treatment includes rest, adequate fluids, and analgesics.

 d. Use a mosquito net to avoid spread of virus.

 e. Danger signs indicating impending progression to DSS include:

 (1) Abrupt resolution of fever with hypothermia, sweating, prostration. Usually occurs on or after the third day of illness.

 (2) Severe/persistent abdominal pain.

 (3) Persistent vomiting.

 (4) Restlessness or severe drowsiness.

 (5) Sharp increase in hematocrit.

 f. Prospectively monitor the hematocrit and platelet count on a daily basis during early illness. Close observation as the fever resolves will identify patients progressing to DHF/DSS. A falling platelet count usually precedes a rise in hematocrit. In patients with shock, thrombocytopenia or an elevated hematocrit, monitor the hematocrit q2-4 hours.

 g. Early and aggressive fluid replacement is essential to maintain blood pressure and urine output. This should be initiated before shock develops, as soon as the hematocrit begins to rise sharply. Initial IV fluid replacement should be with isotonic fluid. For patients presenting in shock, an initial bolus of 10-20 ml/kg should be given. For persistent shock, albumin, plasma substitute or whole blood transfusion may be required. If possible, monitor electrolytes and blood gases for hyponatremia and acidosis.

7. Prognosis

 a. Symptoms resolve in 5-7 days, but full recovery may be prolonged for several weeks due to persistent fatigue.

b. Mortality is variable depending on the severity of disease and the supportive care available, but may range up to 50%.

8. Prevention

a. Elimination of mosquito breeding sites in the domestic environment is essential. Small quantities of water such as may be held in old tires, tin cans and other containers must be eliminated.

b. Larvicides can be used to reduce mosquito breeding in larger bodies of water.

c. In outbreak settings, aerial spraying with mosquito adulticides may be necessary.

d. Personal mosquito protection - 30-35% DEET provides effective mosquito protection. Avoid use in areas of skin that can be placed in the mouth of infants. It is usually recommended that DEET be washed off when indoors but since dengue-carrying mosquitoes often bite indoors, consideration needs to be given to the risk of indoor exposure.

B. Epstein-Barr virus infection - infectious mononucleosis

1. General

a. Infectious mononucleosis is a clinical syndrome characterized by malaise, fever, headache, exudative tonsillitis, and lymphadenopathy.

b. Usually occurs in adolescents and young adults (epidemiology not well known in developing countries). Symptoms tend to be more severe with increasing age at infection.

c. Incubation period is 2-8 weeks.

2. Clinical

a. Malaise, headache, fever, tonsillitis, lymphadenopathy last one to several weeks.

b. Mild transient hepatitis and splenomegaly may occur.

c. Heterophile antibody shows a high titer in adults.

d. Atypical lymphocytosis is usually present.

3. Treatment

a. No specific treatment is necessary or effective. Rest is often prescribed but there are no controlled studies demonstrating its efficacy.

b. Brief courses of prednisone (60 mg/d x4 d) have been effective in shrinking obstructing tonsils and improving airway blockage.

c. Avoid risk of injury (such as contact sports) when splenomegaly present.

C. Herpes simplex, type II (see above, Section VI)

D. Influenza

1. General

a. Acute febrile respiratory illness occurring in annual outbreaks.

b. Highly contagious.

      c. Clinical syndromes include common colds, pharyngitis, tracheobronchitis and pneumonia.

      d. Epidemics occur during the winter months in temperate climates and year-round in the tropics.

  2. Clinical

      a. Influenza syndrome - abrupt onset of fever, chills, headache, myalgia or malaise is characteristic of influenza. Respiratory symptoms, such as dry cough, nasal discharge, hoarseness, sore throat then appear. Respiratory symptoms may persist for 2 weeks or more.

      b. Complications

      (1) Primary influenza pneumonia may occur. Causes fever, cough, dyspnea, hemopytsis, cyanosis. Mortality is high.

      (2) Bacterial superinfection pneumonia with productive cough and consolidation on chest x-ray may occur. Usually responds to antibiotics. *S.aureus* is an important pathogen in this setting.

  3. Treatment

      a. Rimantadine or amantadine 200 mg/d x 5d or the newer neuroaminodase inhibitors (oseltamivir or zanamavir) may shorten the course of the illness by 1-2 days.

      b. Antipyretics - don't use ASA in patients less than 16 years old.

      c. Cough suppressants - avoid in children as they contribute to development of secondary infection by impairing clearance of respiratory secretions.

      d. Antibiotics effective against *S. aureus* should be given if secondary bacterial infection develops (cloxacillin, cephalexin, amoxicillin / clavulanic acid).

  4. Prevention - vaccines are effective and should be prescribed annually before the onset of flu season to individuals at increased risk (including all healthcare workers, whenever possible).

E. Measles (Rubeola)

  1. General

      a. Acute, highly contagious illness characterized by fever, coryza, cough, conjunctivitis, and both an enanthem and an exanthem.

      b. Measles in developing countries is a serious childhood disease with worldwide distribution.

      c. Only one strain of the rubeola virus is known; host factors account for the observed variations in disease severity.

      d. Mortality is variable, but may reach 5-10% in populations with poor nutrition.

      e. The disease is contagious from the fifth day of incubation to the fifth day after the rash appears.

  2. Clinical manifestations

      a. Incubation period is 10-14 days.

b. Prodrome lasts 2-4 days, characterized by fever (to 40°C.), conjunctival injection, cough, coryza, myalgia, headache. Koplik spots (small white spots on the buccal mucosa lateral to the molars) usually appear prior to the rash.

c. The rash develops 2-4 days after onset of the fever (typically on the third day). It begins as a reddish macular rash on the head and neck that spreads to involve the trunk, then the extremities. It rapidly becomes maculopapular, and the lesions may coalesce. The rash fades in the order of its appearance, after 4-5 days, with desquamation.

d. Fever may be elevated to 40°C. Usually subsides by the fourth day, but may persist for up to 6 days. Generalized lymphadenopathy may be present.

3. Complications

a. Secondary bacterial infections - laryngitis, bacterial pneumonia (due to *Strep. pneumonia* or *H. influenza*), or otitis media may occur. Suspect when persistent fever or leukocytosis is present.

b. Stomatitis - may be severe, and interfere with eating.

c. Diarrhea - severe, persistent diarrhea may occur, more commonly in young, malnourished children. Occasionally, bacterial infection (with *Campylobacter* or *Shigella*) may occur.

d. Xerophthalmia due to vitamin A deficiency may be seen.

e. Encephalitis may rarely occur (usually in older children). Manifested by recurrent fever, headache, vomiting, stiff neck, followed by stupor and convulsions.

f. Malnutrition and failure to thrive may occur following severe measles.

4. Treatment

a. Supportive care - adequate hydration and antipyretics. Codeine may be helpful for control of cough and amelioration of headache and myalgia.

b. Appropriate antibiotics for secondary bacterial infections.

c. Vitamin A 100,000 IU po for children <6 months, 200,000 IU po for children >6 months, daily for two days has been shown to significantly reduce morbidity and mortality, especially in children with severe measles.

5. Prevention

a. Prevention of measles is essential to its management.

b. A vaccine, given as MMR (measles, mumps, rubella) is recommended at age 9 months, repeated at 15 months and at 12 years. Monovalent measles vaccine may be given during epidemics to children as young as 6 months.

F. Mumps

1. General

a. Acute systemic viral infection characterized by nonsuppurative parotitis.

b. Usually self-limited, occurring most commonly in school-aged children.

c. Incubation period 14-21 days.

d. Communicable from 7 days before to 9 days after the appearance of swelling.

2. Clinical

a. Usually begins with short prodromal phase with low-grade fever, malaise, headache, anorexia.

b. Parotid tenderness and enlargement then develops, usually unilaterally at first. Bilateral parotitis eventually develops in 70% of patients.

c. Swelling lasts 3 days, then resolves over 7 days.

3. Complications

a. Aseptic meningitis - headache, neck stiffness, lethargy, vomiting and fever develop 4-5 days after onset of parotitis. Course is usually benign.

b. Encephalitis - patients present with obtundation, seizures, high fever.

c. Orchitis - occurs more frequently in postpubertal men. Usually unilateral. Generally develops within 1 week of the parotitis. Characterized by marked testicular swelling and severe pain associated with fever, nausea, headache.

4. Treatment - bedrest, supportive and symptomatic treatment.

5. Prevention - live immunization with MMR at age 12-15 months.

G. Poliovirus

1. General

a. Acute illness causing flaccid asymmetric weakness.

b. Incubation period 4-10 days (may be as long as 4-5 weeks).

2. Clinical

a. Begins with fever and malaise, followed within hours by headache, vomiting and then the development of neck and back stiffness.

b. Paralysis usually begins on the second to fifth day after onset of headache.

c. Children have less intense symptoms than adults.

d. Paralysis is usually asymmetric, more proximal than distal. There are no sensory changes. Affected muscles are flaccid, with absent DTR's.

3. Treatment

a. No specific treatment is available.

b. Motor improvement usually begins within the first few weeks.

c. Bed rest until fever resolves, then active physiotherapy.

d. Avoid intramuscular injections in patients with early symptoms consistent with polio.

4. Prevention - live-attenuated or killed vaccines.

H. Rabies prophylaxis

1. Wound care

a. Immediate, local wound treatment is critically important. The amount of virus present in the wound can be significantly reduced (up to 90%) by optimal wound management.

b. Immediately wash and scrub the wound thoroughly with soap and water. Extensive or deep wounds should be irrigated with povidone iodine (using a 20 cc syringe and 18 gauge or larger plastic IV cannula). After scrubbing and irrigation, apply 1% povidone-iodine solution to the wound (0.1% benzalkonium chloride or 70% alcohol are alternatives if povidone-iodine is not available). For large open wounds, exposure to UV light (sunlight) may help inactivate virus. In small children with extensive wounds, consider general anaesthesia or sedation to permit adequate wound care.

c. Avoid suturing bite wounds unless closure is essential for functional or cosmetic results. Wound closure increases the risk of infection.

d. Give tetanus prophylaxis and antibiotics as indicated.

2. Post exposure rabies prophylaxis

a. Assess risk of rabies exposure

(1) Carefully assess the circumstances of the bite and the behaviour of the animal. Animals exhibiting atypical behaviour (unusually passive or aggressive, difficulty walking, etc.) should be considered as potentially rabid even in the absence of hydrophobia and foaming at the mouth. Rabid animals often stray outside of their usual territory. Bites which occurred when an animal was provoked (interference with the animal's food, young or territory) are considered low risk for rabies.

(2) In some countries, bats are an important cause of rabies. Bat bites are easily over-looked as evidence of a wound is often minimal. If the circumstances of the bite suggest that rabies exposure may have occurred, rabies immune globulin and rabies vaccine should be administered.

b. Rabies immune globulin (RIG)

(1) RIG, a human blood product, is the preferred agent for passive immunization.

(2) Total dose = 20 IU/kg. As much as possible (at least one half of the volume) must be infiltrated around the wound and the remainder administered intramuscularly in the gluteal muscle.

(3) Do not mix in the same syringe as vaccine.

c. Equine antirabies serum

(1) Supplied as 1000 IU/5ml (equine). Dose is 40 IU/kg, infiltrated around the wound and intramuscularly as for RIG.

(2) Be prepared to treat anaphylactic reactions.

d. Rabies vaccine

(1) Vaccination should be initiated at the same time as RIG but must never be administered in the same syringe or into the same muscle as RIG.

(2) Rabies vaccine should be injected intramuscularly into the deltoid muscle (never gluteal). In young children the outer thigh can be used. A variety of different rabies vaccines are available:

Rabies Vaccines			
Vaccine	**Cost**	**Virus grown in:**	**Comments**
Cell Culture Vaccines			
Human Diploid Cell Vaccine (HDCV)	$$$$	Human cells	Intramuscular or intradermal Serum sickness reactions to boosters in ~6% of recipients
Rabies Vaccine Absorbed (RVA)	$$$	Fetal rhesus monkey cells	Intramuscular only
Purified Vero Cell Rabies Vaccine (PVRV)	$$$	Vero Cells	Intramuscular or intradermal
Purified Chick Embryo Cell Vaccine (PCEC)	$$$	Chick fibroblasts	Intramuscular or intradermal
Avian Embryo Vaccines			
Duck Embryo Vaccine	$	Duck embryos	Poor immunogenicity High rate of reactions
Purified Duck Embryo Vaccine (Swiss - Berna)	$$	Duck embryos	Improved efficacy and reduced reaction rate
Neural Tissue Vaccines			
Semple, Pasteur, Fermi NTVs	$	Various brain tissues (rabbit, sheep, goat)	Neuroparalytic reactions: 1:200 - 1:2000 Transmission of prion diseases
Suckling mouse brain vaccine (SMBV)	$	Mouse brain	Neuroparalytic reactions: 1:8000 (reduced myelin contamination)

The cell culture vaccines are all of proven efficacy, with a low risk of serious adverse consequences but are expensive and not universally available. Vaccines derived from virus grown in brain tissue are generally the least expensive but cause a high rate of neuroparalytic reactions and should be used only if other rabies vaccines are unavailable. For most cell culture vaccines the standard regimen is 1.0 ml intramuscularly on Days 0, 3, 7, 14 and 28 (Essen regimen). This regimen provides a reliable degree of immunity but development of protective antibody level is slow and newer mulitsite intradermal regimens may be more effective, particularly with severe exposures. Intradermal post exposure vaccination may be used to reduce cost but care should be taken to use only those vaccines and regimens with proven efficacy. Partially used vials of reconstituted, preservative-free vaccine should be used within 8 hours.

(3) Dosing regimens:

Regimen	Number of Doses (sites)							Vials
Day	**0**	**3**	**7**	**14**	**21**	**28**	**90**	
Essen - Intramuscular	1	1	1	1	-	1	-	5
Zagreb - Intramuscular	2	-	1	-	1	-	-	3
TRC - Intradermal	2	2	2	-	-	1	1	5
Oxford - Intradermal	8	-	4	-	-	1	1	4

Elimination of the day 90 dose in the Oxford and TRC regimens may be associated with a reduced antibody response. If this dose is eliminated, 2 doses should be given on day 28. The Intramuscular Zagreb (2.1.1.) regimen provides limited immunity and should be used only for very minor exposures (minor scratches, abrasions without bleeding, licking of broken skin).
A 2-site, 4-visit intradermal HDCV regimen over 21 days provides only short-term protection and is not recommended.

(4) WHO-recommended vaccines

Vaccines meeting WHO criteria for Post-exposure Intradermal Use		Dose
HDCV	Rabivac	0.1 ml
PVRV	Verorab, Imovax, Rabies vero, TRC Verorab	0.1 ml
PCEC	Rabipur. RabAvert	0.1 ml
PDEV	Lyssaac N	0.2 ml

3. Pre-exposure Prophylaxis

a. For individuals at significant risk of rabies exposure, pre-exposure vaccination should be considered, especially if they live in areas where safe post-exposure prophylaxis cannot be reliably provided. Pre-exposure prophylaxis eliminates the need for RIG (risk of transmission of blood borne pathogens) or equine antiscrum (risk of anaphylaxis). In areas where rabies vaccine is derived from neural tissue, the reduced requirement for post-exposure vaccine lessens the risk of serious neuroparalytic reactions.

b. Pre-exposure vaccination protocols

(1) Neural tissue derived vaccines should not be used for pre-exposure prophylaxis because of the risk of serious adverse reactions.

(2) All of the cell culture derived vaccines provide equivalent pre-exposure prophylaxis when used in recommended intramuscular regimens. Not all vaccine preparations are approved for intradermal use.

(3) The intradermal route should not be used in individuals taking chloroquine or mefloquine for prophylaxis or treatment, as antibody responses are impaired.

(4) Dose: 1.0 ml IM or 0.1 ml intradermally on Days 0,7 and 21 or 28.

      (5) Booster doses every 2-3 years are recommended for individuals at very high risk.

      (6) If a suspect exposure occurs in an individual who has received pre-exposure prophylaxis, post-exposure prophylaxis is still necessary, but requires only two intramuscular or intradermal doses on days 0 and 3, or a single 4-site intradermal booster on day 0.

I. Respiratory syncytial virus (see "bronchiolitis" section, Chapter 13, section IV, C)

J. Rubella (German measles)

  1. General

    a. Acute, usually benign infectious disease characterized by rash, generalized lymphadenopathy and minimal prodromal symptoms.

    b. Causes congenital malformations when the infection occurs in early pregnancy.

    c. Occurs most commonly in children 5-9 years old.

    d. Incubation period is 12-19 days.

    e. Communicable from 7 days before until 5 days after the rash appears.

  2. Clinical

    a. A maculopapular rash appears on the face and spreads rapidly to the trunk and proximal extremities. It usually lasts only 3 days. Infection may occur without rash.

    b. Malaise and sore throat may occur with the rash, as well as fever.

    c. There may be postauricular and suboccipital lymphadenopathy prior to onset of the rash.

    d. Recovery is usually prompt and uneventful.

  3. Treatment

    a. None is available.

    b. Patients rarely need even symptomatic medication.

  4. Prevention - active immunization in childhood (MMR vaccine).

K. Varicella zoster virus

  1. Varicella (chickenpox)

    a. General

      (1) Acute, communicable disease characterized by generalized vesicular rash. It is highly contagious.

      (2) Incubation period of 10-23 days (usually 14).

      (3) Communicable 1 day prior to the appearance of the lesions to 6 days after (or when all the lesions are crusted).

    b. Clinical

      (1) In children, there is little prodrome (24 hours of malaise and fever). Adults may become very ill. May produce severe illness in the immunocompromised patient.

(2) Rash begins with discrete, erythematous macules and papules on the thorax, scalp, mucous membranes. Lesions then progress quickly to clear vesicles surrounded by erythema. They then become umbilicated, cloudy and purulent and form crusts in 2-4 days. Lesions in all stages of development may be seen within one area. Crusts fall off in 1-3 weeks.

c. Treatment

(1) Most patients require only symptomatic treatment.

(2) Itching may be controlled by an antipruritic lotion such as calamine. Antihistamines may also help. Nails should be kept short and hands clean. Children may need to wear gloves to prevent excoriation and scarring.

(3) If cellulitis is present, systemic antibiotics covering Group A *Streptococcus* and *Staphylococcus* should be used.

(4) Severe varicella in adults or immunocompromized patients should be treated with IV acyclovir or oral famcyclovir or valacyclovir. Illness may present as varicella pneumonia with respiratory distress.

(5) Acyclovir 20 mg/kg qid x 5 days orally can be used in immunocompetent children if treatment is considered necessary. Start within 24 hours of onset of rash.

d. Prevention

(1) Varicella vaccine (live virus) is effective and is widely used in developed countries (at or after 12 months of age).

(2) Varicella-zoster immune globulin (VZIG) may be given to individuals at high risk of complications but is very expensive.

e. Complications

(1) Toxic shock syndrome/necrotizing fasciitis can occur in patients who develop colonization of lesions with Group A *Streptococcus*.

(2) Reyes syndrome, with vomiting, irritability, decreasing level of consciousness, is associated with use of aspirin. Aspirin must be avoided in varicella or in febrile illnesses that may represent the prodrome of varicella.

(3) Varicella encephalitis, characterized by decreased level of consciousness, headache, vomiting and seizures is a serious complication, which may be life threatening in adults. Neurologic sequelae persist in 15%.

(4) Acute cerebellar ataxia, with onset from one week to 21 days after onset of rash is a benign complication in children. It resolves over 2-4 weeks.

(5) Varicella pneumonia can be severe. It is more common in adults, pregnant women and immunocompromised hosts. Usually presents 3-5 days after onset of rash.

2. Herpes zoster (shingles)
a. General
- (1) Reactivation of latent varicella virus in the dorsal root or cranial nerve ganglion cells.
- (2) Lesions erupt for several days and are gone in 2-3 weeks. Postherpetic neuralgia is frequently seen in older patients.

b. Clinical
- (1) The appearance of zoster lesions is usually preceded by itching, tenderness or pain. Neurologic changes within the affected dermatome include hypesthesia, dysesthesia or hyperesthesia. The interval between pain and the eruption is usually 3-5 days.
- (2) Zoster lesions appear posteriorly and progress to the anterior and peripheral distribution of the nerve. Erythematous macules, papules and plaques appear first, followed by grouped vesicles within 24 hours. The vesicles become purulent, crust and fall off in 1-2 weeks.
- (3) Zoster appears most often in thoracic and cervical segments.

c. Treatment
- (1) Acyclovir is effective for both localized and disseminated zoster. The dose is 800 mg 5x/d x 7d. It should be started within 48 hours of onset or as soon as possible. Famcyclovir (500 mg tid) and valacyclovir (1 gm bid) are better absorbed and are the treatment of choice, if available.
- (2) Analgesics are usually necessary to control pain.
- (3) Vesicular stage
  - (a) Cool compresses with 1:20 Burrows solution.
  - (b) Paint the lesions with flexible collodion q12h.
  - (c) Apply drying shake lotion (alcohol, menthol and/or phenol).
  - (d) Occlusive dressing (cotton and elastic bandage).
- (4) Use systemic antibiotics if secondary infection is present.
- (5) Systemic steroids may decrease the incidence of postherpetic neuralgia. These should be started as early as possible and only when combined with antiviral treatment (prednisone 40-60 mg qd x 2 weeks).

CHAPTER 2

HIV/AIDS

I. HIV PREVENTION

  A. General - HIV infections must be prevented one person at a time using proven interventions that have been shown to make a difference. The following should be considered:

    1. Education, public awareness, dramatic presentations, and media programs are essential but not sufficient. They are the foundation on which other programs are built. Continuing efforts are necessary to prevent unscientific and unsubstantiated information from being incorporated in these programs. Whenever possible, HIV-positive individuals should be encouraged to provide leadership and participate in these activities. Anecdotes are particularly effective.

    2. Stigma, discrimination and bigotry have characterized attitudes to HIV/AIDS and this has resulted in denial, both for individuals and for societies. Strategies to address discrimination, "mainstream" HIV illness, and change attitudes are essential if prevention is to be effectively addressed.

    3. Poverty, gender inequities, illiteracy, civil unrest, migration, and other health determinants are important to the continuing expansion of the HIV epidemic. These must be addressed wherever possible.

    4. Access to voluntary testing and counseling (VTC) is becoming a "human right" and it also can be an important prevention strategy. About 80% of individuals when properly counseled will alter behavior so that they will not transmit infection to sexual partners. All HIV care programs should have an accessible site for VTC. Confidentiality must be assured. However, within the appropriate cultural and legal contexts, individuals who are known to be positive and who are putting others at risk, may require additional interventions to protect their sexual partners.

    5. Routine screening of blood products and major efforts to reduce needle transmission, both from "medical" needle use and self-administered injections either legal or illegal, must occur with programs to prevent blood-borne transmission.

    6. Occupational risks of HIV infection are significant, particularly in settings of high HIV prevalence. Following substantial hollow bore needle injury where the risk of infection may be as high as 1 in 250, individuals should reduce their risk with a course of anti-retrovirals (risk reduction by about 75%). Although studies have used AZT and begin within the first 12 hours, combinations of AZT with other agents, particularly 3TC, are now commonly used and treatment is empirically prescribed for four weeks. Nevirapine should not be used for prophylaxis following possible exposure because of the risk of serious hepatic injury.

7. Reducing genital inflammation and secretions through treating sexually transmitted infections and other inflammatory processes in the genital tract, reduces excretion of HIV in genital secretions and the infectivity of individuals with HIV. Treating inflammatory genital diseases, particularly ulcers, reduces the risk of individuals acquiring infection (less susceptible) following intercourse with an HIV-positive individual. For both these reasons, controlling sexually transmitted diseases and promoting genital health substantially reduces HIV incidence (a reduction of about 40% in one study).

8. Interventions targeted toward sex workers (prostitutes) and their clients is an effective measure to slow HIV incidence. They are far "upstream" in the HIV/AIDS "river" and efforts to prevent transmission to and from this core group are very cost-effective. In all communities, these individuals merit programs to make condoms accessible, discourage promiscuity, prevent and treat STDs, facilitate peer education, and identify economic alternatives to sex work. This is an intervention that can have a marked effect but requires a sustained commitment.

9. At places of employment, workplace educational programs and peer education can change behavior.

10. Mother-to-infant transmission can be markedly reduced (from 25% to less than 8%) with peripartum prophylaxis with two proven regimens. Breast-feeding results in transmission to a further 10-15% of infants. Breast milk substitutes should be considered but it is recognized that this is a challenge in many societies, expensive, and may in itself result in increased morbidity and mortality (see below). The importance of adolescent programs cannot be over-emphasized. Mentoring, promoting chastity, providing alternate ways for young people to find significance in life are all important initiatives for educational and religious instruction together with peer education and role models. In many countries, the incidence of HIV in women between the ages of 15 and 20 can be 2-5% annually. This must be addressed urgently.

11. Sexual fulfillment and sustained satisfaction within monogamous marital relationships need to be a focus with a commitment from religious and social organizations to teach and encourage this ideal.

12. Reducing viral load with antiretroviral medications could have a major effect on the risk of transmission. This is important for individual relationships, particularly spousal transmission, but it requires more study to know its effect on HIV population incidence.

13. Circumcision protects men from acquiring HIV with a risk reduction of 50-80%. Although more research is needed before circumcision is advocated as a public health intervention, it should be offered to discordant couples if the wife is HIV-positive.

14. Sexual abuse, rape, and other forms of gender inequities often lead to an unhealthy promiscuous and unhappy sexual lifestyle and programs to prevent these should be in place.

15. Other prevention initiatives including Vitamin A supplementation and avoidance of estrogen/progesterone contraception need further study.

B. Preventing mother to child transmission

1. The vast majority of mother to child HIV transmissions can now be prevented, with a reduction of over 95% in well controlled 'resource sufficient' healthcare settings (a reduction from 35-45% to 1-2%). Ideally the following should be considered:

   a. Prevention of infection in women prior to, during and following pregnancy remains the first priority. Primary HIV infection during pregnancy or breast feeding is associated with increased transmission and strategies to address this should be a component of pre-and postnatal care.

   b. Prophylaxis during pregnancy including TMP/SMX, acyclovir and tuberculosis prophylaxis should be prescribed as indicated in the non-pregnant state. Fluconazole and other azoles should be avoided during the first trimester.

   c. During pregnancy, treatment with antiretrovirals (ARVs) to suppress viral load and maintain the mother's health can be continued or initiated. Efavirenz should be avoided in the first trimester and some experts stop all ARV's in the first trimester and restart them together at 14 weeks. d4T and ddI should not be used together due to the occurrence of lactic acidosis which appears to be more common in pregnancy. AZT can be added to the regimen at term regardless of the ARV regimen selected, due to the substantial evidence that this agent prevents mother to child transmission. However, many clinicians would continue with the regimen that has been effective for the mother during pregnancy and not add another drug at delivery.

   d. Caesarean section further reduces the risk of mother-to-child transmission (MTCT) and should be considered in situations of high risk of MTCT (such as when HIV-positive women have not received AZT) and when Caesarean section is feasible and safe. Premature rupture of membranes and premature birth both increase transmission risk and should be prevented, if possible.

   e. The infant should be given AZT or nevirapine--see below.

   f. Women should be counseled on alternatives to breast feeding, with the recognition that 12-18% of infants will be infected by lactation. Strategies to reduce the probability of transmission during lactation are being investigated but none are proven to be effective. When adequate supplies of formula and clean water are available, exclusive formula feeding seems safer than either breast-feeding or mixed breast-milk and formula feeding.

   g. HIV infection in infants cannot be diagnosed with antibody tests until 18 months of age. If it is essential to determine the HIV status prior to that time, viral load measurements or P24 studies are necessary. These are expensive and require sophisticated laboratory expertise.

2. In resource constrained environments, prophylaxis during delivery is now being used routinely along with a prescription for the infant. These regimens are capable of reducing transmission during delivery from about 18-25% to 7-10%. Some regimens used are:

   a. Nevirapine 200mg PO at onset of labor plus 2mg/kg for the infant at 48-72 hours.

   b. AZT 600mg PO at onset of labor and 300mg q3h until delivery plus 4mg/kg q12h for 7 days for the infant.

   c. AZT during the last trimester with 2mg/kg IV at onset of labor followed by 1mg/kg IV/hour until delivery plus 2mg/kg q6h for 6 weeks for the infant (the PACTG 076 protocol).

C. Post exposure HIV prophylaxis for health care personnel (based on USPHS guidelines)

  1. Risk of transmission of HIV - is estimated to be 0.3% for percutaneous exposure and 0.09% for membrane exposure. Risk is lower for exposure through intact skin.

   a. Risk increases with:

    (1) Larger quantities of blood involved in exposure (hollow needle).

    (2) Direct injection into a vessel.

    (3) Deep injury.

    (4) Terminally ill patients - probably reflecting higher viral loads.

   b. Post-exposure prophylaxis may reduce the risk of HIV transmission by about 80%.

  2. Evaluation

   a. Test health care worker immediately to establish baseline HIV status.

   b. Test the exposure source. If negative, no further follow up is necessary.

   c. Evaluate the potential of the exposure to transmit HIV.

    (1) Type of exposure - percutaneous injury, membrane exposure, intact or non-intact skin.

    (2) Amount of exposure - blood, bloody fluid, or body fluids.

  3. Recommendations

   a. Percutaneous injury

    (1) Patient has asymptomatic infection or low viral load (less than 1500 RNA copies/ml) - recommend giving 2-drug regimen.

    (2) Patient has symptomatic infection or high viral load, or exposure is more severe (large hollow bore needle, deep puncture, visible blood on device, or needle used in patient's vessel) - recommend giving 3-drug regimen.

   b. Mucus membrane or non-intact skin exposure

    (1) Small volume exposure (few drops of fluid)

     (a) Patient has asymptomatic infection or low viral load (less than 1500 RNA copies/ml) - consider giving 2-drug regimen (because of drug toxicity, worker may decline).

(b) Patient has symptomatic infection or high viral load - recommend giving 2-drug regimen.
  (2) Large volume exposure (major splash)
    (a) Patient has asymptomatic infection or low viral load -(less than 1500 RNA copies/ml) - recommend 2-drug regimen.
    (b) Patient has symptomatic infection or high viral load - recommend 3-drug regimen.
  c. HIV status of source is unknown - may consider 2-drug regimen if prevalence of HIV is high.

4. Drug selection
  a. Recommendations regarding the specific regimen to use are currently empiric.
  b. Goal is to complete a four week course of anti-retroviral therapy.
  c. Standard combinations of two nucleoside reverse transcriptase inhibitors may be used for two drug regimen (AZT or D4T with 3TC, ddI, or ddC).
  d. In higher risk exposures, a third agent should be added (a non-nucleoside reverse transcriptase inhibitor or protease inhibitor) to the standard 2-drug regimen.
  e. Monitor closely for drug toxicity.

II. HIV/AIDS DIAGNOSIS

A. Clinical case definitions
1. WHO and CDC definitions for an AIDS-defining event are provided in Tables 1 and 2 at the end of the chapter.
2. In addition, CDC uses the CD4 count (below 200) as an additional definition for the transition from HIV infection to AIDS.

B. Testing
1. HIV tests can now be done with finger prick on whole blood with two different tests. These give excellent sensitivity and specificity (>99%) in populations in which the prevalence exceeds 2%. A second rapid test should be done to confirm a positive test but may not be necessary routinely for a negative result.
  a. These tests are simple to perform and interpret and can be carried out in the office setting by nurses or other individuals who have had 1-2 hours of training.
  b. Pre-test counseling followed by a rapid test, with the availability of results and post-test counseling, all occurring in 1-2 hours, seems to be acceptable in most cultures for most individuals. It ensures that individuals who choose to be tested are not left in a state of worry for several days and allows all individuals who opt for a rapid test to receive the information.
  c. Frequently in these situations, a further post-test counseling session, often with a spouse, should be carried out within a few days.

2. Ideally, all patients with HIV infection should have surrogate markers for determination of disease status. The analogy of the train headed towards a disaster continues to be a useful framework for understanding disease markers. The distance between the train and the upcoming accident is represented by the CD4 count (particularly as it falls below 300/cu mm); the speed of the train by the viral load (particularly when it is above 30,000 RNA copies/ml). The lower the CD4 count (closer to the accident) and the higher the viral load (increasing train speed), the less time before an AIDS-defining illness can be anticipated to occur. However, in most situations in resource-poor countries, the CD4 counts and viral load measurements will not be available. There are no other well-tested surrogate markers for treating HIV infection with antiretroviral therapy (ART). Presumably other less expensive tests will be identified in the future.

III. PREVENTING/TREATING OPPORTUNISTIC INFECTIONS (OI'S)
A. General
1. Few studies have been carried out in resource poor societies.
2. OI's begin to occur as CD4 count falls below 400 and become increasingly frequent and severe as it falls below 200.
B. Presenting/defining illnesses in Africa
1. Respiratory infections occur in 30% of patients.
   a. Pneumococcal pneumonia is common.
   b. *Pneumocystis carinii* (PCP) represents less than 10% of pneumonias. In children, PCP is more common and has been found in up to 30% of individuals at post-mortem. In the developed world, almost one-half of the initial presenting infections are PCP.
2. Oropharyngeal /esophageal candidiasis in 15% of patients.
3. Wasting syndrome - diarrhea, fever, and wasting (greater than 10% loss of body weight) in 25% of patients.
4. Herpes zoster in 10% of patients.
5. Soft tissue and skin infections in 5% of patients.
6. Skin rash, especially pruritic folliculitis that on biopsy demonstrates eosinophils.
7. Toxoplasmosis, cryptococcosis, and other life-threatening CNS infections in 3-4% of patients.
8. Tuberculosis is common.
   a. One-fifth of respiratory infections are tuberculosis.
   b. Occurs in resource poor countries in many individuals with CD4 counts between 200 and 400.
   c. Extra-pulmonary tuberculosis is the presenting illness in 3-5% of patients.
C. Prophylaxis
1. The duration of illness in Africa and presumably in other resource poor

countries without access to effective anti-retroviral therapy (ART) is usually between 6 and 12 months after an AIDS-defining event, if the presenting illness is survived. However, some patients may survive for several years.

2. Routine prophylaxis should include:

a. TMP/SMX for common bacterial infections, PCP and some protozoal infections. In adults in West Africa, TMP/SMX prolongs life by an average of about six months when prescribed three times weekly, presumably due to prevention of bacterial infection. This remains controversial as it may promote resistance and has been less successful in some studies.

b. Tuberculosis prophylaxis should be routine in patients who have no evidence of active disease. A chest x-ray should be done first to exclude pulmonary tuberculosis. Unfortunately, new *M. tuberculosis* infections occur commonly among HIV infected individuals in many resource poor settings and, although prophylaxis is effective in preventing reactivation (reduces the incidence of reactivated TB from about 12% to 5%), it will not prevent subsequent new infections once prophylaxis is stopped. Patients are treated with standard regimens. See Chapter 1, VIII, D.

c. Fluconazole or one of the other azoles may need to be given continuously once an individual has recurrent severe oropharyngeal/esophageal candidiasis.

d. Toxoplasmosis is prevented with oral TMP/SMX prophylaxis. If the clinical diagnosis of toxoplasmosis is made, life-long treatment (secondary prevention) is necessary with pyrimethamine. See Chapter 1, IV, D,4.

e. Pneumococcal vaccine did not prevent pneumococcal infections in one study in Uganda.

f. Studies in children in resource poor countries are completely inadequate. However, it appears that MMR is safe; killed (rather than live) polio vaccine should be used if possible. BCG should not be given. Other immunizations should occur on schedule.

g. Patients with recurring salmonellosis may require prolonged (life-long) therapy with a quinolone.

D. Treatment of opportunistic infections

1. General

a. OI's in HIV-positive patients should be treated early and as aggressively as possible if individuals are to survive the initial infection.

b. As noted earlier, individuals even without antiretroviral therapy may have many months of quality life and surviving the "AIDS-defining" illness is a worthwhile goal.

2. Acute respiratory infections (ARI)

  a. Tuberculosis must always be ruled out and can present acutely (about 10% of acute pneumonias). Patients with re-activation tuberculosis usually present with fever, cough, weight loss and night sweats, which have persisted for more than one week. Tuberculosis is discussed in Chapter 1, VIII.

  b. Empiric treatment for respiratory infection should include *Pneumocystis carinii* even though this diagnosis is less common in developing countries.

    (1) PCP more commonly presents with a history of exertional dyspnea, interstitial infiltrates, tachypnea at rest, and an LDH over 400.

    (2) An initial regimen of TMP/SMX (1 DS tid in adults) and amoxicillin, 500 mg tid is inexpensive and will be effective in 90% or more of non-tuberculous ARIs.

    (3) Studies for bacterial pathogens are usually not helpful.

  c. In children, lymphoid interstitial pneumonia (LIP) also needs to be considered and responds to corticosteroids.

  d. *Mycobacterium avium intracellulare* (MAI) is a common cause of fever, sometimes with respiratory infiltrates in patients with very low CD4 counts (<50) in Western countries. It is unusual in developing countries probably because individuals with severe immunosuppression rarely survive.

3. Diarrheal disease

  a. Many pathogens have been associated with both acute and chronic diarrhea in HIV-infected individuals and diarrhea is often a part of the wasting syndrome.

  b. Pathogens

    (1) *Shigella*, GI viruses, and toxigenic *E. coli* are all isolated from acute diarrheal illnesses and should be managed as in non-HIV-infected patients.

    (2) *Salmonella* infections are particularly frustrating, as they tend to recur. *S. typhosa* (typhoid fever) is more severe in HIV-infected individuals.

    (3) Other *Salmonella* spp., if they relapse multiple times, may need long-term suppressive therapy.

    (4) Chronic diarrhea can be due to parasites (*Cryptosporidia, Strongyloides, Isospora, Giardia,* and *Microsporidia*), bacteria (*M. tuberculosis*, MAC, *Salmonella*), and viruses (CMV is particularly common in the late stage of AIDS patients).

  c. Specific therapy depends upon an exact diagnosis, which is difficult to make if cultures are not available.

  d. An empiric trial of TMP/SMX is an appropriate initial approach, perhaps followed by a trial of anti-tuberculous treatment if studies are negative for intestinal parasites. Could consider a trial of a course of a fluoroquinolone first before resorting to TB trial.

4. **Candidiasis**

    a. Candidiasis (oral thrush) usually responds to fluconazole, 100 mg daily.

    b. Recurrent candidiasis may be treated with twice weekly fluconazole.

    c. Oral troches with clotrimazole are also effective.

    d. Ketoconazole 200mg daily can also be used but is less effective and occasionally causes hepatitis.

    e. Nystatin and gentian violet can be effective in one-half to two-thirds of patient but should only be used if there are no alternate regimens.

    f. Esophageal candidiasis can cause dysphagia and wasting and usually requires continuous (life-long) suppressive therapy with fluconazole, if possible.

    g. Herpes infections including zoster and simplex ideally should be managed initially with acyclovir, famciclovir, or valacyclovir. Herpes simplex in particular is a recurrent illness and long-term (life-long) suppressive therapy may be needed.

5. **Skin and soft tissue infections**

    a. Skin and soft tissue infections are usually due to *S. aureus* and *Group A Strep* but occasionally can be due to Gram-negative rods.

    b. Antibiotic therapy should be started immediately after diagnosis and surgical incision and drainage should be done, if necessary. Cloxacillin, cephalexin or clindamycin may be used as first line agents. If there is a poor response to treatment, addition of ciprofloxacin or TMP/SMX may be considered to provide Gram negative coverage.

6. **Extrapulmonary tuberculosis**

    a. Tuberculosis outside the respiratory tract is common and should be considered when patients have prolonged fever, weight loss, and generalized symptoms.

    b. Biopsy of involved lymph nodes, liver biopsy, or imaging may identify a site and cultures of urine or stool may permit a more exact diagnosis.

    c. If a definite diagnosis of tuberculosis is suspected but unable to be proven, a trial of empiric therapy is indicated. The trial should continue for at least three weeks. If the patient is responding with improved appetite, weight gain, and fever resolution, therapy should be continued for a full course of treatment. If there is no improvement, other etiologies of the symptom complex should be considered.

7. **CNS infections**

    a. CNS infections are usually fatal.

      b. Bacterial meningitis should be treated as in non-HIV patients (see Chapter 1, III). TMP/SMX or pyrimethamine may be prescribed for possible toxoplasmosis; amphotericin and/or fluconazole for possible cryptococcal meningitis.

      c. CNS toxoplasmosis presents as a space occupying lesion. Treatment usually results in prompt improvement, evident within 1-2 weeks. All patients presenting with features of a space-occupying lesion deserve a trial of therapy for toxoplasmosis (as below). Failure to respond to anti-toxo therapy within 2 weeks makes the diagnosis unlikely and increases the likelihood of an alternative diagnosis (TB, primary CNS lymphoma, etc.).

        (1) Pyrimethamine 200mg stat, then 75-100 mg/day + sulfadiazine 1-1.5 g q6h + folinic acid 10-15 mg/day x 3-5 weeks. In patients with severe sulfa allergy, sulfadiazine can be replaced by clarithromycin 1gram bid or clindamycin 600 mg q6h.

        (2) TMP/SMX (10 mg TMP/50 mg SMX/kg/day in two doses) x 30 days.

        (3) After completing the initial treatment phase, lifelong secondary prophylaxis with TMP/SMX is required.

   8. Drug toxicities

      a. In 15-20% of patients, TMP/SMX produces fever, pruritus, skin rash, and occasionally a Stephens-Johnson-like syndrome. In most instances, patients can be maintained on the regimen and be treated "through" this side effect unless bullae or vesicles are present or the rash is becoming more extensive.

      b. A number of agents, particularly ketoconazole and rifampin, interact with antiretroviral drugs.

IV. ANTIRETROVIRAL TREATMENT

  A. General

   1. The use of anti-retrovirals (ARV's) in resource poor countries is rapidly becoming possible due to reduced prices and drug donations. The research necessary to know how these drugs should be used in these populations is still underway. However, the increased availability of drugs and their positive impact on HIV illness will almost certainly lead to their increased use in the future.

   2. The following are some generalizations that must be kept in mind:

      a. Everyone agrees that ARV's should be given, if possible, once an AIDS-defining event has occurred and when the CD4 count falls below 200. Otherwise, treatment initiation is controversial and long-term perspective studies are necessary. Although unproven, it is possible that treatment during primary infection within the first three months of acquiring the virus, may lead to "long-term" viral suppression by the immune system without continuous therapy. For most other indications, once the patient begins on therapy, it should be life-long.

b. In developed countries the goal of therapy has been viral suppression (below 400 RNA copies/ml) together with a rising CD4 count that may return to normal values. The return of the CD4 count protects patients from OI's and prophylactic therapies become unnecessary when CD4 counts exceed 200 for at least 3 months.

c. Immune reconstitution illnesses have become common as patients recover their immune function and these can be severe, even life-threatening.

    (1) Tuberculosis, in particular, as well as other pathogens can be associated with a very significant "inflammatory" response with "pneumonia", fever and other manifestations that reflect a host recovery response to the pathogen.

    (2) The treatment of immune reconstitution diseases is with corticosteroids as well as specific targeted antimicrobial treatment.

    (3) These diseases are difficult to diagnose but should be considered whenever patients deteriorate during the first 4-6 weeks of ARV's despite an improving immune system.

d. ARV's must always be used in combination and except for peripartum prophylaxis, the goal is to use three or four drugs. Although 2 NRTIs have been used with short-term improvement, they have not usually allowed long-term viral suppression. Three-drug treatment is necessary in order to prevent rapid emergence of resistance and treatment failure. Patients must understand this and agree to be compliant. Usually this means taking over 95% of their medications correctly.

e. Strategies to make drug use more patient-friendly include combining agents in one pill and developing once daily therapies. Both of these are occurring and will likely be the standard of treatment within 1-2 years.

f. With excellent compliance (over 95% of drugs taken) together with a triple drug regimen, naive previously untreated patients respond in about 80% of instances. Most patients with CD4 counts above 100 will have a long-term (3-5 years) response or longer.

g. Resistance will emerge in patients who are not compliant and in about 20% of patients who appear to be compliant. Once resistance emerges (rising viral load above 15,000; falling CD4 count; new OI's), treatment should be altered to an entirely different regimen.

h. Genotyping involves determining the exact genetic basis of resistance and is now being used routinely in patients who fail therapy in developed countries. It is expensive (>$150 U.S.) and requires very specialized expertise. However, it does offer important information in order to select the optimal treatment regimen.

B. Choosing anti-retrovirals (ARVs)

1. Table 3 has a list of the current marketed ARV's in the U.S.

   a. Initial therapy has consisted of AZT and 3TC, 2 nuclease reverse transcriptase inhibitors (NRTI) together with nelfinavir, a protease inhibitor (PI). However, other NRTIs can be combined with any protease inhibitor as an initial regimen.

   b. A second line regimen, chosen either because of availability, failure or toxicity, in most instances would include either two different NRTIs plus a non-nucleoside reverse transcriptase inhibitor (NNRTI) such as efavirenz, nevirapine, or delavirdine or one NRTI plus a PI together with an NNRTI. Always choose at least three.

   c. Several studies have now shown that three NRTIs specifically abacavir with two other NRTIs can provide equivalent therapy to either regimen 1 or 2 when used in treatment-naive patients.

   d. Double PI's (using ritonavir plus another PI) are particularly effective due to the longer half-life of the PI secondary to the effect of ritonavir on cytochrome P450 enzymes that delay the metabolism of most PI's. Ritonavir in a dose of 100mg can be combined with any PI and is currently marketed in combination with lopinavir. The combination of ritonavir plus lopinavir may enable once daily therapy.

   e. Once daily therapy may permit ARVs to be given as directly observed therapy (DOT).

   f. Monitoring ARV therapy traditionally is done with viral loads and CD4 counts every 4-6 months together with liver enzymes and blood counts.

   g. The complexities of these regimens with their adverse effects and interactions at times can appear to be overwhelming. Close monitoring for side effects of therapy is essential. Table 3 lists common side effects/adverse events. Patients need a great deal of counseling and other support when they start on ARV's and initiation of treatment must never be done haphazardly.

   h. Never change one medication if the entire regimen is failing. For a failing regimen all agents need to be replaced. If the patient is having toxicities presumably from one of the three agents, stop all of them, let the patient recover over 5-10 days from the side effects and then restart three agents choosing an alternative to the one considered most likely to be responsible for the toxic side effect.

   i. Ensure that patients know to stop all ARV's (not just one or two) if problems appear to be occurring. They must be educated to not start and stop ARV's whenever they choose without medical input. This will result in rapid emergence of resistance and treatment failure.

TABLE 1
WHO CLINICAL STAGING

STAGE 1	No clinical symptoms Normal activity May have lymphadenopathy
STAGE 2	Weight loss < 10% Minor skin rash Herpes zoster Recurrent upper respiratory infections Symptomatic but still normal activity
STAGE 3	Weight loss >10% Chronic diarrhea >1 month Recurrent fevers >1 month Oral thrush Pulmonary tuberculosis Bedridden <50% of time for past month
STAGE 4	Cryptococcal meningitis Toxoplasmosis, central nervous system Kaposi sarcoma Dementia Bedridden 75% for past month

TABLE 2
CDC CLASSIFICATION

A	Asymptomatic Persistent generalized lymphadenopathy Acute (primary) HIV illness
B	Vulvovaginal candidiasis > 1 month, persistent Candidiasis, oropharyngeal Constitutional symptoms - fever, diarrhea > 1 month Cervical dysplasia, severe or carcinoma in situ
C	Candidiasis, esophageal, tracheal, bronchial Coccidiomycosis, extrapulmonary Cryptococcosis, extrapulmonary Cervical cancer, invasive Cryptosporidiosis, chronic (diarrhea > 1 month) CMV retinitis, GI, CNS HIV encephalopathy Herpes simplex with ulcers > 1 month Isosporosis, chronic > 1 month Kaposi sarcoma Lymphoma, Burkitt's immunoblastic, CNS *M. Avium, M. Kansasii*, extrapulmonary *M. tuberculosis* pulmonary and extrapulmonary *Pneumocystis carinii* pneumonia Recurrent pneumonia (> two episodes/year) Progressive multifocal leukoencephalopathy Salmonella bacteremia, recurrent Toxoplasmosis, cerebral Wasting syndrome

TABLE 3
Antiretroviral Agents

Generic Name	Trade Name	Usual Dose	Major Adverse Effects
Nucleoside Reverse Transcriptase Inhibitors			
Zidovudine (ZDV, AZT)	Retrovir	300mg bid.	Anemia (1%), granulocytopenia (2%), nausea (50%), headache (60%), insomnia
Lamivudine (3TC)	Epivir	150mg bid.	Well tolerated, fatigue (20%), headaches (20%)
Stavudine (D4T)	Zerit	40mg bid	Peripheral neuropathy (15%), pancreatitis (1%), nausea (5%)
Didanosine (ddI)	Videx	400mg qd	Pancreatitis (6%), diarrhea (25%), peripheral neuropathy (20%), rash (9%)
Zalcitabine (ddC)	Hivid	0.75mg tid	Peripheral neuropathy (30%), oral ulcers (13%), rash (8%)
Abacavir	Ziagen	300mg bid	Hypersensitivity (5%), can be fatal (myalgia, edema, rash, GI upset)
Non-Nucleoside Reverse Transcriptase Inhibitors			
Delavirdine	Rescriptor	400mg tid.	Rash (18%)
Efavirenz	Sustiva	600mg qd	CNS, insomnia, nightmares (60%), rash (28%)
Nevirapine	Viramune	200mg bid	Hepatic necrosis (1%), rash (30%), severe rash (Stevens - Johnson 1%)
Protease Inhibitors*			
Saquinavir	Fortovase	1200mg tid	Well tolerated 50% GI
Ritonavir	Norvir	600mg bid	Many drug interactions, circumoral paresthesias (6%)
Nelfinavir	Viracept	1250mg bid	Diarrhea (30%)
Indinavir	Crixivan	800mg tid	Kidney stones (2-5%), nausea (10%)
Amprenavir	Agenerase	1200mg bid	Rash (25%), nausea (30%), paresthesias (30%)
Lopinavir/ Ritonavir	Kaletra	400/100mg bid	Diarrhea (15%), nausea (10%)

*All protease inhibitors can cause a metabolic syndrome with insulin resistance, lipodystrophy (central obesity, wasting of face and limbs, and increased cholesterol)

CHAPTER 3

CARDIOLOGY

I. HYPERTENSION

A. Classification

Classification of Hypertension		
	Diastolic BP	**Systolic BP**
Normal	< 85 mm Hg	< 130 mm Hg
High-normal	85-89 mm Hg	130-139 mm Hg
Mild (Stage I)	90 - 99 mm Hg	140 - 159 mm Hg
Moderate (Stage II)	100 - 109 mm Hg	160 - 179 mm Hg
Severe (Stage III)	>110 mm Hg	> 180 mm Hg
Isolated systolic hypertension	< 90 mm Hg	> 140 mm Hg

B. Definitions

1. **Hypertensive urgency** - clinical situation in which BP is significantly elevated, but the patient is asymptomatic. BP should be lowered in 24 hours. Accelerated hypertension is markedly elevated BP which may be associated with hemorrhages and exudates but without papilledema or other evidence of evolving end-organ dysfunction.
2. **Hypertensive emergency** - clinical situation in which the BP must be lowered within 1 hour due to the presence of target organ damage.
   a. Malignant hypertension - a hypertensive emergency with hemorrhages, exudates and papilledema associated with a significant rise in the patient's baseline blood pressure. Diastolic BP is usually in the range of 120-140 mmHg.
   b. Hypertensive encephalopathy - headache, alteration in consciousness and other CNS dysfunction associated with sudden and marked elevation in BP and hemorrhages and exudates with or without papilledema. Reversible by rapid reduction of BP.

C. General

1. The rationale for treatment of hypertension is to prevent the complications of stroke, heart failure and renal disease. The blood pressure must be controlled over a long period of time for treatment to be beneficial. It is especially important to aggressively treat hypertension in patients with other risk factors for cardiovascular disease, such as diabetes, smoking and hyperlipidemia.
2. Educate the patient. Emphasize the rationale of low salt diet, weight loss, alcohol reduction and medical treatment. Explain potential drug side effects.
3. Keep the drug regimen as simple and economical as possible, using the fewest drugs possible and giving them no more than twice daily, if possible.

D. Evaluation

1. Diagnosis
   a. Be sure of the diagnosis before initiating drug therapy. If possible, obtain at least three readings prior to initiating treatment.
   b. Use an appropriately sized (cuff should cover 50% of the length and 80% of the circumference of the upper arm) and calibrated blood pressure cuff.

2. Primary (essential) hypertension
   a. Represents 95% of cases.
   b. Onset between ages 20-50 yrs.
   c. Positive family history frequently present.

3. Secondary hypertension
   a. Suspect when patient presents with severe or difficult to control hypertension, when patient presents with target organ damage, when onset is before age 20 or after age 50.
   b. Common causes of secondary hypertension include:
       (1) Primary renal disease - serum creatinine is elevated. Most common cause of secondary hypertension.
       (2) Primary hyperaldosteronism - hypokalemia and metabolic acidosis are frequently present.
       (3) Renovascular - difficult to detect without adequate radiologic testing. Diagnosis suggested with disproportionate response to ACE-inhibitors.
       (4) Other considerations - oral contraceptives, pheochromocytoma, sleep apnea, Cushing's syndrome, coarctation of the aorta or heavy alcohol use.

4. Determine the presence of end-organ damage - premature cardiovascular disease, heart failure, LVH, stroke and intracerebral hemorrhage, or renal insufficiency.

5. Identify other cardiovascular risk factors such as diabetes, cigarette smoking, or elevated cholesterol.

6. Physical exam - look for arteriolar narrowing, retinal hemorrhages or papilledema. Determine BP in both arms, look for signs of LVH on cardiac exam (displacement of PMI, 3rd or 4th heart sound). Check for abdominal masses or bruits and peripheral edema.

7. Laboratory - check CBC, U/A, glucose, BUN, creatinine, and ECG.

E. Treatment

1. The goal of treatment - is a diastolic pressure of <90 mmHg, and a systolic pressure of <140 mmHg. Maximum benefit is obtained by lowering the diastolic blood pressure to < 85 mm Hg.

2. High normal blood pressure
   a. Observation only - recheck in 3-6 months.
   b. Begin non-pharmacologic treatment - weight reduction, salt restriction, alcohol reduction, exercise, relaxation and stress reduction.

3. Mild hypertension

a. May initially try non-pharmacologic treatment.

b. If the response is inadequate, begin treatment with a moderate dose of a diuretic, ß-blocker, methyldopa or reserpine. If available, ACE-inhibitors or calcium channel blockers may be used.

c. Re-evaluate the patient in 4-8 weeks. Expect a decrease of 10-15 mmHg in systolic and diastolic BP.

d. If the response is inadequate, consider increasing the dose, adding a diuretic, or changing to a different class of drugs.

4. Moderate hypertension

a. Needs to be treated aggressively.

b. Begin with a diuretic plus a second drug.

c. Evaluate the patient in 2-4 weeks. Increase the dosage, if necessary.

d. If the response is inadequate, add a third drug or change to a new class of drugs.

5. Severe hypertension and malignant hypertension

a. Hospitalization is usually necessary.

b. Look for renal disease or other causes of secondary hypertension.

c. Treat initially with diuretics, IV hydralazine. Add oral agents to maintain control of BP.

6. Isolated systolic hypertension

a. Benefits of treatment are the same as for diastolic hypertension.

b. Goal of treatment is systolic BP <140 mm Hg while maintaining the diastolic BP > 65 mm Hg.

c. Begin treatment with diuretics; add ß-blockers, or calcium channel blockers as necessary.

7. Associated disease processes - consider the following suggestions for treatment of hypertension when associated with other medical problems:

Associated Disease	Preferred Drugs	Drugs to Avoid
Congestive heart failure	Diuretics ACE-inhibitors ß-blockers	-
Diabetes mellitus	ACE-inhibitors Ca-channel blockers	ß-blockers
Renal failure	Diuretics (loop) Hydralazine Ca-channel blockers	ACE-inhibitors
Angina pectoris	Nitrates ß-blockers Ca-channel blockers (long-acting only)	Hydralazine

II. VALVULAR HEART DISEASE
A. Aortic stenosis

1. Common acquired valvular lesion. Most develop as a consequence of congenital bicuspid valvular anatomy. Rheumatic fever may cause aortic stenosis but seldom without evidence of mitral valve disease. Idiopathic sclerosis occurs in the elderly.
2. Cardinal symptoms are dyspnea, angina and exertional syncope, but most patients remain asymptomatic for long periods of time.
3. Physical examination reveals a normal first heart sound followed by a harsh systolic murmur that radiates to the neck. Carotid artery upstroke is delayed.
4. Once symptomatic, life expectancy is reduced. Surgical valve replacement is the only treatment.

B. Aortic regurgitation

1. Chronic aortic regurgitation may be due to congenital bicuspid aortic valve, rheumatic fever, endocarditis, syphilis or connective tissue disease.
2. Most patients are asymptomatic at the time of diagnosis.
3. Physical examination shows bounding peripheral pulses with widened pulse pressure, laterally displaced, hyperdynamic apex impulse and high-pitched, blowing diastolic murmur heard best along the left sternal margin.
4. Patients with chronic aortic regurgitation eventually develop heart failure. Vasodilator therapy may help preserve ventricular function if valve replacement is not an option. Hydralazine and nifedipine show better results than ACE-inhibitors.
5. Acute aortic regurgitation may develop with infective endocarditis, aortic dissection or trauma. The characteristic bounding pulses and loud murmur may not be present in these cases.

C. Mitral stenosis

1. Most commonly found as a sequela to rheumatic fever. There is usually a long asymptomatic period of many years after the episode of rheumatic fever. Symptoms may first occur during periods of stress, such as pregnancy.
2. Dyspnea is the primary symptom associated with mitral stenosis. Episodes of pulmonary congestion may occur during febrile illnesses, anemia or pregnancy. Atrial fibrillation is often present as well.
3. Physical examination shows accentuation of S1, an opening snap in early diastole followed by a low-pitched diastolic rumble. The murmur is best heard with the bell of the stethoscope applied over the apex. Having the patient lie on their left side may help accentuate it. There may also be a systolic lift along the lower sternal edge.
4. Atrial fibrillation may be treated with digoxin for control of the ventricular rate. Low dose calcium channel blocker or ß-blocker may be helpful also. Systemic embolization is common and anticoagulation with warfarin should be considered, if available.

D. Mitral regurgitation

1. Causes include mitral valve prolapse, ruptured chordae tendineae, rheumatic fever, papillary muscle ischemia or infarction and endocarditis. Functional mitral regurgitation may develop as a consequence of left ventricular dilation.

2. Clinical course is variable and depends on the etiology, acuity and severity of the regurgitation. In chronic mitral regurgitation, the left atrium dilates, due to regurgitant blood volume. In acute situations, the left atrium is noncompliant and pulmonary edema occurs.

3. Physical examination reveals an enlarged apical impulse which is displaced downward and to the left. S1 is accentuated and is followed by a high-pitched, holosystolic murmur which radiates to the axilla. A prominent S3 gallop may be present.

4. Treatment is valve replacement. Vasodilator therapy is of no benefit in non-hypertensive patients.

E. Mitral valve prolapse

1. Most patients are asymptomatic. Common complaints are chest pain and palpitations. The chest pain is not typical for angina.

2. The hallmark of prolapse is the mid to late systolic click, which is present only in half the cases. There may be a brief midsystolic or late systolic murmur present also. Standing and Valsalva maneuver will cause the click/murmur to occur earlier in systole. Leg elevation or deep knee bend will displace the click/murmur later into systole.

3. The presence of a murmur or mitral regurgitation on echocardiogram indicates a higher risk for endocarditis and antibiotic prophylaxis is recommended.

4. Symptomatic dysrhythmias may be treated with ß-blockers.

III. HEART FAILURE

A. General

1. Clinical syndrome resulting from cardiac decompensation and characterized by signs and symptoms of volume overload and/or inadequate tissue perfusion.

2. Identify and treat the underlying etiology. In developing countries, rheumatic heart disease is a major cause of CHF, especially in young patients. Hypertension may cause both diastolic and systolic heart failure. Ischemic heart disease is less common in less developed countries, but the incidence is increasing.

B. Evaluation

1. Symptoms - cough, shortness of breath, orthopnea, paroxysmal nocturnal dyspnea, exertional dyspnea, malaise, fatigue, loss of appetite.

2. Signs - rales, tachycardia, cardiomegaly, gallop rhythm (left-sided failure). Neck vein distention, hepatomegaly, ascites, edema (right-sided failure).

3. Chest x-ray - look for cephalization, Kerley B lines, alveolar infiltrates, or pleural effusions. With a normal-sized heart on chest x-ray and signs of CHF suspect diastolic dysfunction, due to long-standing hypertension. An enlarged cardiac silhouette suggests systolic dysfunction, with a dilated left ventricle.
4. ECG - look for arrhythmias, left ventricular hypertrophy (S in V1 + R in V5-6 $\geq$ 35 mm), evidence of ischemic disease (q waves).
5. Other laboratory studies which may be helpful include CBC (look for anemia), creatinine (to evaluate renal function), electrolytes (monitor with diuretic therapy).

C. Treatment

1. Treat the underlying conditions (hypertension, ischemic disease, valvular disease, alcohol abuse).
2. Restrict salt to < 2gm per day. Water restriction may be helpful if the patient has hyponatremia.
3. Monitor the patient's weight.
4. Bedrest is usually necessary during acute episodes of heart failure. Otherwise, regular mild exercise is beneficial.
5. Drug treatment
   a. Diuretics
      (1) Use for volume reduction. Improve symptoms.
      (2) Thiazides are good for mild CHF, loop diuretics for severe CHF.
      (3) Use combinations of loop and thiazide diuretics if the patient is unresponsive to single agents.
      (4) Avoid hypokalemia and intravascular volume depletion with over-vigorous diuresis.
   b. ACE-inhibitors
      (1) ACE-inhibitors decrease the rate of development of overt CHF in patients with left ventricular dysfunction. They improve symptoms and decrease mortality in patients with CHF.
      (2) They are considered first line therapy in CHF, reducing both pre-load and after-load. Use the highest dose tolerated by the patient.
      (3) The combination of nitrates and hydralazine produce much the same effect as ACE-inhibitors, if ACE-inhibitors are unavailable or not tolerated.
   c. Beta Blockers
      (1) Have been shown to improve survival in patients with mild to moderate heart failure.
      (2) More effective when used in combination with ACE-inhibitors.
      (3) CHF symptoms may worsen initially.
      (4) Begin at very low doses (metoprolol 6.25 mg bid) and gradually increase as tolerated.
   d. Spironolactone
      (1) Has been shown to improve survival in heart failure.
      (2) Use 25-50mg/day

e. Digoxin
  (1) Improves exercise tolerance and symptoms in systolic heart failure. Digoxin does not improve survival.
  (2) Use in symptomatic patients with systolic ventricular dysfunction. The presence of an S3 is a major correlate of response to digoxin.
  (3) May be used to treat heart failure in infants and children. (see Ch 14, section V)
  (4) Digitalizing dose in adults is usually 1 mg. Give 0.25-0.5 mg slowly IV, then 0.25 mg q 6 hrs. until full dose is given. Onset of action is 15-30 minutes. In less urgent situations, the same dose may be given P.O. Maintenance dose is usually 0.125-0.25 mg per day. Dosage must be reduced in patients with renal insufficiency.
  (5) Watch for digoxin toxicity in patients on long term treatment.

D. Pulmonary edema

1. Severe CHF manifests itself as pulmonary edema (severe dyspnea, rales, gallop rhythm, edema, chest x-ray with cardiomegaly and perihilar infiltrates). This is a medical emergency.
2. Administer high flow oxygen (10-15L/min.), if available.
3. Furosemide 40mg IV if the patient has not previously been on diuretics; otherwise, give twice the patient's usual daily dose IV.
4. Morphine 2-5 mg IV q 15 min. Improves anxiety and dyspnea. Helps relieve chest pain and discomfort.
5. Nitrates may be useful. Use NTG 1/150gr. SL or topical nitroglycerin paste 1/2-1 inch. If available, nitro drip 5-50mg/min. may be used until symptoms improve. Nitrates also help relieve chest pain associated with cardiac ischemia.
6. Digoxin should be given (0.25-0.5mg po or IV in adults).
7. If all else fails, phlebotomy may be done. Remove 1-2 units of blood from the patient, and transfuse back as packed cells. This is especially effective in patients with renal failure, where dialysis cannot be performed immediately.

IV. ENDOCARDITIS

A. Prevention

1. No controlled human studies to demonstrate that antibiotic prophylaxis prevents endocarditis.
2. Use of prophylactic antibiotics in individuals with underlying cardiac abnormalities undergoing bacteremia-inducing procedures is common practice.
3. High risk patients include those with prosthetic valves, previous bacterial endocarditis, or complex cyanotic congenital heart disease.
4. Moderate risk patients include other congenital cardiac malformations, acquired valvular dysfunction, hypertrophic cardiomyopathy, and mitral valve prolapse with murmur.

Endocarditis Prevention		
Dental/respiratory tract procedures	Oral	Amoxicillin 2gm (50mg/kg) PO 1h prior to procedure. No subsequent doses are necessary. PCN-allergic: clindamycin 600 mg (20mg/kg), cephalexin 2 gm (50mg/kg), or azithromycin 500 mg (15mg/kg) PO 1 hr prior to procedure.
	Parenteral (if unable to take oral)	Ampicillin 2gm (50mg/kg) IM/IV 30min. prior to procedure PCN-allergic: clindamycin 600 mg (20mg/kg) IV or cefazolin 1gm (25mg/kg) IM/IV 30 min. prior to procedure.
Gastrointestinal or genitourinary procedures	Moderate risk	Amoxicillin 2gm (50mg/kg) PO 1 h prior to procedure or ampicillin 2gm (50mg/kg) IM/IV 30 min. prior to procedure PCN-allergic: vancomycin 1gm (20mg/kg) IV over 1-2h, complete infusion within 30min. of starting procedure.
	High risk	Ampicillin 2gm (50mg/kg) IM/IV + gentamicin 1.5mg/kg IM/IV within 30 min. of starting the procedure. 6 hours later, ampicillin 1gm (25mg/kg) or amoxicillin 1gm (25mg/kg) PO. PCN-allergic: Vancomycin 1gm (20mg/kg) IV over 1-2h + gentamicin 1.5mg/kg IM/IV. Complete infusion within 30 min. of starting procedure.

B. Infective endocarditis

1. Difficult to diagnose in settings where blood cultures are not available. It should be considered in patients with pre-existing valvular heart disease, persistent fevers, new onset of CHF, or signs of systemic embolization.
2. Classification
   a. Acute form - fulminant course with high fever, systemic toxicity, leukocytosis.
   b. Subacute form - slow, indolent course with low-grade fever, night sweats, weight loss, vague systemic complaints. Usually occurs in patients with prior valvular disease.
3. Signs and symptoms vary. Fever occurs in 95%. Nonspecific symptoms such as anorexia, weight loss, malaise, fatigue, chills, weakness and night sweats are common. Heart murmurs are present in most patients, but changing murmurs are uncommon.
4. CHF is the leading cause of death. Major embolic episodes are the second most common complication.
5. Empiric treatment
   a. Acute (usually staph) - nafcillin /oxacillin 2gm q4h IV or cefazolin 2gm q8h IV x 4-6 weeks + gentamicin 1.0mg/kg q8h IV x 3-5 days.
   b. Subacute (strep viridans or enterococci) - penicillin G 12-18 million units/d or ampicillin 12gm/d given q4h IV plus gentamicin 1.0-1.5mg/kg/d given q8h IV x 4-6 weeks.

V. PERICARDITIS
A. Acute pericarditis
1. Most frequent etiology is viral. In developing countries consider TB or rheumatic fever.
2. Examination
   a. Listen for a pericardial friction rub. Measure the pulsus paradoxus (drop in systolic BP with inspiration). Suspect tamponade if greater than 10mm Hg.
   b. Suspect effusion if the cardiac silhouette is large on chest x-ray, or the ECG shows decreased voltage. If ultrasound is available, the diagnosis can be confirmed by finding fluid in the pericardial space. If ultrasound is not available, and effusion is suspected, a pericardiocentesis can be performed and fluid removed for analysis. Pericardial fluid secondary to TB is usually exudative and bloody.
3. Treatment
   a. Viral or rheumatic fever - treatment is symptomatic with aspirin or NSAIDs. Steroids may be used if there are signs of pancarditis or CHF associated with rheumatic fever. They should not be used in the acute phase of viral myocarditis.
   b. Treatment of tamponade is emergent drainage of the pericardial space by pericardiocentesis.
   c. Tuberculous pericardial effusions usually respond very rapidly to TB treatment, with significant decrease in heart size on chest x-ray after 2-3 weeks.
   d. Steroids are recommended during the initial stages of treatment, to decrease the development of chronic constrictive pericarditis (prednisone 40-60mg/d or 1mg/kg/d).

B. Chronic constrictive pericarditis
1. Frequent sequela to TB pericarditis. May be prevented by the use of steroids in the acute treatment.
2. Definitive treatment requires pericardiectomy.
3. Symptoms of venous congestion may be helped with salt restriction and diuretics.

VI. CARDIAC DYSRHYTHMIAS
A. Palpitations
1. The subjective feeling of palpitations are usually due either to premature atrial beats or premature ventricular contractions. An ECG may demonstrate the arrhythmia, and reveal any underlying cardiac disease, such as LVH, ischemic heart disease, atrial enlargement, etc.
2. Ectopic beats do not generally require treatment unless they are very bothersome to the patient. ß-blockers, especially propranolol, are effective in low doses.

B. Supraventricular tachycardia

1. Diagnosis - regular rhythm, rate 150-220/min. with narrow QRS, unless a bundle branch block is present.

2. Treatment

   a. Vagal maneuvers - carotid sinus massage (in absence of carotid bruit only), Valsalva.

   b. Adenosine may be used, if available.

   c. Digoxin may be given IV (will take 30-60 minutes to work).

   d. Verapamil or diltiazem IV will control the arrhythmia acutely, if available.

   e. Treat the underlying cause (hypoxia, CHF).

   f. Use oral ß-blockers, digoxin or verapamil for long-term suppression.

C. Atrial flutter

1. Diagnosis - flutter waves present with atrial rate of 240-360/min., usually with 2:1 block.

2. Treatment

   a. Digoxin 0.5mg IV to slow the rate (will take 30-60 min. to work). May be dangerous in patients with WPW.

   b. Verapamil or diltiazem IV work faster, if available.

   c. Oral digoxin for maintenance or prevention.

D. Atrial fibrillation

1. Diagnosis - irregular ventricular rhythm, absent P waves, rate is 160-180/min when uncontrolled.

2. Treatment

   a. Therapy is aimed at controlling the ventricular rate. IV digoxin is preferred for immediate treatment, to slow down the ventricular response. If available, IV diltiazem or verapamil are also very effective. Oral digoxin, verapamil or ß-blockers can then be used for chronic rate control.

   b. Patients with atrial fibrillation > 1 year and large left atrial size have low likelihood of staying in normal sinus rhythm. Attempts should not be made to convert them to normal sinus rhythm, either electrically or medically.

   c. Patients with atrial fibrillation have a risk of ischemic stroke at least 5x that of persons in normal sinus rhythm, even in the absence of valvular heart disease. Long-term anticoagulation with warfarin, if available, should be considered in these patients.

E. Premature ventricular contractions

1. Diagnosis - irregular wide complex beats that occur independent of p waves, and are followed by a compensatory pause. Of more concern when occurring in groups (three or more = ventricular tachycardia), multifocal, when closely coupled (R on T). Look for hypoxia, electrolyte abnormality, or drug toxicity.

2. Treatment

   a. No treatment indicated if the heart is structurally normal.

   b. If patient experiences palpitations, ß-blockers may be used.

c. With more complex patterns, or in the presence of LV dysfunction, other anti-arrhythmics may be used. Monitor closely due to their pro-arrhythmic potential.

VII. CORONARY ARTERY DISEASE
A. General
1. The incidence of coronary artery disease in the developing world is much lower than in western countries, however with changes in diet, exercise patterns, and cigarette smoking, the incidence is rising.
2. The absence of diagnostic facilities makes evaluation of CAD difficult.
3. Definitions
   a. Stable angina - history of ischemic chest pain that is not changing in frequency, intensity, or duration.
   b. Unstable angina - angina that is new in onset, or increasing frequency, duration or intensity, or occurring at rest is considered unstable and at high risk of progressing to an acute infarct.
   c. Myocardial infarction - diagnosis requires two of the following:
   (1) Prolonged episode of chest pain.
   (2) ECG changes that are consistent with myocardial ischemia.
   (3) Elevated cardiac enzymes.
B. Evaluation
1. History
   a. Typical symptoms of ischemic heart disease
   (1) Chest pain with exertion, relieved with rest.
   (2) Pressure or heaviness in the anterior chest/substernal area.
   (3) Radiation to the left arm or jaw.
   (4) Associated with diaphoresis, nausea, shortness of breath.
   b. Atypical symptoms (may be angina equivalent)
   (1) Epigastric pain.
   (2) Radiation to the right arm or other areas.
   (3) Lightheadedness, nausea, shortness of breath without associated pain.
   c. Risk factors associated with coronary artery disease include smoking, hypertension, diabetes, hyperlipidemia, and positive family history.
2. Physical examination
   a. Exam is not diagnostic.
   b. Patient may be hemodynamically labile with hypertension or hypotension.
   c. With left ventricular dysfunction, new murmurs may be heard, or pulmonary congestion may develop.
3. Cardiac enzymes
   a. Creatine kinase (CK) - especially the MB fraction, has high sensitivity of diagnosis of myocardial damage. Levels rise by 3 hours following onset of symptoms, and remain elevated for > 24 hours.

        b. Troponin - currently the most sensitive test for myocardial injury. Levels rise in 3 hours after onset of symptoms, peak at 24 -48 hours, and gradually decline over about one week.

        c. AST - older test which is less specific, but more readily available in developing countries. Levels become elevated at 8-12 hours, peak at 24-48 hours, and fall to normal in 5-7 days.

        d. The WBC and sed rate are both elevated in acute MI, usually within 24 hours.

    4. ECG

        a. May be normal with ischemia and early infarct.

        b. Ischemia usually presents as ST depression and/or T-wave inversion over the involved area of myocardium.

        c. Acute ST segment elevation suggests myocardial injury.

        d. Development of new Q waves is generally diagnostic of acute MI.

C. Treatment

    1. Stable angina pectoris

        a. Begin aspirin 325mg PO qd.

        b. Give anti-anginal agents - nitrates, ß-blockers.

        c. Patients may use SL NTG for episodes of chest pain not relieved with rest.

    2. Unstable angina

        a. Hospitalization is warranted. Cardiac monitoring, if available.

        b. Keep at bedrest, give soft diet, oxygen, if available.

        c. Begin aspirin 325mg PO qd, nitrates (oral or topical).

        d. Morphine may be given for pain.

        e. Consider heparin, if available.

    3. Myocardial infarction

        a. If thrombolytics or coronary angiography with angioplasty are available, these are the recommended treatment modalities for patients presenting with an acute MI.

        b. If not available, the following interventions are helpful:

           (1) Aspirin 325mg PO immediately on admission and qd.

           (2) Oxygen until pain is relieved.

           (3) Morphine 2-5 mg SQ or IV prn to control pain.

           (4) Nitroglycerin tablets or ointments. Drip, if available. Titrate to control pain. Monitor BP.

           (5) ß-blockers - adjust the dose to maintain normal heart rate.

           (6) Full heparin anticoagulation for 24-48 hours, if available.

           (7) ACE-inhibitor for Q wave MI or signs of CHF.

CHAPTER 4

PULMONARY DISEASE

I. ASTHMA
A. General
1. Etiology
a. Asthma is a disorder in which the airways have increased responsiveness to various stimuli, resulting in decreased airflow and bronchospasm.

b. Chronic inflammation of the airway plays a central role in the development of the symptoms of asthma.

2. Symptoms
a. Vary with the severity of the attack. Classic symptoms include cough, wheezing, shortness of breath and chest tightness. Symptoms occur episodically.

b. In children, recurrent episodes of cough, wheezing, and, sometimes, respiratory distress, are usually due to asthma. It can also present as recurrent cough, especially at night or with viral respiratory infection (cough-variant asthma). There is often a personal or family history of atopy.

c. Ask about the following: duration and severity of symptoms, underlying disease history, previous use of medication, provocative factors (viral infection, environmental allergens, exercise, drugs).

3. Signs
a. Tachypnea, tachycardia, prolonged expiratory phase and expiratory wheezing are usually present. With increasing airway obstruction, the patient may be unable to lie down and may use accessory muscles of respiration. A child may show retractions.

b. With severe disease, the patient has difficulty speaking, respirations become difficult and shallow and cyanosis may be present. Wheezing may become less audible because of poor air movement. The child in respiratory distress is uncomfortable and may have trouble drinking, feeding or talking.

4. Laboratory
a. CBC and chest x-ray may be helpful if pneumonia is suspected. Chest x-ray should also be considered if this is the first episode of wheezing.

b. Measurement of oxygen saturation is helpful in severe disease, if available.

5. Differential diagnosis - remember all that wheezes is not asthma. Exclude the following:
a. Bronchiolitis - swelling and obstruction of small airways from inflammation due to viral infection. Usually in infants < 2 years old. May occur in adults.

b. Croup - usually has inspiratory stridor rather than expiratory wheezing.

c. Gastroesophageal reflux.

d. Endobronchial tuberculosis.

e. Congestive heart failure with pulmonary edema - dyspnea is usually worse lying down.

f. Foreign body in the airway

B. Management of acute asthma exacerbations

1. Supplemental oxygen - to maintain oxygen saturation, improve respiratory distress.

2. Hydration - po or IV.

3. Inhaled bronchodilators - give q 20 min. up to 1 hour (may be given continuously in a severe attack):

    a. Albuterol (salbutamol) 0.5-1.0cc in 2cc NS by nebulizer or two puffs by metered dose inhaler with spacer. Same dosage for children.

    b. Ipratropium (Atrovent) 0.5mg may be added to inhaled ß-agonists for increased efficacy.

4. Steroids

    a. Any of the following may be given IV or IM: dexamethasone (Decadron) 4mg q12h (0.1mg/kg), hydrocortisone (Solu-Cortef) 100-200mg q 4-6 hrs (4mg/kg), methylprednisolone (Solu-Medrol) 125mg q 4-6 hours (1mg/kg).

    b. Prednisone 60-80mg/d po (1-2 mg/kg/d) is as effective as IV steroids; onset of action is less rapid. Give once daily for 5-7 days for acute exacerbations.

    c. No need to taper steroids if used less than 2 weeks in non-steroid-dependent patients.

5. Injectable ß-agonists

    a. Epinephrine 1:1000 0.01cc/kg (adult 0.3cc) SQ q20-40 min. x 3 doses. Sus-Phrine 0.005cc/kg may be given if epinephrine was effective. It lasts several hours.

    b. Terbutaline 0.25mg SQ; repeat after 30-60 min.

    c. Injectable ß-agonists have no advantage of over inhaled forms. Use in life-threatening situations or if inhaled drugs are not available.

6. Aminophylline

    a. Considered second line therapy to ß-agonists and steroids. Use if other treatments are not available, or patient is not improving.

    b. Loading dose - 5mg/kg IV over 15-20 minutes, then maintenance infusion (0.5mg/kg/hr IV) or intermittent boluses (3-5mg/kg IV q6h). Decrease dose for CHF, liver disease. Increase dose for smokers, adolescents.

7. Antibiotics - use only if bacterial infection is demonstrated or suspected.

8. Consider admission for the following:

    a. Patients who continue to have wheezing or respiratory distress after bronchodilator treatment or those who improve initially and then deteriorate.

b. Patients with cyanosis.

c. Patients who are unable to drink or appear dehydrated.

d. Suspected pneumonia.

C. Chronic asthma management by disease severity

Classification of asthma based on symptoms		
Category	**Symptoms**	**Night symptoms**
Mild intermittent	< 2 X per week	< 2 X per month
Mild persistent	> 2 X per week	> 2 X per month
Moderate persistent	Daily	> 1 X per week
Severe	Continuous	Frequent

1. **Classification of asthma** - based on the frequency of symptoms during normal daytime activities, night time asthma symptoms, and symptoms during exercise. Record the amount of bronchodilator medication used, and measure peak expiratory flow rates when possible.

2. **Treatment** - based on the severity of symptoms

   a. Inhaled ß-agonists are first line therapy for asthma. Use intermittently in mild disease, on a scheduled basis with moderate or severe disease (1-2 puffs qid). Efficacy is significantly improved with the use of a spacer device, even with children. Albuterol (salbutamol) is most commonly used.

   b. Inhaled steroids should be used in all patients with moderate and severe disease, if available. These are given on a scheduled basis 1-2 puffs bid. During an acute asthma exacerbation, increased use of inhaled steroids is not helpful. Oral steroids (prednisone) may be added to the regimen for an acute exacerbation. Long-term oral steroids should be avoided.

   c. Long acting ß-agonists (salmeterol) are very useful, and are generally added to regimens if inhaled steroids fail to control symptoms.

   d. Inhaled anticholinergics such as ipratropium (Atrovent) may be added to ß-agonists.

   e. Inhaled cromolyn sodium may be used prophylactically 1 capsule (20mg) qid or before exercise, especially in patients with allergic triggers.

   f. Oral ß-agonists are usually used only in young children, or where inhalers are not available. Oral ß-agonists have more side effects than inhaled.

Dosage of Oral ß-Agonists			
Drug (generic)	**Drug (brand)**	**Adult dose**	**Pediatric dose**
Albuterol (salbutamol)	Proventil, Ventolin	2-4mg po tid	0.1mg/kg/dose po tid
Metaproterenol	Alupent	20mg po tid or qid	0.3-0.5mg/kg/dose q6-8h
Terbutaline	Brethine	2.5-5.0mg po tid	0.05mg/kg/dose up to 5mg tid

g. Oral theophylline is not recommended as first line therapy, but can be used if other medications are not available. The therapeutic range is narrow, and the patient must be monitored for toxicity (GI, cardiac, CNS). The following dosages of theophylline may be used:

Theophylline Dosage	
Age	Dose
1 - 9 years	24mg/kg/d
9 - 12 years	20mg/kg/d
12 - 16 years	18mg/kg/d
Adults	13mg/kg/d (600-900mg/d)

h. In pregnant patients, use ß-agonists and inhaled steroids first. If not well controlled, may use oral steroids and theophylline. Avoid epinephrine. Treat infections with penicillin or erythromycin.

II. COPD
A. Definition
1. Chronic airway obstruction due to a combination of the following:
   a. Emphysema - characterized by air trapping secondary to destruction of pulmonary parenchyma with enlargement of the distal air spaces.
   b. Chronic bronchitis - characterized by excess mucous production. Defined by the presence of cough on most days at least 3 months a year for two consecutive years.
   c. Asthma - chronic inflammation of the airway with increased responsiveness to various stimuli.
2. Obstruction may be partially reversible with bronchodilators.
B. Evaluation
1. **History** - cigarette smoking is most commonly associated with the development of COPD, usually after >20 pack/years of smoking. Patients experience increased cough and sputum production with increased frequency of respiratory infections. Dyspnea is gradual in onset, but progressive. In late stages, the patient may develop cor pulmonale.
2. **Physical exam** - prolonged expiration frequently with wheezes and rhonchi. In severe disease, the breath sounds are diminished. There is increased resonance on percussion of the chest.
3. **Chest x-ray** - may be normal in early disease. In advanced disease, films show hyperinflation with increased AP diameter, and flattened diaphragms.
4. **Other findings**
   a. With severe disease, the hemoglobin may be increased suggesting chronic hypoxia.
   b. Spirometry shows decreased FEV1 and FEV1/FVC.

C.Treatment
1.Acute exacerbation of COPD
  a. Clinical findings
- (1) Change in cough from baseline (increased quantity and purulence of sputum).
- (2) Increased shortness of breath with wheezing and chest tightness.

  b. Evaluation
- (1) Document degree of respiratory distress (able to speak full sentences, pursed lip breathing, retractions, etc.)
- (2) CBC, sputum Gram stain and chest x-ray may be helpful if pneumonia is suspected.
- (3) Measure pulse oximetry or ABGs, if available.

  c. Treatment
- (1) Low flow oxygen, 2-4L/min. (to avoid CO_2 retention).
- (2) Inhaled ß-agonists using inhaler with spacer or nebulizer. Repeat q 20-30 minutes.
- (3) Anticholinergic agents - ipratropium inhaler given 5 minutes after the ß-agonist inhalation, if available. If giving by nebulization, add 0.5mg of ipratropium to albuterol and NS.
- (4) Steroids - oral are as effective as injectable. Prednisone 60-80mg po qd, dexamethasone 4mg IV or IM q12h (0.1mg/kg), hydrocortisone 100-200mg IV/IM q 4-6 hrs (4mg/kg), methylprednisolone 125mg IV/IM q 4-6 hours (1mg/kg) may be used. Continue for several days until improved, then taper quickly. No additional benefit to use of steroids beyond 2 weeks.
- (5) Antibiotics - use if there is increased volume or purulence of sputum (TMP/SMX, amoxicillin, doxycycline, or ciprofloxacin).
- (6) Theophylline - no longer mainstay treatment, but may be given if no improvement with other meds. Load with 5mg/kg IV (aminophylline) over 15 minutes, followed by 0.5mg/kg/hr IV.

2.Chronic treatment of COPD
  a. Encourage smoking cessation.

  b. Inhaled agents:
- (1) ß-agonists (albuterol or salbutamol).
- (2) Inhaled anticholinergics (ipratropium) are considered first line as bronchodilators, but are expensive.
- (3) Steroid inhalers are useful only in the minority of patients with asthma/COPD.

  c. Chronic theophylline 200-300mg po q12h. Observe for toxicity.

  d. Chronic oral steroids should be avoided, if possible. Use only in patients with severe disease who fail to respond to above medications. Use the smallest dose possible, and switch to alternate day administration or inhaled steroids when possible.

  e. In chronically hypoxic patients, continuous oxygen therapy improves symptoms and prolongs survival but may not be available.

    f. Immunize for pneumococcus and influenza, when possible.

3. Cor pulmonale

    a. Right sided heart failure secondary to pulmonary disease, usually pulmonary hypertension.

    b. Development of cor pulmonale is a poor prognostic sign in COPD.

    c. Symptoms - may be associated with increased dyspnea on exertion, fatigue and occasionally syncope.

    d. Signs - JVD, hepatomegaly, and peripheral edema usually are present without signs of left heart failure.

    e. Treatment

        (1) Oxygen therapy, when possible.

        (2) Diuretics - begin with low doses of furosemide. Avoid excessive diuresis, which may result in decreased cardiac output and azotemia.

    f. Digoxin is useful only if biventricular failure is present.

    g. Vasodilators (nifedipine) may be tried cautiously. Begin with a low dose (30 mg/day) and titrate upward. Monitor for decreased cardiac output.

    h. Consider phlebotomy for patients with hematocrit >55-60%.

III. RESPIRATORY TRACT INFECTIONS

A. Acute bronchitis

1. General

    a. Infectious disorder of the respiratory tract usually caused by viruses, but sometimes due to mycoplasma, pneumococcus, haemophilus.

    b. Cigarette smokers develop recurrent and persistent tracheobronchitis infections.

2. Symptoms

    a. Cough - dry cough suggests viral etiology, cough productive of purulent sputum suggests bacterial.

    b. URI symptoms - coryza, sore throat, myalgias may be present.

    c. Fever and chills may occur.

3. Physical examination

    a. Patients appear only mildly ill.

    b. Chest exam is normal unless COPD is present.

4. Laboratory

    a. Chest x-ray is normal.

    b. CBC and sputum are not usually necessary.

5. Treatment

    a. Symptomatic treatment is usually sufficient - analgesics, cough suppressants, decongestants.

    b. Inhaled bronchodilators (albuterol) are useful if wheezing is present.

    c. Antibiotics are only rarely useful. Use if the patient is febrile or has underlying lung disease (erythromycin or other macrolides, amoxicillin, TMP/SMX, doxycycline).

B. Acute pneumonia (see Chapter 14, section IV, B)
  1. Etiologic agents
    a. Adults < 60 y.o., no underlying disease
      (1) *Strep pneumoniae*
      (2) *Mycoplasma pneumoniae*
      (3) Respiratory viruses
      (4) *Chlamydia pneumoniae*
      (5) *M. catarrhalis, H. influenzae* in smokers.
    b. Adults > 60 y.o. and/or underlying disease (COPD, diabetes, heart failure, alcohol abuse)
      (1) *Strep pneumoniae*
      (2) Respiratory viruses
      (3) *H. influenzae, M. catarrhalis*
      (4) Gram negative bacilli
      (5) *Staph aureus*
      (6) *Legionella*
  2. Clinical
    a. Acute inflammation of the pulmonary parenchymal tissue.
    b. May be alveolar (exudative material in the alveoli) with patchy or lobar infiltrates on chest x-ray, or interstitial (material in the interstitium), with diffuse reticular or reticulonodular infiltrates.
    c. Community-acquired pneumonias in adults can be classified as typical or atypical, based on their symptoms (has limited clinical usefulness)
      (1) Typical - cough productive of yellow or green sputum, sometimes streaked with blood, dyspnea, pleuritic chest pain, fever with shaking chills. Examination of the chest shows signs of consolidation (dullness to percussion, bronchial breath sounds with egophony). Chest x-ray shows lobar consolidation. Typical presentation favors bacterial etiology.
      (2) Atypical - low-grade fever with dry, hacking cough, dyspnea, rhinorrhea, malaise. Chest exam may reveal a few crackles but no signs of consolidation. Chest x-ray typically shows a diffuse infiltrate which appears worse than the clinical examination would suggest. Sputum is scant and Gram stain unremarkable. Consider *Mycoplasma, Chlamydia pneumoniae*, or viral etiologies.
      (3) Lung abscess - presents with fever, consolidation and cough, typically productive of foul smelling sputum. Often occurs in a setting in which aspiration may have occurred.
    d. Community acquired pneumonia in patients with underlying illnesses (such as COPD, diabetes, heart failure, alcohol abuse) and/or age >60, may present as a more severe illness, with uncommon pathogens. Smokers are at particular risk of infection with *H influenza*. Alcoholic patients may develop *Klebsiella pneumonia*. *Staph aureus* may cause

a severe necrotizing pneumonia in postoperative, diabetic or debilitated patients and in children recovering from measles. Tuberculosis should always be considered in the differential diagnosis of patients with pneumonia, especially when there is associated malnutrition and weight loss.

3. **Diagnosis/assessment of severity**
   a. Do a thorough history and physical exam. Obtain the following laboratory studies: CBC with differential, sputum Gram stain (if the patient is producing sputum and is ill enough to require hospital admission), and chest x-ray. Do sputum culture for very ill patients, oxygen saturation or arterial blood gas, if available. An AFB smear should be done if tuberculosis is a possibility. Do thoracentesis if a pleural effusion is present.
   b. Suspected etiologic agent should be determined, based on the patient's overall health status, presentation, clinical findings and laboratory tests.

4. **General treatment guidelines**
   a. Treatment of pneumonia is basically empiric, since the etiologic agent is found in less than 50% of cases, even under optimal conditions.
   b. Consider hospitalization for the following patients:
      (1) Elderly adults with heart failure, COPD, or other comorbid problems.
      (2) Clinical findings of hypotension, respiratory distress, confusion or decreased level of consciousness.
      (3) Laboratory findings of WBC <4000 or >30,000, multilobar pneumonia, pleural effusion, abnormal renal function, severe anemia.
   c. General treatment measures - oxygen (if hypoxia present), hydration, cough suppressants or expectorants.
   d. Duration of treatment
      (1) *Strep. pneumonia* - 7 days.
      (2) *H. influenza* - 10 days.
      (3) *Staph. aureus* - 2 weeks parenteral followed by 1-3 weeks po.
      (4) *Mycoplasma* or *Chlamydia pneumoniae* - 7 days.

5. **Outpatient antibiotic therapy**
   a. Adults < 60 y.o. and no underlying diseases
      (1) Probable bacterial pneumonia - oral amoxicillin, TMP/SMX, new fluoroquinolones. Smokers should have coverage for *H. influenzae* (TMP/SMX, amoxicillin, tetracycline, amoxicillin/clavulanate, new fluoroquinolones).
      (2) Probable atypical pneumonia - erythromycin po x 14-21d. Alternative is tetracycline, doxycycline, azithromycin, or clarithromycin.
   b. Adults >60 y.o. and/or underlying disease

    (1) Erythromycin + amoxicillin, or TMP/SMX or new fluoroquinolones.

    (2) If available, a second-generation cephalosporin may be used.

6. Hospitalized adults

    a. Any of the following may be given parenterally: Penicillin G, ampicillin, chloramphenicol, cefazolin.

    b. Use IV second-generation cephalosporin, if available.

    c. Add aminoglycoside if severely ill or debilitated and a macrolide if *Legionella* infection is considered.

    d. Use nafcillin or cloxacillin IV if staph pneumonia is suspected (abscesses, etc.). An aminoglycoside may also be added.

    e. Change to oral antibiotics when afebrile >24h and clinically improving.

7. Follow-up

    a. Repeat chest x-ray does not need to be done prior to discharge on patients who are doing well clinically. It may take up to 4 weeks for pneumococcal pneumonia to resolve radiologically and even longer for atypical pneumonias, or in patients with pre-existing illnesses.

    b. Follow-up visit is recommended 6 weeks after discharge with repeat chest x-ray if symptoms persist. Consider tuberculosis in patients with un-resolving infiltrates or worsening clinical status.

IV. OTHER PULMONARY PROBLEMS

A. Pleural effusion

1. Definition - abnormal accumulation of fluid in the pleural space.

2. Classification

    a. Transudate

        (1) Fluid protein <3.0 or pleural protein/serum protein ratio <0.5.

        (2) Causes include heart failure, ascites, hypoalbuminemia, postpartum.

        (3) Treatment involves treating the underlying disease process.

    b. Exudate

        (1) Fluid protein >3.0 or pleural protein/serum protein ratio >0.5.

        (2) Causes include neoplasms, infection (especially tuberculosis), connective tissue disease.

        (3) Treatment - consider a trial of tuberculosis treatment for all patients with exudative pleural effusion, unless another etiology is clearly established. Malignant effusions may need multiple therapeutic thoracenteses for relief of dyspnea.

3. Clinical

    a. Patients generally have dyspnea, tachycardia and orthopnea if the effusion is large.

    b. Onset of symptoms may be gradual (tuberculosis, cancer) or abrupt (heart failure).

     c. Decreased breath sounds and dullness to percussion will be found if the effusion is >300cc.

4. Diagnosis

     a. Chest x-ray will show blunting of the costophrenic angles with effusions >300cc. Lateral decubitus views can detect 100-200cc of fluid.

     b. Diagnostic thoracentesis should be done on patients with new pleural effusions. Fluid should be sent for cell count and differential, total protein, Gram stain and AFB smear. Obtain cultures, if available.

5. Special considerations

     a. Chronic transudates may show protein concentrations >3gm.

     b. Heart failure is the most common cause of transudative effusions. Most are bilateral or right-sided. They are rare on the left side alone.

     c. Pericarditis may give a unilateral left-sided effusion.

     d. Effusions due to metastatic cancer are usually bilateral. Breast cancer is the most common metastatic tumor causing effusion.

B. Aspiration pneumonia

     1. Acute aspiration may be silent or the patient may show signs of hypoxemia minutes to hours afterward, with tachypnea, tachycardia and cyanosis. Physical exam may show wheezes, rales or rhonchi. Frothy, bloody sputum may be present.

     2. Chest x-ray may show either a lobar infiltrate or diffuse alveolar and interstitial infiltrate. The right lower lobe is most frequently involved in aspiration. Patients with chronic aspiration may have repeated episodes of pneumonia.

C. Lung abscess

     1. Definition - cavitation in the pulmonary parenchyma. Periodontal disease is important in the formation of anerobic lung abscess (rare in edentulous people).

     2. Anerobes and aerobes are present. Consider other causes of cavitary lung disease, such as tuberculosis.

     3. Clinical signs include cough productive of fetid sputum, fever, chest pain, dyspnea, weakness, weight loss. CBC usually shows leukocytosis with left shift and anemia.

     4. Chest x-ray reveals a cavity with an air-fluid level. Usually occurs in the posterior segment of the right upper lobe or superior segment of the right lower lobe. Cavitation develops 1-2 weeks after aspiration.

     5. Treatment

     a. Postural drainage may be helpful.

     b. Clindamycin is the drug of choice, if available, 600-900mg IV q8h until the patient is afebrile for 5 days, then 300mg po qid x 6-8 weeks. Penicillin G 6-12 million units/day IV may be given if clindamycin is not available, followed by 500mg po qid x 6-8 weeks plus metronidazole 500mg po qid. Where available, amoxicillin/clavulanic acid can also be used.

c. Continue treatment until the cavity closes.

D.Empyema

1. Definition - collection of purulent material in the pleural space. It develops secondary to pneumonia or rupture of a lung abscess into the pleural space.
2. Etiologic agents include *Staph aureus*, Gram negative rods and anerobes.
3. Clinical signs include dyspnea, fever, chills, and pleuritic chest pain.
4. Diagnosis is established by performing a thoracentesis.
   a. With empyema, the aspirated fluid shows a high WBC count, Gram stain shows the presence of bacteria, pleural fluid glucose is <20mg/dl and the pH<7.2.
   b. In parapneumonic effusions, the glucose is >20mg/dl and pH >7.2. These generally resolve with treatment of the pneumonia.
5. Treatment
   a. Closed chest tube drainage if empyema is present. The tube may be withdrawn when drainage is <50cc/d and the cavity is <50cc.
   b. Use antibiotics specific for the organisms found on Gram stain or culture of the fluid.
   c. Evaluate for possible tuberculosis.

CHAPTER 5

GASTROENTEROLOGY

I. ESOPHAGEAL DISORDERS
A. Gastroesophageal reflux disease (GERD)
1. **Definition** - esophageal inflammation that develops as a result of gastric secretions refluxing into the esophagus. Reflux occurs because of transient or chronic relaxation of the lower esophageal sphincter. GERD can be either erosive (erosions and inflammation seen on endoscopy) or non-erosive (normal endoscopy).
2. **Symptoms**
   a. Heartburn (pyrosis) - intermittent, substernal burning, usually quickly relieved by antacids.
   b. Regurgitation (reflux of sour or bitter material into the mouth when lying down or bending over) and water-brash (filling of the mouth with clear, salty fluid).
   c. Dysphagia - difficulty swallowing. May be due to stricture or inflammation and edema.
   d. Odynophagia - painful swallowing. May accompany severe esophagitis, especially with ulceration.
   e. Chest pain - atypical presentation. Difficult to distinguish from cardiac chest pain; angina before assuming symptoms are due to GERD.
   f. Chronic cough and asthma may be associated with esophageal reflux. These symptoms may improve when the reflux is treated.
   g. Night sweats have been associated with reflux in some patients. The sweating is usually mild. These patients may not have typical symptoms of heartburn.
3. **Management**
   a. Patients with typical symptoms of GERD may be treated empirically.
   b. Diagnostic testing should be done in those patients not responding to treatment and those with symptoms suggesting serious disease (dysphagia, odynophagia, hematemesis, weight loss, anemia, or heme-positive stools). EGD is the preferred diagnostic procedure, however up to 1/3 of patients may have normal appearing mucosa, requiring biopsy for diagnosis. UGI may be performed for diagnosis, but is difficult to interpret.
   c. Life style modification
      (1) Discontinue smoking.
      (2) Avoid high fat foods, chocolate, and alcohol, which lower esophageal sphincter tone. Avoid foods which aggravate symptoms.
      (3) Avoid overeating or lying down with food in the stomach.
      (4) Elevate the head of the bed on 6 inch blocks.
   d. Drug treatment
      (1) Antacids 1 and 3 hours after meals and at bedtime.

(2) H2 blockers bid (cimetidine, ranitidine, famotidine). High-dose regimens and long courses (12-16 weeks) may be needed for healing. Maintenance regimens at full dose are often required to prevent recurrences.

(3) Proton-pump inhibitors (omeprazole, lansoprazole) more effectively relieve symptoms and heal esophagitis faster than H2 blockers. Usually given for 4-8 weeks.

(4) Prokinetic drugs (bethanechol, metoclopramide) increase esophageal sphincter tone and promote gastric emptying. Give with acid reducing therapy. These drugs have a higher incidence of side effects.

e. Surgery (Nissen fundoplication) may effectively relieve severe symptoms that are refractory to medical treatment.

f. Esophageal stricture may occur in the distal esophagus. Fibrosis develops as a result of long standing inflammation secondary to chronic reflux. The stricture is smooth, in contrast to the irregular stricture of carcinoma. Treatment is with bouginage, balloon dilatation, or surgery.

g. Bleeding due to esophageal ulcers rarely is massive, and usually responds to medical therapy.

h. Barrett's esophagus - replacement of the normal squamous epithelium of the distal esophagus with metaplastic columnar epithelium. Dysplasia and adenocarcinoma may develop over time. Treatment is as above for GERD with endoscopic biopsy monitoring every 1-2 years, when possible.

B. Infections

1. Candida esophagitis

a. Common in patients with HIV. May also occur in patients with neoplasms, diabetes, chronic renal failure and other conditions with immune incompetence.

b. Odynophagia or dysphagia when associated with oral candidiasis is very suggestive. May treat empirically; if no improvement in 5-7 days, endoscopy is recommended.

c. UGI may show ragged mucosa, or deep ulcerations.

d. EGD shows whitish-yellow exudate with erosive esophagitis and marked inflammation. Diagnosis is confirmed by biopsy.

e. Treatment options:

(1) Nystatin tablets or suspension 0.5-1 million units tid x 10-14d. If severe, the patient may use q2h.

(2) Ketoconazole 200mg/d (3-6mg/kg/d) x 10d. Double the dose in AIDS patients.

(3) Fluconazole 200mg po loading dose (10mg/kg), then 100mg po qd (3-6mg/kg/d) x 3 weeks or at least 2 weeks after symptoms gone.

2. Viral esophagitis (herpes, cytomegalovirus)

   a. Most commonly seen with HIV. CMV is more common than herpetic esophagitis.

   b. Patients present with substernal pain, odynophagia and dysphagia.

   c. UGI and EGD show superficial ulcerations of the esophagus (giant ulcers suggest CMV).

   d. Treatment

     (1) Herpes - may resolve spontaneously, or treat with acyclovir 400 mg po five times daily for 14-21 days or 5 mg/kg IV q 8 hrs for 7-14 days, if patient is unable to swallow.

     (2) CMV - treat with ganciclovir or foscarnet for two weeks.

II. GASTRIC DISORDERS

A. Gastritis

1. General

   a. Inflammatory response of the gastric mucosa to injury.

   b. Symptoms - dyspepsia (epigastric pain) is the primary symptom. Nausea and vomiting may commonly occur.

   c. Difficult to distinguish from functional dyspepsia without endoscopy.

2. Types

   a. Erosive/hemorrhagic gastritis

     (1) Usually due to alcohol, aspirin, NSAIDs.

     (2) Often asymptomatic.

     (3) May present with massive GI bleeding. EGD may show hemorrhages or erosions.

   b. Helicobacter pylori - induced gastritis

     (1) Superficial inflammation of the gastric mucosa, consistently involving the antrum, with variable involvement of the body and fundus.

     (2) High prevalence of infection in developing countries, at a young age.

   c. Atrophic gastritis

     (1) Associated with pernicious anemia and vitamin B12 deficiency.

     (2) Usually involves atrophy of the mucosa of the fundus with minimal superficial inflammation.

     (3) Achlorhydria is common.

3. Treatment

   a. Antacids and H2 blockers may be tried initially.

   b. Discontinue the causative agent, if identified.

   c. H. pylori treatment may be tried if anti-ulcer treatment is ineffective.

B. Peptic ulcer disease

1. Etiology

a. H. pylori infection is present in the majority of patients with peptic ulcer disease, especially in developing countries, and is considered the primary cause of PUD. Eradication of the infection reduces the incidence of ulcer recurrence to 10-20% per year.

b. Aspirin, NSAIDs, or alcohol use account for much of the H. pylori-negative PUD.

c. Hypersecretory state (Zollinger-Ellison syndrome) is an uncommon cause of PUD.

2. Symptoms

a. The most common symptom of PUD is non radiating epigastric pain. The pain of duodenal ulcer classically occurs 2-5 hours after a meal, improves with food or antacids and may awaken patients at night. Symptoms usually improve with time, but recur frequently (up to several times a year).

b. Gastric ulcer pain is similar but may worsen with food. Response to a meal cannot reliably distinguish gastric ulcers from duodenal ulcers.

c. Pain radiating to the back suggests either a penetrating ulcer or acute pancreatitis.

d. Pain which is acutely worse and associated with signs of an acute abdomen suggests perforation.

3. Diagnosis

a. Most young patients with dyspepsia require no diagnostic studies. They may be started on empiric therapy.

b. UGI or EGD (preferable) should be performed on patients with dyspepsia who have not responded to treatment and those with complicating factors (age >45 years, GI blood loss, weight loss, signs of obstruction, or severe, persistent pain).

c. Hospitalize patients with
   (1) Severe persistent vomiting (gastric outlet obstruction).
   (2) GI bleeding.
   (3) Symptoms of penetrating or perforated ulcer.

4. Treatment

a. Nonpharmacologic therapy
   (1) Avoid aspirin, NSAIDs, alcohol, cigarettes.
   (2) No specific dietary restrictions are necessary. Avoid foods which cause dyspepsia.

b. Acid reduction treatment
   (1) H2-receptor antagonists (cimetidine, ranitidine, famotidine) - give at full dose for 4-6 weeks. May keep on maintenance dose thereafter to reduce recurrence (single dose at bedtime).
   (2) Antacids in moderate to high dose are effective in relieving the symptoms of PUD and may help in healing (similar efficacy to H2-receptor blockers). They should be given one hour after meals and at bedtime, or as needed for symptoms.

(3) Sucralfate is thought to protect the gastroduodenal mucosa. It is given as 1 gram qid before meals and at bedtime. It is effective for healing ulcers and in preventing relapse (twice daily dosage).

(4) Proton-pump inhibitors - reserved for patients who do not respond to H2-blockers.

c. H. pylori treatment

(1) All patients with H. pylori-associated PUD should be treated with therapy to eradicate the infection. Treatment improves healing rates for ulcers, decreases complications, and lowers recurrence rates. Inexpensive test kits are available for H. pylori testing.

(2) Treatment regimens

(a) Bismuth 525 mg qid, plus metronidazole 250mg qid, plus tetracycline 500mg qid or amoxicillin 500 mg qid - all for 14 days.

(b) Adding a proton pump inhibitor significantly improves cure rates (omeprazole 20 mg bid).

(c) Substituting clarithromycin 500 mg bid for metronidazole improves cure rates due to high rates of metronidazole resistance.

5. Complications of peptic ulcer disease

a. Bleeding (see Section D, GI bleeding)

b. Obstruction

(1) In some countries, gastric outlet obstruction may be the initial manifestation of PUD. Characterized by periodic vomiting of large quantities of undigested food and liquid. Most patients have a long history of peptic ulcer pain. Early satiety, bloating and epigastric fullness may be present before the vomiting begins.

(2) A "succussion splash" may be heard in the epigastrium when the abdomen is shaken from side to side. Weight loss and signs of dehydration may be present.

(3) Diagnosis is confirmed by UGI or EGD.

(4) Obstruction may improve with NG suction and H2-blocker therapy. If gastric retention persists, surgery is indicated.

c. Perforation

(1) Characterized by the onset of sudden, severe abdominal pain starting in the epigastrium and then becoming more diffuse. It may radiate to the lower abdomen or be referred to the shoulders. Nausea and vomiting may occur.

(2) Physical exam shows a diffusely tender abdomen with signs of peritonitis (guarding, rebound tenderness or rigidity).

(3) Upright abdominal or lateral decubitus x-ray may show free air under the diaphragm.

      (4) Immediate surgical exploration is required. An NG tube should be placed and IV fluids given while awaiting surgery. IV H2 blockers are helpful, if available.

C. Gastric cancer

1. General

a. The incidence of gastric cancer is much higher in other countries than in the US. Many are advanced by the time of diagnosis. Consider EGD (or UGI) on all patients >40 years of age with new GI symptoms.

b. Patients with gastric cancer may have some improvement in their symptoms with H2-blockers, so empiric therapy is not helpful in ruling out malignancy.

c. All gastric ulcers seen on EGD should be biopsied initially, if possible, and a repeat endoscopy should be performed in 2-3 months to evaluate the degree of healing. Surgery is generally recommended for gastric ulcers which do not heal, even in the absence of malignancy on biopsy.

2. Diagnosis

a. Symptoms are similar to PUD. May also include persistent abdominal pain, weight loss, anorexia, early satiety, and GI bleeding.

b. With advanced disease, look for periumbilical or supraclavicular lymph nodes, epigastric mass, enlarged liver or ascites.

3. Treatment

a. Overall prognosis is poor.

b. Surgery for cure may be attempted in early disease.

c. Surgery for palliation of obstruction or bleeding may be considered in more advanced cases.

D. GI bleeding

1. General

a. Acute GI bleeding presents with hematemesis, melena or hematochezia.

b. Chronic bleeding is characterized by iron deficiency anemia or guaiac-positive stool.

2. Initial management

a. Initial assessment - check volume status (VS, orthostatic BP, urine output, rate of blood loss). Stabilize with IV fluids (NS or RL) or blood. If the patient is actively bleeding, start two large IV lines. Follow VS carefully.

b. The patient's general appearance is important. Note whether the patient is pale or jaundiced. Look for cachexia, adenopathy or abdominal masses suggestive of malignancy. Jaundice, palmar erythema and ecchymoses suggest liver disease. Rectal exam is valuable in evaluating for melena, bright red blood or occult blood in the stool.

c. Check Hgb, type and crossmatch blood, if available.

d. Insert NG tube - bright red blood suggests active bleeding in the stomach or duodenum. The presence of coffee-ground material suggests an UGI source of bleeding which is less acute. Heme negative NG aspirate which contains significant bile makes lower GI source of bleeding likely. NG may be removed once aspirate is evaluated. There is no evidence that gastric lavage helps to stop active bleeding or prevent recurrence. It may be helpful to cleanse the stomach prior to endoscopic examination.

3. Upper GI bleed

a. Diagnosis - endoscopy should be done within the first 24h, if possible, to identify the source of bleeding. Most common causes of UGI bleeding are PUD, esophageal varices, Mallory-Weiss tears, and tumors.

b. Management

(1) Most patients with UGI hemorrhage will stop bleeding with only supportive therapy.

(2) H2 blockers (give IV, if available) are usually given. Efficacy is uncertain.

(3) Omeprazole at high dose (40 mg bid) decreases rebleeding from PUD.

(4) Bleeding from Mallory-Weiss tears is usually self-limited.

(5) Surgery is indicated for severe bleeding (>5 units of blood in 24 hours), or rebleeding from gastric or duodenal ulcer, requiring transfusion in the same hospitalization.

(6) Oral propranolol may help prevent recurrent GI bleeding in patients with cirrhosis and esophageal varices in otherwise good condition. Give dose to reduce heart rate by 25%.

(7) Endoscopic therapy (thermal coagulation, saline or epinephrine injection) are effective where available.

4. Lower GI bleed

a. Diagnosis - generally made by doing digital rectal exam and NG aspirate. Hematochezia is usually indicative of a lower GI source, since it takes a large amount of blood to cause hematochezia from an upper GI source, and hemodynamic instability is usually present. Non-bloody bile on NG aspirate is also suggestive of a lower GI source of bleeding. If available, a colonoscopy may be done to identify the source of bleeding. It should be done emergently when bleeding is active. If bleeding has stopped, or occult blood is found, colonoscopy can be done on an elective basis.

b. Management is according to the etiology

(1) Rectal source (anal fissure or hemorrhoids) - small amounts of bright red blood on the surface of the stool or toilet paper. May drip from the anus following bowel movement.

    (2) Colonic polyp or tumor - blood loss depends on size and location of lesion. Right sided lesions produce greater blood loss. Bleeding (hematochezia or melena), abdominal pain, or change in bowel habits are the most common presenting symptoms of colon cancer. Therapy is surgical removal of lesion.

    (3) Diverticular disease - most common cause of large volume lower GI bleeding in western populations. Right-sided diverticula are the most common site. Usually presents without other symptoms. If recurrent, consider colectomy.

    (4) Angiodysplasia - represents a significant source of bleeding, especially in the elderly. If recurrent, consider colectomy.

III. OTHER INTESTINAL DISORDERS

A. Anorectal disorders

1. Hemorrhoids

a. Hemorrhoids represent dilated anorectal veins. They are associated with pregnancy, portal hypertension, and constipation. Rarity in Africa is probably due to high-residue diets.

b. Types

    (1) Internal hemorrhoids - located proximal to (above) the dentate line. Not usually palpable or visible (unless prolapsed). Often associated with bleeding and prolapse.

    (2) External hemorrhoids - located distal to (below) the dentate line. Located at the anal verge and can be seen at external inspection. Often manifest with thrombosis.

c. Classification

    (1) First degree - may cause bleeding.

    (2) Second degree - prolapse on high pressure (defecation) but return spontaneously.

    (3) Third degree - prolapse with defecation and must be manually reduced.

    (4) Fourth degree - prolapse and are not reducible.

d. Symptoms

    (1) Bleeding - usually limited, occurring with defecation. May cause chronic blood loss. Usually caused by internal hemorrhoids.

    (2) Pain - usually associated with thrombosed external hemorrhoids.

    (3) Prolapse - may cause pruritus ani and mucous discharge. If prolapse cannot be reduced, the hemorrhoid may become thrombosed (usually external hemorrhoids).

e. Treatment

    (1) Hot Sitz baths 15 minutes tid and after each bowel movement relieve pain and edema.

    (2) Bulk laxatives, such as psyllium seed compounds or stool softeners. Avoid laxatives causing liquid stools. Add fiber to diet.

(3) Topical anesthetics and hydrocortisone cream or suppositories may help relieve pain and discomfort.

(4) If thrombosis is acute and painful, the clots can be excised by making an elliptical incision in the overlying skin after infiltration with a local anesthetic. Bleeding is controlled by leaving a small piece of gauze in the wound for a few hours and applying a pressure dressing. Sitz baths may be started 6-12 hours after the procedure.

2. Anal fissure

a. Clinical

(1) Linear tear of the anal canal.

(2) Most common cause of painful rectal bleeding.

(3) Often associated with swelling of the surrounding tissues.

(4) Usually occur in the midline posteriorly.

(5) Most common symptom is pain during and immediately after a bowel movement. Pain then subsides between movements. Bleeding is minimal.

b. Treatment

(1) Hot Sitz baths 15 minutes 3-4x/d and after each bowel movement.

(2) Add bran and fiber to the diet.

(3) Meticulous anal hygiene.

(4) Analgesic ointment and steroid creams don't aid healing, but may help symptomatically.

(5) Surgery in chronic or refractory cases.

3. Anorectal abscesses

a. General

(1) Perianal abscesses are the most common anorectal abscess.

(2) Pus spreads between the internal and external sphincters to form a painful, tender, erythematous swelling at the anal verge (usually midline posteriorly).

(3) Can have ischiorectal and deeper abscesses.

b. Symptoms

(1) Progressively worsening rectal pain, worse immediately before defecation, persists between bowel movements. Pain and tenderness eventually interferes with walking or sitting.

(2) On rectal examination, a tender mass or induration is present. The patient may be febrile.

c. Treatment - surgical drainage in the OR.

4. Fistula in ano

a. Tract leading from the rectal lumen to the perianal skin.

b. These are usually non-tender, but may have persistent drainage of blood, pus or mucous.

c. If the tract becomes blocked, recurrent abscesses may form.

d. May be associated with ulcerative colitis, Crohn's disease or tuberculosis.

e. The only definitive treatment is surgical excision.

5. Rectal prolapse

    a. Definition - protrusion of part or all layers of the rectum through the anal canal.

    b. Types

        (1) Prolapse involving the rectal mucosa only. Most common in children <2 years old.

        (2) Prolapse involving all layers of the rectum.

        (3) Intussusception of the upper rectum into and through the lower rectum (apex of the intussusception protrudes through the anus).

    c. Symptoms

        (1) Most patients note the presence of a mass after defecation or with strenuous activity. If severe, it may be present with standing or walking.

        (2) Irritation of the mucosa may cause a mucous discharge and bleeding.

    d. Treatment is usually manual reduction and prevention of constipation. Surgery may be indicated in adults with recurrent prolapse.

6. Pilonidal sinus

    a. Clinical

        (1) Occurs in the midline in the upper part of the natal cleft overlying the lower sacrum and coccyx.

        (2) Infected pilonidal cysts may be mistaken for perirectal abscesses.

        (3) Usually a chronic and recurring disease. Forms by the penetration of the skin by an ingrowing hair. Infection then develops.

        (4) Patients present with swelling, pain or persistent discharge. An abscess will cause a tender mass.

    b. Treatment

        (1) Immediate incision and drainage of abscesses.

        (2) Surgical excision of the sinus system.

B. Tropical sprue

    1. Chronic malabsorptive disorder of unknown etiology, possibly secondary to an infectious agent. Inflammatory changes in small intestinal villi are thought to produce malabsorption.

    2. Common in some areas of the tropics (countries of the Caribbean, and Far East, but uncommon in Africa).

    3. Symptoms include chronic diarrhea, abdominal symptoms (gas, bloating, cramps), weight loss, anemia, and sequelae of nutritional deficiency.

    4. Often have deficiencies of B12 and folate, giving a megaloblastic anemia.

    5. Diagnosis is by exclusion

        a. Check for intestinal parasitic infections, HIV, intestinal lymphoma, and other causes of malabsorption.

b. Small bowel biopsy demonstrating villous atrophy is suggestive but is also seen with celiac disease and HIV enteropathy.

6. Treatment
   a. Vitamin B12 1000μg IM weekly.
   b. Folate 5mg qd x 2-4 weeks.
   c. Tetracycline 250mg qid x 3-6 months.

IV. GALLBLADDER DISEASE
A. Cholelithiasis and acute cholecystitis
1. Cholelithiasis
   a. Risk factors include increasing age, females>males, obesity, pregnancy, chronic hemolytic states. Incidence in Africa is much lower than in western countries.
   b. Most patients with cholelithiasis are asymptomatic. About 20% will develop symptoms over time. The most common presentation is biliary colic. This is a steady, intense pain in the right upper quadrant. Laboratory studies are normal and most cases resolve spontaneously. 10-20% of patients go on to develop complications, such as acute cholecystitis, cholangitis and gallstone pancreatitis.
   c. Patients with diabetes and sickle cell disease have a higher incidence of stones and of complications, but prophylactic cholecystectomy is not recommended.

2. Acute cholecystitis
   a. Acute inflammation of the gallbladder, usually as a result of a stone impaction within the cystic duct.
   b. Most patients have a history of biliary colic. The pain associated with cholecystitis is similar, but more severe and persistent. May be associated with nausea and vomiting. Often precipitated by ingestion of fatty foods. Symptoms last more than six hours and may be associated with fever.
   c. Physical examination shows tenderness in the RUQ with a positive Murphy's sign (increased tenderness on palpation in the RUQ with deep inspiration).
   d. Laboratory
      (1) Leukocytosis is common. LFTs may be slightly elevated.
      (2) Abdominal ultrasound shows stones and gallbladder wall thickening.
   e. Management
      (1) Depends on the severity of disease and the patient's surgical risk.
      (2) Patients with mild disease and low surgical risk should receive supportive treatment (IV fluids, narcotic analgesics), and early cholecystectomy. Antibiotics (ampicillin and gentamicin) may be given.
      (3) High risk patients should receive percutaneous cholecystostomy and IV antibiotics with delayed cholecystectomy.

    f. Complications of untreated cholecystitis include gangrenous cholecystitis and perforation of the gallbladder.

B. Ascending cholangitis

    1. Represents bacterial infection of the biliary tract resulting from obstruction of the common bile duct (usually from a stone or stricture of the common bile duct).

    2. Charcot's triad is frequently present (RUQ pain, fever, jaundice). Patient is acutely ill and may be septic.

    3. Laboratory

        a. WBC is elevated with a left shift.

        b. Alkaline phosphatase is elevated showing a cholestatic pattern. Transaminases may be mildly elevated.

    4. Management

        a. Broad spectrum parenteral antibiotics - ampicillin, gentamicin. In seriously ill patients, add chloramphenicol or metronidazole.

        b. Emergent surgical drainage.

V. Hepatic Disease

A. Acute viral hepatitis

Acute Viral Hepatitis Classification					
Hepatitis Virus	Transmission	Incubation	Prevention	Fulminant Hepatitis	Sequelae
A	Oral-fecal	2-7 wks Ave. - 4 wks	IGG, Hep A vaccine	0.1%	None
B	Injection, sexual, vertical	4-16 wks Ave. - 10 wks	HBIG, Hep B vaccine	0.1-1%	High rate of chronic infection when infected at young age (90%)
C	Injection	2-20 wks Ave. - 8 wks	None	0.1%	High incidence of chronic infection (50-70%)
D	Injection	4-24 wks Ave. - 10 wks	Hep B vaccine	5-20%	Requires hepatitis B for infection to occur. May produce chronic hepatitis
E	Oral-fecal	2-8 wks Ave. - 6 wks	Uncertain	1-2%	None

    1. **Clinical phases** (similar for all types)

        a. Prodromal phase

            (1) May be present for 1-2 weeks prior to onset of icteric phase.

            (2) Common symptoms - anorexia, nausea, vomiting, malaise, low grade fever.

            (3) Less common symptoms - arthralgias, myalgias, rash.

        b. Icteric phase

(1) Clinical jaundice appears. Prodromal symptoms diminish.

(2) Liver becomes enlarged and tender, urine becomes dark, stools become light colored. Jaundice peaks at two weeks.

(3) A significant proportion of patients do not develop jaundice.

c. Recovery phase - constitutional symptoms disappear.

2. Differential diagnosis

a. Other viral illnesses - especially mononucleosis and CMV.

b. Other infectious diseases - toxoplasmosis, leptospirosis, brucellosis, tuberculosis.

c. Other non-infectious causes of hepatitis - alcohol, drugs.

3. Laboratory

a. ALT, AST increased to > 1-2000 IU (ALT> AST).

b. Alkaline phosphatase may be mildly elevated.

c. Bilirubin elevated to >10 mg%.

d. Prothrombin time may be elevated in severe disease (indicates poor synthetic function).

e. Check specific hepatitis antibodies to determine the type of hepatitis, if possible.

4. Management

a. Strict attention to hygiene by patients and medical attendants is crucial to avoid spread.

b. Rest according to symptoms of fatigue.

c. Anti-emetics - hydroxyzine, prochlorperazine.

d. Avoid hepatotoxins (alcohol, paracetamol, acetaminophen).

e. Pruritus may be treated with cholestyramine 4gm po tid.

5. Post exposure prophylaxis

a. Hepatitis A

(1) Immune serum globulin may be given to close contacts as soon as possible (effective if given within 2 weeks of exposure). Dose is 0.02cc/kg up to 5cc.

(2) Hepatitis A vaccine provides good protection at 4 weeks post vaccination. When given post-exposure, produces a significant reduction in risk of infection and attenuates clinical disease but is not as effective as immune serum globulin.

b. Hepatitis B

(1) Transmission is via sexual contact or needle puncture, but attention to hygiene is still important and should be emphasized to patients and staff.

(2) Acute intense exposure to hepatitis B (needle stick, sexual partner, oral ingestion) requires HBIG 0.06cc/kg (5cc in adults) and hepatitis B vaccine 1cc IM at 0, 1 and 6 months for post-exposure prophylaxis. Should be given within 14 days of exposure.

(3) Infants exposed to hepatitis in the perinatal period need HBIG 0.06cc/kg within 12 hours of birth and HBV vaccine 0.5cc IM within 7d. Repeat HBV vaccine at 1 and 6 months to complete the course.

(4) Postexposure prophylaxis is difficult when serologic testing is unavailable. If the source material has high risk of being HBsAg-positive, and the exposed person has never previously been immunized, HBIG and HBV vaccine should be given, as above.

B. Fulminant hepatitis

1. Most common with hepatitis D - requires coinfection with hepatitis B virus either acutely or chronically.
2. Watch for and hospitalize patients with severe nausea and vomiting, elevated prothrombin time, encephalopathy or bleeding.
3. Treatment is supportive
   a. Provide adequate hydration.
   b. Give neomycin (or lactulose, if available) to treat encephalopathy.
   c. Steroid administration has not been shown to be useful.
4. Follow-up - check AST, pro-time, bilirubin, albumin/globulin, HBsAg (if available) at onset, 2 and 12 weeks. Then q 4 weeks if still abnormal. Refer for biopsy if LFTs still abnormal 6-12 months after onset.

C. Chronic hepatitis

1. General
   a. Inflammation of the liver lasting more than 6 months.
   b. Occurs secondary to chronic viral hepatitis, autoimmune liver disease, drugs and toxins (including alcohol), malnutrition, hemosiderosis, biliary cirrhosis, or chronic CHF.
   c. Classification is based on etiology, degree of inflammation and necrosis, and extent of fibrosis.
   d. Earlier age of infection predicts development of chronic hepatitis.
2. Clinical
   a. Symptoms - most patients are asymptomatic. Most common complaint is fatigue and mild RUQ pain.
   b. Examination - no findings or stigmata of chronic liver disease. Some patients have RUQ tenderness.
3. Laboratory
   a. Low grade elevation of ALT and AST are common. Occasionally, marked increases are seen. Levels of chronic enzyme elevation provide an estimate of disease severity.
   b. Decreased synthetic function occurs with advanced disease (low serum albumin, prolonged PT).
4. Complications
   a. Increased risk for hepatocellular carcinoma.
   b. May progress to cirrhosis.

    c. Immune complex disease may occur with development of arthritis, membranous nephropathy (presents as nephrotic syndrome), vasculitis (polyarteritis nodosa) and cryoglobulinemia.

5. Treatment

    a. Hepatitis B - interferon alpha, lamivudine.

    b. Hepatitis C - interferon alpha, ribavirin.

    c. Autoimmune hepatitis - steroids.

6. Hepatitis C, HIV virus co-infection increases the risk of rapid disease progression from both hepatitis C and HIV.

D. Cirrhosis and chronic liver failure

1. Causes - same as for chronic hepatitis.

2. Clinical

    a. Symptoms often depend on the underlying cause of cirrhosis, and reflect the sequelae of the disease. Patients may be asymptomatic or may present with GI bleeding, ascites and signs of portal hypertension or encephalopathy and coagulation abnormalities. Pruritus is common.

    b. The liver is usually small by the time it becomes cirrhotic. Spider angiomas, palmar erythema and ascites are common.

    c. LFTs may be normal or elevated, hypoalbuminemia is common and coagulation abnormalities (elevated PT and bleeding time) are unresponsive to vitamin K.

    d. Liver biopsy establishes the diagnosis.

3. Sequelae of cirrhosis

    a. Portal hypertension - bleeding esophageal varices, congestive gastropathy, splenomegaly with hypersplenism.

    b. Ascites - abdominal hernia, spontaneous bacterial peritonitis.

    c. Hepatorenal syndrome

    d. Hepatic encephalopathy

    e. Coagulopathy

    f. Hepatocellular carcinoma

    g. Feminization

4. Treatment

    a. Pruritus - cholestyramine 4 gm po with meals.

    b. Vitamin deficiencies

      (1) Vit K 10 mg SQ q 4 weeks.

      (2) Vit D 50,000 units po 2-3x/week or 100,000 units IM q4wk.

      (3) Vit A 25,000 units po qd.

      (4) Calcium 1 gm po qd.

      (5) Zinc sulfate 220mg/d.

    c. Ascites - salt and water restriction, diuretics, paracentesis.

    d. Encephalopathy

      (1) Restrict protein to 30-40gm/d.

      (2) Neomycin 1gm po bid (or metronidazole 250mg q8h)

    (3) Lactulose 15-30cc po q4-6h (to give 2-3 stools/d).

  e. Coagulation abnormalities - Vitamin K 10mg SQ qdx3d.

  f. Bleeding varices - propranolol (titrate dose to reduce resting heart rate by 25%). Perform sclerotherapy, or surgical shunting when possible.

E. Ascites

1. Etiology

  a. Cirrhosis - accounts for 80% of ascites.

  b. Other causes - cancer, tuberculosis, heart failure, pancreatic disease.

2. Evaluation

  a. Ultrasound may be done to confirm the presence of ascites especially when small amounts of fluid are present, and may suggest an etiology.

  b. Diagnostic paracentesis should be done on all patients as part of the initial evaluation for new onset ascites or in those patients with known ascites who have a change in their clinical status.

    (1) Remove 30-50cc of fluid.

    (2) Obtain cell count and differential and Gram stain. Do AFB smears if there is a preponderance of lymphocytes or exudative fluid.

    (3) Obtain albumin level from serum and ascites, if possible. Calculate serum albumin/ascites gradient by subtracting the ascites albumin value from the serum albumin value.

      (a) Gradient > 1.1 g/dl is consistent with cirrhosis, alcoholic hepatitis, CHF, and hepatic metastases.

      (b) Gradient < 1.1 g/dl is seen with peritoneal TB or carcinomatosis, pancreatitis, and nephrotic syndrome.

    (4) Use ascitic fluid protein if albumin is not available.

      (a) Transudate (protein < 3gm/100ml or ratio of ascitic fluid protein/total protein <0.5) is consistent with portal hypertension, CHF.

      (b) Exudate (protein > 3gm/100ml or ratio of ascitic fluid protein/total protein > 0.5) is found with infection, especially TB, and carcinomatosis.

3. Treatment

  a. Treat the underlying cause, if possible.

  b. Ascites due to portal hypertension

    (1) Salt restriction to less than 2 gm per day is imperative.

    (2) Diuretics - spironolactone 100 mg and furosemide 40 mg in combination once daily, doubling the dose to a maximum of 400 mg and 160 mg respectively. Goal is to have to patient lose 1 kg/d if edema is present, 1/2 kg/d if ascites without edema.

    (3) Large-volume paracentesis may be done in patients who are very uncomfortable or in those who have not responded to diuretics.

  c. Tuberculosis - see Chapter 1, VIII, B, 3, g

  d. Peritoneal carcinomatosis

(1) Treat the underlying cancer.

(2) Provide symptomatic relief with repeated paracenteses.

4. Spontaneous bacterial peritonitis (SBP)

  a. Suspect in patients with fever, abdominal pain or tenderness, or mental status change.

  b. Diagnostic paracentesis should be done. >250 PMN/mm3 of ascitic fluid is suggestive of SBP.

  c. Organisms include *E. Coli, Klebsiella, Strep pneumoniae*, other Strep species.

  d. Treat with parenteral ampicillin and gentamicin or third generation cephalosporin x 5d.

VI. PANCREATIC DISORDERS

A. Acute pancreatitis

1. Etiology

  a. Alcohol use and gallstones are the most common causes.

  b. Other causes include hypertriglyceridemia, hypercalcemia, drugs, HIV and other viral infections, ascaris infection.

2. Symptoms

  a. Steady epigastric or RUQ pain with radiation to the back, made worse with food.

  b. Usually associated with nausea and persistent vomiting.

3. Signs

  a. Physical signs are usually less than expected from the level of pain.

  b. Epigastric tenderness and guarding may be present.

  c. Pancreatic pseudocyst may be palpated as an epigastric mass.

  d. With hemorrhage (1%), flank ecchymosis may be seen.

4. Laboratory diagnosis

  a. Elevated serum amylase and lipase (more specific but less sensitive).

  b. Amylase returns to normal in 1-2d, lipase remains elevated for 5-10d.

  c. Height of the amylase level does not correlate with severity of disease.

5. Treatment

  a. Identify and treat the underlying cause, if possible.

  b. Patients with mild pain and no vomiting may be treated as outpatients with pain medication, clear liquid diet until improved.

  c. Inpatient treatment

    (1) NG drainage until pain improves and the patient is able to tolerate fluids, then advance diet as tolerated.

    (2) IV fluids are usually needed, as significant third-space losses may occur.

    (3) Narcotic analgesics and antiemetics to control pain and vomiting.

    (4) H2-blockers of no proven benefit.

    (5) With severe necrotizing pancreatitis, broad spectrum antibiotics (2nd or 3rd generation cephalosporins) may reduce mortality.

6. **Pancreatic pseudocysts**
   a. Collections of necrotic tissue, fluid and blood that develop in or near the pancreas, usually during a severe episode of acute pancreatitis.
   b. Persistence of an elevated serum amylase level for more than a week after the onset of pancreatitis may suggest formation of a pseudocyst.
   c. May cause pain.
   d. If >5cm, consider surgical drainage.
   e. Complications of the cyst include infection, perforation and hemorrhage.

B. **Chronic pancreatitis**
   1. **Symptoms**
      a. Characterized by bouts of mild to severe recurrent epigastric pain, nausea and vomiting. 80% occur in alcoholic patients.
      b. Pancreatic insufficiency with weight loss and steatorrhea may occur.
      c. Pancreatic cancer should be considered.
   2. **Diagnosis**
      a. Serum amylase and lipase levels may be slightly elevated, but are frequently normal.
      b. The patient may also have occasional episodes of acute pancreatitis.
      c. KUB may reveal pancreatic calcifications.
      d. Ultrasound to look for associated gallstones.
   3. **Treatment**
      a. Treat acute exacerbations as above.
      b. Patient may need chronic pain medication.
      c. Small, low fat meals may be helpful.
      d. Eliminate alcohol.

C. **Pancreatic insufficiency**
   1. **Exocrine insufficiency**
      a. Manifested by weight loss and steatorrhea (frequent, greasy bowel movements).
      b. Treat with oral pancreatic enzymes (Pancreatin or Viokase 6-8 tablets with each meal). May work better when given with antacids or H2 blockers.
      c. High calorie diet, rich in carbohydrate and protein, low in fat may decrease steatorrhea.
   2. **Endocrine insufficiency**
      a. Patients with destruction of the pancreas may develop diabetes.
      b. Treat with insulin.

CHAPTER 6

RENAL DISEASE

I. ACUTE RENAL FAILURE
A. Classification
1. **Prerenal** - renal hypoperfusion usually secondary to extracellular volume depletion. Patient may be hypotensive. If renal function was previously normal, urine should be concentrated with elevated specific gravity, and low urine volume. The BUN is elevated out of proportion to the creatinine with a ratio of >20:1.
2. **Postrenal** - impaired excretion of urine (usually due to ureteral or urethral obstruction).
3. **Intrinsic renal** - abnormality of the renal parenchyma (includes vascular, glomerular or tubular injury). Extracellular volume is normal or increased. BUN and creatinine are elevated proportionately.

B. Complications
1. Complications include pulmonary edema, hyponatremia, hyperkalemia, acidosis, hyperphosphatemia, anorexia, nausea, vomiting and other uremic symptoms.
2. The consequences of acute renal failure are more severe than those of chronic renal failure due to lack of time to activate adaptive mechanisms.

C. Treatment
1. Correct reversible causes
   a. Prerenal - improve renal blood flow with hydration, correction of hypotension, treatment of CHF, etc.
   b. Postrenal - catheter to relieve obstruction, ultrasound to look for hydronephrosis.
   c. Renal - investigate cause (drugs, trauma, hypotension, sepsis). Try to convert oliguric to nonoliguric ARF. If edema is present, give furosemide 2-10mg/kg. If no edema is present, give NS 500cc IV fluid challenge. If there is no response, restrict further fluids.
2. Closely monitor fluid balance (I/O, daily weights, BP measurement). Avoid overhydration. Restrict fluids to replacement of losses plus 500cc/d.
3. Monitor renal function and electrolytes, especially potassium. Limit dietary intake of potassium and phosphates. Oral aluminum hydroxide antacids may be used to absorb dietary phosphates. Kayexalate may be used to treat hyperkalemia.
4. Avoid nephrotoxic drugs such as NSAIDs, aminoglycosides, or x-ray contrast agents
5. Patients who fail to improve should be considered for peritoneal or hemodialysis.

II. CHRONIC RENAL FAILURE
A. Causes
1. **Renal parenchymal disease** - chronic glomerulopathies, hypertension, diabetes.
2. **Infection** - chronic pyelonephritis, schistosomiasis.
3. **Chronic outlet obstruction** - stricture, BPH.

B. Clinical
1. Symptoms are usually minimal until the disease has progressed to the uremic stage. Symptoms of uremia include fatigue, anorexia, nausea, vomiting, pruritus, altered mental status.
2. Signs of chronic renal failure are variable. They may include hypertension, peripheral edema, peripheral neuropathy, pericarditis, GI bleeding, asterixis, lethargy.
3. Laboratory findings include elevated BUN and creatinine, acidosis, normochromic/normocytic anemia, hyperkalemia.

C. Treatment
1. Correct aggravating factors - volume depletion, outlet obstruction, infection, hypertension, nephrotoxins.
2. Treat complications of uremia
   a. Hyperkalemia - dietary potassium restriction. Monitor electrolytes and treat hyperkalemia if severe. (see VI.C.)
   b. Sodium and fluid balance - restrict intake of salt and water, but avoid volume depletion. Diuretics (furosemide or thiazides) may be used for volume overload.
   c. Hypertension - usually volume dependent, and will respond to diuretics. Other agents may be necessary as well.
   d. Anemia - iron supplements should be given.
   e. Renal osteodystrophy and acidosis can be treated with calcium carbonate and sodium bicarbonate.
   f. Pruritus may be helped by phosphate restriction or oral antihistamines.
3. Dietary management - give high calorie, low protein diet. Restrict sodium if hypertension or edema are present. Restrict potassium if urine output is <1 liter/d. Vitamins B, C and folic acid may be given.
4. Overall prognosis for these patients is poor without dialysis.

III. GLOMERULONEPHRITIS
A. Acute nephritis
1. Characterized by inflammatory and/or necrotizing lesions within the glomeruli, resulting in hematuria.
2. The presence of RBC casts in the urinary sediment provides evidence of the glomerular origin of hematuria.

B. Causes
1. **Post-streptococcal glomerulonephritis** - common in children (peak age 7 years), less common in adults. Follows streptococcal infections (pharyngitis, pyoderma or impetigo).

2. IgA nephropathy - most common cause of glomerulonephritis worldwide. Usually presents with gross or microscopic hematuria. Common in young adults following acute infections, most commonly viral.

3. Rapidly progressive glomerulonephritis - due to immune complex disease or anti-basement membrane antibodies (Goodpasture disease).

4. Membranoproliferative glomerulonephritis - often associated with nephrotic syndrome.

C. Manifestations

1. Mild glomerulonephritis syndromes - cause hematuria with RBC casts, mild proteinuria, minimal azotemia, no edema or hypertension.

2. Severe glomerulonephritis syndromes - cause hematuria with RBC casts, proteinuria (sometimes nephrotic range), loss of renal function, hypertension and edema.

D. Treatment

1. Supportive - salt restriction, antihypertensives, diuretics. Patients may develop CHF, seizures or strokes in the acute phase of the disease.

2. Look for treatable causes

a. A course of antistreptococcal antibiotics (penicillin or erythromycin) should be given in suspected post-streptococcal glomerulonephritis.

b. Consider the use of steroids and immunosuppressive agents.

E. Outcome

1. Post-streptococcal glomerulonephritis - 90% completely recover within a short time. Urine abnormalities may persist (hematuria and proteinuria). Rarely, rapidly progressive disease may develop.

2. Other causes have a higher incidence of chronic renal failure.

IV. Nephrotic Syndrome

A. General

1. Characterized by abnormal loss of protein, predominantly albumin, usually due to noninflammatory lesions of the glomerulus.

2. Any disorder that affects the glomerulus can cause nephrotic syndrome.

B. Causes

1. Minimal change disease (nil disease, lipoid nephrosis)

a. Cause of nephrotic syndrome in 75% of children, 15-20% of adults.

b. Patients usually present with periorbital and peripheral edema, due to severe proteinuria.

c. One third of adults have hypertension and microscopic hematuria (RBC casts are absent).

2. Focal segmental glomerulosclerosis

a. May be idiopathic or secondary to sickle cell disease, HIV disease, chronic reflux.

b. Patient presents with either asymptomatic proteinuria or edema. The degree of proteinuria will vary.

      c. Hypertension and microscopic hematuria are common. Renal function is decreased in 30% of patients.

   3. Membranous nephropathy

      a. Most commonly idiopathic, but may be associated with infections (*Plasmodium malaria, Schistosoma mansoni*, hepatitis B and C, syphilis, leprosy), systemic lupus, solid neoplasms, and drugs.

      b. Typically presents with proteinuria and edema.

      c. Hypertension and microscopic hematuria may be found. Renal function is usually normal initially.

   4. Systemic diseases - diabetes, amyloidosis.

C. Manifestations

   1. Massive proteinuria (>3gm/d), hypoalbuminemia (serum albumin <3gm/dl), edema (may cause ascites and anasarca), hyperlipidemia.

   2. The patient is usually normotensive, unless nephritis is associated.

D. Treatment

   1. Treat infection and hypertension aggressively.

   2. Salt restriction (2-4gm/d), diuretics.

   3. Look for underlying causes.

   4. Steroids are especially helpful in patients with minimal change disease and should be tried in all patients presenting with nephrotic syndrome. Children respond more rapidly than adults. 90% respond to steroids initially, but 50% relapse within one year.

      a. Prednisone 1-2mg/kg/d (maximum of 60mg) in divided doses is given for 4-8 weeks, then decreased to qod dosing if proteinuria is resolved, and tapered over several months.

      b. Relapse requires starting steroids again and tapering more slowly. Some patients require long term steroids.

      c. Consider the patient to be steroid-resistant if they fail to respond after 16 weeks of treatment.

   5. Cytotoxic agents (cyclophosphamide 2mg/kg/d x 8 weeks) may be useful for patients not responsive to steroids (especially adults), or those who appear to be steroid-dependent.

E. Outcome

   1. Prognosis probably is worse in developing countries, though data is poor.

   2. With minimal change disease, up to 90% achieve long-term remission. With membranous nephropathy, up to 50% develop progressive disease.

V. TESTS FOR EVALUATION OF RENAL FUNCTION

A. Urinalysis

   1. Most important routine test for evaluating renal disease.

   2. Urine color

      a. Color varies from pale yellow to dark depending on concentration.

b. Red color is usually due to the presence of blood. Hematuria is present if RBCs are found in the urine sediment and the supernatant is clear after centrifugation.

c. Red supernatant with a urine dipstick positive for heme indicates the presence of hemoglobinuria or myoglobulinuria. Rare causes of red urine include ingestion of beets or porphyria.

3. Proteinuria

    a. Urine protein usually consists of albumin, but may include other clinically important proteins including light chains.

    b. Daily protein excretion should be less than 150 mg/24 hrs but may reach >20 gm per day in nephrotic syndrome.

    c. Urine dipsticks are insensitive for detecting microalbuminuria, requiring >3-500mg/24 hrs of protein excretion before becoming positive. They only detect albumin.

    d. Sulfosalicylic acid (SSA) detects all types of protein in the urine. A positive SSA test with a negative urine dipstick is most commonly found in multiple myeloma.

4. pH

    a. Alkaline urine (pH > 7.0) is associated with infection with urea splitting organisms.

    b. Strongly acidic urine (pH < 5.3) is seen in metabolic acidosis. When the pH is persistently low, consider renal tubular acidosis.

5. Specific gravity

    a. Measures the amount of solute in the urine. Large molecules such as glucose or contrast material increase the specific gravity. Specific gravity must be correlated with the clinical setting.

    b. High specific gravity is seen in dehydration. Low specific gravity can be found in conditions where there is inability to concentrate urine.

6. Urine sediment

    a. Examined after centrifuging urine for 3 minutes, decanting the supernatant, and placing a small amount of the sediment on a covered glass slide.

    b. Bacteria - commonly represents contamination.

    c. Epithelial cells - presence of > 3-5 squamous epithelial cells indicates contamination of the urine during collection.

    d. Pyuria - >3-5 WBC/high power field or positive leukocyte esterase dipstick is significant, indicating possible infection.

    e. Hematuria - urine dipsticks are very sensitive, detecting the equivalent of 2-3 RBC/hpf. Microscopic hematuria with >2-3 RBC/high power field in spun urine sediment is significant.

    f. Casts

        (1) Hyaline casts - usually seen in dehydration with a concentrated urine. They have no pathological significance.

        (2) RBC casts - finding even small numbers suggests a glomerular source of bleeding.

    (3) WBC casts - seen in pyelonephritis and renal tubular disease.
B. Serum chemistries
   1. Electrolytes - see below.
   2. Serum creatinine
      a. Accurately reflects changes in the patients GFR (doubling of the serum creatinine generally reflects a 50% fall in the GFR).
      b. Calculate an estimated creatinine clearance with the following formula:

$$\text{CC (ml/min)} = (140\text{-age}) \times \text{wt (kg)} / \text{Serum Cr (mg\%)} \times 72.$$

       In women, multiply by 0.85 to correct for smaller muscle mass.
   3. Serum BUN
      a. Reflects GFR less accurately than serum creatinine.
      b. May be increased by hypovolemia, bleeding (esp GI), trauma, high protein diet.
      c. May be decreased in liver disease, low protein diet.
C. Abdominal ultrasound
   1. Imaging test of choice in renal failure (no IV contrast).
   2. Useful in evaluating renal size, presence of renal obstruction (hydronephrosis), or renal masses.
D. Intravenous pyelogram
   1. Visualizes the entire urinary system.
   2. Useful in the evaluation of hematuria to localize larger lesions and in the evaluation of stone disease.
   3. Involves IV contrast (risk of allergy, acute renal failure).

VI. FLUIDS AND ELECTROLYTES
A. Adult fluid requirements
   1. Average fluid requirement per day for an adult = 2000-3000cc. This should produce a urine volume of 1000-2000cc/d.
   2. Electrolytes needed daily
      a. Sodium - 50-150mEq
      b. Potassium - 20-60mEq
   3. Average maintenance IV fluid regimen = 2000cc of D5/.45NS with 20mEq KCl/L.
   4. Additional IV fluids are needed to replace any ongoing losses (GI, urinary, insensible).
B. Hypokalemia
   1. Causes
      a. GI loss - NG suction, vomiting, diarrhea.
      b. Renal loss - diuretics, hyperaldosteronism, Bartter's syndrome, RTA type IV.
      c. Chronic metabolic alkalosis.
   2. Symptoms
      a. Weakness, decreased reflexes, paresthesias.

b. ECG - flat or inverted T waves, prominent U waves, depressed ST segments.

3. Treatment

   a. Prefer oral route - diet can give 40-60mEq/d.

   b. IV - give at a rate <10mEq/hour.

   c. If K <2.0, can give up to 40mEq/hour in concentrations up to 60mEq/liter with cardiac monitoring. Give with NS, since glucose can cause K to decrease.

   d. Maximum 200 mEq/d.

C. Hyperkalemia

  1. Causes

   a. Acidosis

   b. Acute renal failure

   c. Adrenal insufficiency

   d. Tissue breakdown

  2. Symptoms

   a. Bradycardia, hypotension, ventricular fibrillation and cardiac arrest.

   b. ECG - tall, peaked T waves, depressed ST segments, tall R waves, prolonged PR, wide QRS.

  3. Treatment

   a. Calcium - calcium gluconate (5-10 ml of 10% solution) IV over 2 minutes. Repeat after 5 minutes if ECG unchanged. Effect lasts only 1 hour.

   b. Glucose/insulin - 1 amp D50W (25gm dextrose) IV over 5 minutes, 5-10 units regular insulin IV. Effect in 30-60 minutes. Lasts several hours.

   c. NaHCO3 - give 1 amp NaHCO3 (44mEq) IV over 5 minutes and repeat after 10-15 minutes. Onset occurs in 15 minutes. Duration 1-2 hours. Don't use NaHCO3 if CHF or hypernatremia are present.

   d. Cation-exchange resins (Kayexalate) 20-50gm in 100-200cc of 20% sorbitol solution. Repeat orally q 3-4 hours up to 4-5 doses/d. 50gm Kayexalate, 50gm sorbitol in 200cc water may be given as a retention enema, as often as once per hour. 1mEq K removed per gram of resin.

D. Hypocalcemia

  1. Causes

   a. Hypoparathyroidism

   b. Renal tubular acidosis

   c. Vitamin D deficiency

   d. Magnesium deficiency

  2. Symptoms

   a. Circumoral paresthesias, carpopedal spasm, positive Chvostek's and Trousseau's signs.

   b. ECG - prolonged QT.

3. Treatment
a. Acute - 10-20cc of 10% calcium gluconate IV over 10-15 minutes or IV drip with 600-800mg Ca/1000 cc D5W.

b. Chronic - 1500-3000mg/d oral calcium, with vitamin D.

E. Hypercalcemia

1. Causes - hyperparathyroidism, cancer, thiazides, immobilization, sarcoidosis, hyperthyroidism, adrenal insufficiency.

2. Symptoms - anorexia, nausea, vomiting, constipation, polyuria, dehydration, obtundation, psychosis.

3. Treatment
a. Saline hydration - alternate NS with 0.45NS at 250-500cc/h. Give furosemide 20-40mg IV q 2 hours to prevent volume overload.

b. Steroids are useful in hypercalcemia secondary to neoplasms. Give hydrocortisone 250-500mg IV q 8 hours initially, then prednisone 10-30mg/d. Onset of action is slow.

c. Calcitonin - skin test with 1 MRC unit (0.1cc of 1:10 dilution of calcitonin SQ). If no reaction, give 4 units/kg SQ or IM q12-24 hours. Use only if rehydration ineffective.

d. Phospate - use only if phosphate is low. Phospho-soda (600mg phos/5cc) 1 tsp. tid-qid. Neutra-Phos (250mg phos/cap) 2-3 cap tid-qid or 100cc retention Fleet enema bid.

F. Hypomagnesemia

1. Causes - malabsorption, alcoholism, severe diarrhea, NG suction.

2. Symptoms - weakness, tremors, personality changes, vertigo, seizures.

3. Treatment
a. 1-2gm MgSO4 as a 10% solution IV over 15 minutes. Then 1 gm IM q4-6 hours. Hold if reflexes are absent.

b. Magnesium oxide 10g tablets (35mEq) 1-2 tabs/d orally.

G. Hyponatremia

1. Assess the patient's volume status.

a. If edema is present - treat with water restriction and diuresis.

b. Normovolemia - suggests SIADH. Treat with fluid restriction (1000-1500 ml/day). With severe hyponatremia, give IV furosemide; replace urine output with NS.

c. Volume depletion - replace deficit with NS.

2. Patient is usually asymptomatic until Na <120-125.

H. Hypernatremia

1. Results from a free water deficit.

2. Replace deficit with hypotonic fluids IV 1/2NS or D5W or increase oral intake, if possible.

3. Rapid correction of serum sodium may be dangerous.

CHAPTER 7

ENDOCRINOLOGY

I. DIABETES MELLITUS

A. General
1. The incidence of diabetes is increasing at an alarming rate in the developing world secondary to changes in socioeconomic status and lifestyle.
2. Management remains difficult due to lack of regular access to monitoring devices and treatments.
3. The ongoing challenge is to design cost effective treatment regimens that provide adequate glycemic control.

B. Classification
1. **Type I** - insulin dependent, ketosis-prone. Insulin production is deficient. Occurs secondary to autoimmune destruction of the pancreatic islet cells. Usual onset is in the first two decades of life, but it can occur at any age.
2. **Type II** - characterized by insulin resistance and variable degrees of relative insulin deficiency. May develop ketosis with stress. Usual onset is after age 40, but can occur at any age also. Most common form of diabetes, with some genetic predisposition.
3. **Atypical diabetes mellitus** - some patients (especially blacks) may be difficult to classify initially. They may present with ketosis and require insulin initially, but later revert to a more typical type II pattern.
4. **Fibrocalculous pancreatic diabetes** - described as a possible subtype of diabetes specific to developing countries. Occurs in chronic pancreatitis secondary to protein-calorie malnutrition or micronutrient deficiency.
5. **Gestational diabetes** - glucose intolerance developing during pregnancy. Occurs in 2% of pregnancies but may be higher in some racial groups. Many (up to 50%) later develop overt diabetes.

C. Definitions (based on plasma glucose, PG)
1. Normal - fasting PG <110 mg% (6.1 mmol/L).
2. Impaired fasting glucose - FPG between 110 and 125 mg% (6.1-6.9 mmol/L). These patients are at increased risk of diabetes.
3. Diabetes mellitus - diagnosed by any one of the following:
   a. Unequivocal symptoms (polyuria, polydipsia, unexplained weight loss) and casual plasma glucose ≥200mg% (11.1mmol/L).
   b. Fasting plasma glucose ≥126mg% (7mmol/L).
   c. 2-hour plasma glucose ≥200mg% (11.1mmol/L) during oral glucose tolerance test.
   d. HbA1c values are not currently considered in the diagnosis of DM.

D. General treatment information
1. **Diet** - general principles
   a. Avoid excessive refined sugars and alcohol.
   b. Encourage a nutritionally balanced diet with total daily calories consisting of 10-20% protein, <30% fat and the rest carbohydrate.

177

      c. Consistent and evenly spaced food intake throughout the day is more important in intense management programs.

      d. If obese, attempt weight loss by restricting total calories and increasing exercise.

  2. Exercise - regular, moderate, aerobic exercise (20-30 minutes three times per week) helps reduce weight, reduce insulin resistance, and improves overall well being.

  3. Glucose monitoring

      a. Urine glucose monitoring is not helpful.

      b. Blood glucose values should be monitored, when possible.

      c. Home glucose monitoring, using portable fingerstick glucose monitors, should be used, if available.

  4. Oral hypoglycemic agents

      a. General

        (1) The only oral hypoglycemic agents listed in the WHO Essential Drug List (revised 12/99) are glibenclamide and metformin. Since these are likely to be the most commonly available medications in the developing world, discussion will be limited to these agents.

        (2) The following chart gives a summary of other oral antidiabetic agents which may be available in certain settings:

Generic name	Brand name	Dosage range (mg/d)	Duration (hours)	Dosing freq. per day
Sulfonylureas				
Acetohexamide	Dymelor	250-1500	12-18	Twice
Chlorpropamide	Diabinese	100-500	60	Once
Glimepiride	Amaryl	1-8	16-24	Once
Glipizide	Glucotrol	2.5-20	12-24	Twice
Glyburide, glibenclamide	DiaBeta, Micronase	1.25-20	16-24	Twice
Tolazamide	Tolinase	100-1000	12-24	Twice
Tolbutamide	Orinase	500-3000	6-12	2-3 times
Meglitidinides				
Nateglinide	Starlix	120-180	½-2	3 times
Repaglinide	Prandin	1.5-16	½-2	3 times
Biguanide				
Metformin	Glucophage	1000-2500	5-6	2-4 times
a-Glucosidase inhibitors				
Acarbose	Precose	150-300	6	3 times
Miglitol	Glyset	75-300	6	3 times
Thiazolidinediones				
Pioglitazone	Actos	15-45	24+	Once
Rosiglitazone	Avandia	2-8	24+	1-2 times

b. Glibenclamide (glyburide)
   (1) Indicated only in type 2 diabetes.
   (2) Usual starting dose is 5mg daily, but may use less in the elderly. Maximum dose is 20mg/d. Half-life is 12 hours.
   (3) Most important side effect is hypoglycemia secondary to the relatively long half-life. Avoid in the presence of hepatic or renal disease, or in pregnant or breast-feeding females. Use with caution in the elderly.

c. Metformin
   (1) Initial drug of choice in obese diabetics. May be used alone or in combination with glibenclamide or insulin. Hypoglycemia is not usually associated with metformin use.
   (2) Starting dose is 500 mg 1-2 times daily. Titrate the dose to the maximum tolerated or 2500 mg per day.
   (3) Avoid in situations that predispose to development of lactic acidosis (eg: renal insufficiency, CHF, severe dehydration). GI side effects are common but may resolve with continued use.

5. Insulin

Type	Onset	Peak	Duration
Regular	1/2hr	2-4hr	8-12 hr
NPH	1-2hr	6-12hr	20-22 hr
PZI	6-8hr	14-24hr	36+hr
Lente	1-2hr	6-12hr	18-28hr

E. Treatment regimens
1. Type I DM
   a. The usual daily insulin requirement is 0.5 - 1.0 unit/kg/day.
   b. Patient may be started on 0.2-0.4 units of intermediate insulin (NPH) and the dose increased daily. Dosage adjustments are made according to multiple daily glucose measurement (fasting, before meals and at bedtime). Once control is achieved, the glucose may be monitored once daily in the morning.
   c. If good control cannot be achieved (all blood sugars <150 pre-prandial) with a once daily dose of intermediate insulin, twice daily dosing with a mixture of NPH and regular insulin should be tried. Two-thirds of the total dosage is given before breakfast and one-third before supper. The insulin is given 30 minutes before breakfast and supper. The ratio of NPH to regular insulin is 2:1. (For example, if the total insulin requirement is 60 units/d, it should be given as 30u NPH + 15 u reg. Q AM, 10 u NPH + 5 u reg. Q PM).
   d. A more intensive regimen involves giving NPH insulin once or twice daily with regular insulin 30 minutes before meals according to blood glucose values. This is impractical in most settings unless frequent blood glucose self-monitoring is available.

2. Type II DM

a. Patients with Type II DM whose glucose is not adequately controlled with weight loss, diet and exercise should be started on an oral hypoglycemic agent. Begin with a low dose of a sulfonylurea (glibenclamide) and titrate to the maximum dose.

b. If blood glucose control is inadequate, metformin may be added to the regimen. Titrate to the maximum dose of both drugs. In obese patients metformin should be used as the initial therapy. Avoid metformin in the presence of CHF or hepatic or renal insufficiency.

c. A once daily injection of an intermediate insulin may adequately control a patient with Type II DM, if oral agents are not effective.

d. A combination of intermediate insulin at bedtime, and a sulfonylurea or metformin during the day may be effective in patients who are poorly controlled with either regimen alone. Adjust the insulin dose based on fasting blood glucose and oral hypoglycemic agent dose based on noon and evening blood glucose. If the blood sugar remains uncontrolled, switch to twice daily NPH or NPH + regular insulin.

3. Surgery

a. Patients undergoing surgery should receive 1/3 - 2/3 their usual dose of insulin on the morning of surgery as intermediate-acting insulin.

b. D5W should be given at 150cc/hr during surgery.

c. Monitor glucose every 4 hours and supplement with insulin as needed.

4. Gestational diabetes

a. Screen all pregnant patients at 24-28 weeks using 50g oral glucose tolerance test. If the 1 hour glucose is >140mg%, perform a 100g glucose tolerance test. If two or more of the following values are present, treatment for gestational diabetes is indicated:

(1) FBG $\geq$ 105mg% (10.5mmol/L)

(2) 1 hr glucose $\geq$ 190 mg% (10.6mmol/L)

(3) 2 hr glucose $\geq$ 165 mg% (9.2mmol/L)

(4) 3 hr glucose $\geq$ 145 mg% (8.1mmol/L)

b. Treatment

(1) Goal is a FBG 60-90mg% (3.3-5.0mmol/L) and one hour postprandial glucose 70-140mg% (3.9-7.8mmol/L). Maintain euglycemia to prevent macrosomia in the fetus.

(2) Do not use sulfonylureas or metformin in pregnancy.

(3) Begin a diabetic diet.

(4) Give bedtime NPH to control fasting hyperglycemia, and regular insulin before meals to control post-prandial hyperglycemia.

c. Monitor blood glucose closely with a goal of normalizing values.

F. Ketoacidosis

1. General

a. Usually occurs only with type I diabetes. Characterized by severe hyperglycemia, ketonemia and acidemia, and volume depletion.

b. Symptoms include nausea and vomiting, polyuria and thirst, abdominal pain, somnolence and visual disturbances. Physical findings include tachycardia, hypotension, hyperpnea or Kussmaul's breathing, impaired consciousness, weight loss, and fruity breath odor (ketones).

c. Look for an acute precipitating factor, especially underlying infection. Give broad-spectrum parenteral antibiotics to febrile patients (ampicillin plus gentamicin).

d. Assess degree of dehydration (most patients with DKA are at least 5-10% dehydrated).

e. Measure CBC, urinalysis, blood glucose, and BUN. Monitor electrolytes, blood gases , serum acetone, if possible.

f. Monitor urine output. Keep a flow sheet (intake and output, glucose, potassium, insulin).

2. Fluids

a. Start an IV immediately.

b. Give normal saline 10-20cc/kg in children, 1 liter in adults over the first hour. If hypotension or shock persists, repeat the same quantity of NS in the next hour.

c. Once stabilized, give fluids to replace half the estimated deficit in 8 hours, the rest in the next 16-20 hours. Maintenance fluids for adults are 150-200cc/hr.

3. Insulin

a. 5-10 units of regular insulin (0.1units/kg) should be given as a bolus IV, followed by an insulin drip of 2-10units/hr (0.1units/kg/h). Try to decrease the glucose 75-100mg%/hr down to 300mg%. IV fluids and insulin need to be continued until acidemia is corrected and food is tolerated.

b. When the glucose is 200-300mg%, change IV fluids to D5/.45NS. When serum ketones are negative, give 10units regular insulin SQ and discontinue the insulin drip ½ hour later.

c. Begin a weight-based regimen of short acting insulin q4-6 hours when patient is able to resume eating. Give 0.1 units/kg with an additional 1 unit for each 50mg% above 150mg%. Reduce the dose if the glucose is <90 mg%.

d. If IV access is not able to be obtained, intermittent IM regular insulin (better absorption than SQ) may be given as 10 units IM (0.1units/kg) q2-3h until the glucose is <300mg%.

4. Potassium replacement

a. Most patients with DKA are potassium-depleted.

b. Potassium should be added to the IV fluids after the first liter of fluid is infused and the patient has voided. Average 20mEq KCl/liter IV fluids.

c. Serum potassium levels should be monitored, if possible. Try to keep K in the 4-5 mEq range.

d. ECG can be used to guide therapy if serum K levels are unavailable.

5. Bicarbonate therapy should be given as 1-2 mEq/kg IV only if the patient is in shock (2 amps of 5% solution or 100mEq NaHCO3 per liter 0.45NS in adults as an infusion, not bolus).

G. Hyperosmolar hyperglycemic nonketotic syndrome

1. General

a. Characterized by severe hyperosmolarity, hyperglycemia and dehydration.

b. Usually presents with insidious onset over several weeks in elderly patients with mild or undiagnosed type II DM.

c. Plasma glucose levels are usually higher than in DKA. BUN and creatinine are usually elevated as well.

2. Management

a. The primary treatment is fluid replacement. Give 1 liter NS in the first 30-60 minutes, followed by another liter over the next hour. Further fluids should be given based on electrolyte and glucose levels. Total fluid deficit may be > 8 liters. Change to D5/1/2NS when the glucose falls to 250-300mg%.

b. Insulin should be given at 3-4 units/hr initially. Glucose levels should be followed every hour.

c. Potassium should be given as 20mEq/L. Follow serum K+ levels and supplement as needed. Potassium deficit is less than in DKA.

H. Complications of diabetes mellitus

1. Diabetic retinopathy

a. A leading cause of blindness. Lesions include microaneurysms, retinal hemorrhages, exudates and macular edema.

b. Treatment requires access to laser therapy for photocoagulation.

c. Excellent blood pressure control with use of ACE inhibitors is helpful in slowing progression.

2. Diabetic nephropathy

a. Onset is marked by development of microalbuminuria; may progress to nephrotic syndrome and end-stage renal disease.

b. The major risk factors for the development or progression of diabetic nephropathy are poor glycemic control and the presence of hypertension.

c. Strict control of glucose and blood pressure, use of ACE inhibitors and dietary protein restriction have been shown to slow the rate of decline of renal function. Intervention should be started at the first sign of microalbuminuria (albumin excretion rate of 30-300mg/d).

3. Diabetic neuropathy

a. Peripheral sensory neuropathy is common in the distal upper and lower extremities. Amitriptyline may be helpful in controlling the pain.

b. Peripheral motor neuropathy in the hands and feet may occur.

    c. Autonomic neuropathy may cause symptoms such as impotence, neurogenic bladder, diarrhea, incontinence, or postural hypotension.

    d. Gastroparesis may be manifested by nausea and vomiting. Metoclopramide 10mg taken 30 minutes before meals and at bedtime may be helpful.

4. Diabetic foot problems

    a. Result from sensory neuropathies and peripheral vascular disease, common problems in diabetic patients.

    b. Ulcers develop frequently and easily become infected, leading to cellulitis and, occasionally, osteomyelitis. Staph and strep are most common, but Gram-negative and anaerobic bacteria may be involved.

    c. Treatment involves hospitalization, IV broad spectrum antibiotics, and aggressive surgical debridement.

5. Atherosclerosis of the coronary and peripheral arteries

    a. Common in diabetic patients with disease longer than 10 years.

    b. Coronary artery disease, myocardial infarction and peripheral vascular disease are common. Cardiovascular disease is a major cause of death in patients with diabetes.

    c. Efforts should be directed at prevention through risk factor reduction (treating hypertension, hyperlipidemia, and smoking cessation). Aspirin therapy may also be beneficial for primary and secondary prevention.

II. THYROID DISEASE

A. Endemic goiter (iodine deficiency)

1. Goiter is defined an enlargement of the thyroid gland.

    a. The most common cause in the developing world is iodine deficiency due to lack of iodine in the soil.

    b. The presence of goitrogens in the diet may also result in goiter.

    c. When more than 10% of the population is affected, it is termed endemic goiter.

2. Clinical manifestations

    a. Goiter develops early in life, and may result in progressive enlargement of the thyroid gland. Occasionally this may lead to symptoms of airway obstruction due to tracheal compression.

    b. The majority of patients with endemic goiter remain euthyroid. Hypothyroidism may occasionally develop; hyperthyroidism is less common.

    c. Chronic iodine deficiency produces subtle intellectual and neuromuscular disabilities.

3. Treatment

    a. Iodine supplements should be given. Patient should use iodinated salt or Lugol's solution (1 drop/day is more than sufficient). High dose iodine supplements may result in either hypo or hyperthyroidism, especially in patients >45 years old.

    b. Patients with goiters should avoid foods containing goitrogens, if possible. In Africa, this includes cassava and millet, which contain thiocyanate, which inhibits uptake of iodine by the thyroid.

    c. Use of thyroxine may slow or prevent further thyroid enlargement. Start with 100µg/d (50µg/d in elderly).

    d. Surgery is indicated to relieve symptoms of airway obstruction. More commonly, it is performed for cosmetic reasons. The goiter may recur unless total thyroidectomy is performed. The patient should be euthyroid before surgery.

B. Hypothyroidism

1. Clinical

    a. Etiology is most commonly due to Hashimoto's thyroiditis. May be transiently present due to subacute thyroiditis. The acquired form is secondary to surgical or radioiodine ablative treatment.

    b. Characterized by apathy, dry skin, hypothermia, constipation, coarse, sparse hair, delayed reflexes.

2. Diagnosis

    a. Clinical diagnosis of mild disease is difficult.

    b. Obtain thyroid function tests when possible. T3, T4 and FTI are low, T3RU is low and TSH is elevated (rarely, the TSH is low if the defect is in the pituitary or hypothalamus).

3. Treatment

    a. L-thyroxine is the drug of choice. Starting doses are as follows:

        (1) Newborn - 25-50 µg/d.

        (2) 4 week - 1 year - 50-75 µg/d (5-6 µg/kg/d).

        (3) Children - 3-6 µg/kg/d. Start with 1/4 daily dose and increase at weekly intervals.

        (4) Adults - 25-50 µg/d initially. Increase q 4 weeks up to 100-150 µg/d (1.5-3 µg/kg/d). In the elderly, use 75% of usual dose.

    b. Follow with TSH levels, when possible. Don't over-treat, since this may lead to osteopenia.

    c. Wait a minimum of 4-6 weeks after each dosage change to re-check labs.

4. Myxedema coma

    a. Clinical - patients in myxedema coma have signs of hypothyroidism, with nonpitting edema of the lower extremities, stuporous or comatose mental status, and hypothermia.

    b. Treatment

        (1) L-thyroxine 300-500µg (2µg/kg) IV over 5-10 minutes initially, and 100µg IV q 24 hours thereafter.

        (2) Cover with corticosteroids due to the possibility of adrenal insufficiency (hydrocortisone 100mg IV bolus, then 25mg q6h as a continuous IV drip or dexamethasone 6mg IV, then 4mg IV q6h).

(3) IV fluids as determined by glucose, electrolytes and hydration status.

(4) Vigorous treatment of infection and other associated conditions.

(5) Do not rewarm externally.

C. Hyperthyroidism (thyrotoxicosis)

1. Causes

a. Graves disease (symmetric goiter) is responsible for 90% of hyperthyroidism in patients < 40 years old.

b. Toxic multinodular goiter (asymmetric goiter) is the most common cause of hyperthyroidism in middle-aged and elderly patients. Common in areas of iodine deficiency.

c. Toxic adenoma - single toxic nodule.

d. Autoimmune thyroiditis (high thyroid antibodies) - Hashimoto's thyrotoxicosis.

e. Subacute thyroiditis (transient hyperthyroidism) - de Quervain's thyroiditis. Sed rate is usually elevated in this condition.

2. Clinical signs

a. Symptoms include nervousness, palpitations, heat intolerance, insomnia, weight loss, sweating, diarrhea, tremor, and hair loss.

b. Physical examination may show warm moist skin, tachycardia, hyperdynamic precordium, brisk reflexes, proximal muscle weakness, and thyroid enlargement. Eye findings include widened distance between upper and lower eyelids, lid lag, proptosis and frequent blinking.

3. Diagnosis

a. Confirm diagnosis with thyroid tests, if possible.

b. Typical pattern shows undetectable TSH, elevated free T4, elevated FTI.

4. Treatment of Graves disease

a. Acute treatment of the hyperthyroidism

(1) Antithyroid drugs

  (a) Start carbimazole 30-60mg/d, methimazole 20-30mg/d or PTU 100-150mg tid. Increase dose after 3-4 weeks, if no improvement is noted. When the patient appears clinically euthyroid, obtain TSH, if possible.

  (b) After the patient is euthyroid for several months, the carbimazole may be decreased to 5-15mg/d, methimazole to 5-10mg/d, or PTU to 50-100mg/d.

  (c) Follow q 2-3 months for a total of 6-12 months. Check for remission at that time (10-50% have remission and will no longer need treatment).

  (d) Most important side effect is agranulocytosis.

(2) ß-Blockers

  (a) Propranolol 20-40mg q4-6h may be given for symptomatic improvement.

    (b) Avoid in patients with CHF or asthma.

b. Second phase of treatment

    (1) Antithyroid drugs for 6-18 months.

        (a) If the thyroid becomes smaller and the amount of drug needed is lower, remission is probable.

        (b) Stop treatment and repeat TFTs in 4 weeks, if available. If normal, follow q 2 months for 1 year, then less often.

    (2) Surgery

        (a) Indicated in large, obstructing glands or nodular glands.

        (b) Give antithyroid drugs for 1-2 months before surgery.

        (c) Give SSKI 2 drops tid or Lugol's solution 5 drops tid for 7-10 days prior to surgery, to decrease gland vascularity.

    (3) Radioactive iodine

        (a) Very effective, if available.

        (b) Stop anti-thyroid drugs 4 days prior to I^{131} uptake.

        (c) After treatment, check monthly to assure the patient is euthyroid. Allow 6 months before consideration of a second dose.

        (d) Avoid pregnancy for 6 months after treatment.

5. Treatment of other causes of hyperthyroidism

  a. Toxic multinodular goiter - either I^{131} or surgery.

  b. Solitary toxic nodule - treat with I^{131} (elderly), surgery (young).

  c. Subacute thyroiditis - may use aspirin 650mg qid or prednisone 40mg qd, with taper over 2 weeks. May give ß-blockers if symptomatic.

  d. Pregnant patients - use anti-thyroid drugs to keep free T4 high normal. May use ß-blockers and iodides short-term. Consider surgery during the second trimester if uncontrolled despite medication.

6. Thyroid storm (mortality 20-40%)

  a. Clinical signs

    (1) Exaggerated signs and symptoms of hyperthyroidism.

    (2) High fever, tachycardia, atrial fibrillation, change in mental status are often present.

    (3) Vomiting and diarrhea leading to dehydration and electrolyte abnormalities may occur.

  b. Treatment

    (1) IV fluids, according to electrolyte needs.

    (2) PTU 400mg po or NG q8h.

    (3) Sodium iodide 250mg q6h po or IV, 1-2gm in 1 liter NS/day IV infusion or SSKI 5 drops q8h po or NG. Do not begin until 2 hours after first dose of PTU.

    (4) Dexamethasone 4-6mg IV q6h.

    (5) Paracetamol (acetaminophen) 300-600mg q4-6h for fever (do not use aspirin).

(6) Propranolol 10-40mg po q4-6h (patients without asthma, CHF, chronic bronchitis). Patients with hyperthyroidism may need higher doses than normal.

(7) Oxygen, if available.

D. Solitary thyroid nodule

1. Etiology

a. Patient is usually euthyroid.

b. Malignancy is unusual (3-4%).

c. Some are actually dominant nodules in multinodular goiter.

2. Clinical manifestations

a. Usually present with an asymptomatic mass in the neck. May be detected on routine exam.

b. Suspect malignancy when the following are present:

(1) Nodule is solitary and hard, >2cm in size.

(2) Age is >40 years or <20 years.

(3) Recurrent laryngeal nerve paralysis is present.

(4) Adenopathy is present.

(5) Positive family history of thyroid cancer.

(6) History of previous neck irradiation.

3. Management

a. All nodules should be carefully measured and documented on the record so that changes in size will serve as an alert to the presence of malignancy.

b. If the clinical exam suggests a benign process and the patient is euthyroid, needle aspiration should be attempted using a 25g needle.

(1) If colloid material is obtained, indicating a cyst, the nodule should be completely aspirated. If it re-accumulates, it may be aspirated again twice more. Then, surgery or sclerosis with tetracycline (100mg of the parenteral preparation) should be considered.

(2) If the lesion is solid, the aspirate should be placed on a slide, air-dried and stained (Wright's stain is often adequate). If available, it should be read by a pathologist. The need for surgery should then be based on cytology results. If malignant, surgery is indicated. If benign, the patient may be started on thyroxine replacement and followed every 6 months.

c. Surgery should be considered for nodules in males, patients <20 years of age or those with positive family history of thyroid carcinoma.

d. If aspiration and cytology is not available and the patient does not have signs suggestive of malignancy, a trial of thyroxine replacement may be given for 3-6 months. Continuing enlargement is an indication for surgery. If the nodule remains stable, the patient may continue to be followed.

e. If the patient is clinically hyperthyroid and has a nodule, they should be treated with antithyroid medication, followed by surgery or I^{131}, if available

CHAPTER 8

HEMATOLOGY

I. ANEMIA
A. General principles
1. History
    a. Symptoms are related to the rate of development of the anemia.

    b. Acute blood loss (e.g. massive GI bleeding) does not allow time for compensatory adjustment of intravascular volume to occur, leading to postural hypotension, decreased cardiac output, sweating, restlessness, thirst.

    c. Chronically developing anemia causes nonspecific symptoms such as dyspnea on exertion, dizziness, palpitations, easy fatigability, headache, anorexia and, sometimes, weight loss.

2. Physical exam
    a. With severe anemia there will be pallor, tachycardia, systolic ejection murmurs. In acute blood loss, hypotension may be present.

    b. Look for splenomegaly.

    c. Evaluate hydration status.

3. Laboratory
    a. Check CBC with differential, MCV, platelets and peripheral smear (evaluate RBC morphology if RBC indices not available).

    b. If indicated, check reticulocyte count, sickle cell screen, stool for ova and parasites and occult blood, malaria smear.

4. Assessment
    a. Evaluate Hgb levels according to the patient's age.

    b. Determine the mechanism of the anemia (using patient history, RBC morphology and reticulocyte count)

       (1) Decreased marrow production

       (2) Bleeding

       (3) Hemolysis (increased destruction)

    c. Classify the anemia

       (1) Microcytic (small RBCs)

       (2) Macrocytic (large RBCs)

       (3) Normocytic (normal RBCs)

5. Pediatric considerations
    a. Anemia affects up to half of all children in developing countries and can have life-long effects on health and cognitive development. Both individual and community interventions are needed to adequately combat anemia.

    b. Community interventions to prevent/treat anemia:

       (1) Dietary - encourage breastfeeding. Use of cow's milk is associated with intestinal blood loss in many infants (especially in those <1 year of age). Encourage iron-rich weaning foods.

       (2) Supplementation - consider iron supplementation for premature babies and infants in high-risk areas.

(3) Hygiene - encourage use of shoes to avoid hookworm infection. Encourage use of latrines to avoid spread of hookworm.

(4) Medical - consider periodic screening for children. Consider presumptive iron therapy for any anemic child.

B. Microcytic anemia (MCV < 80fl)

1. Iron-deficiency

a. Most common cause of anemia. Up to 50% of pregnant women and preschool children in developing countries are iron deficient.

b. Causes

(1) Nutritional - cereal-based diets have low iron content, in poorly absorbable form.

(2) Excessive blood loss - usually menstrual, GI (hookworm, PUD, trichuriasis, schistosomiasis) or GU (schistosomiasis).

c. Evaluation

(1) Peripheral smear shows hypochromic, microcytic RBCs in advanced anemia (normocytic with mild disease).

(2) Sore tongue (glossitis), atrophy of the lingual papillae, erosions at the corner of the mouth (angular stomatitis), brittle, fragile fingernails and spooning of the nails (koilonychia) may be seen on physical exam.

d. Oral therapy

(1) Peds - FeS04 30mg/kg/d in 3 doses (10mg/kg/dose), elemental iron 6mg/kg/d.

(2) Adults - FeS04 200-300mg tid, elemental iron 60mg tid.

(3) Maximal reticulocytosis occurs 7-10 days after initiation of treatment. Hgb level rises in 2-2 1/2 weeks and returns to normal after 2 months.

(4) Treat for 6 months to 1 year to replenish stores.

e. Parenteral therapy

(1) Indicated if any of the following conditions are present: small or large bowel inflammation, rapid transit GI problems, malabsorption, noncompliance with oral therapy.

(2) IM iron dextran may be given as Imferon (50mg of iron/ml) at 0.1mg/kg/dose to a maximum of 2ml/dose. Total dosage is given over 2-3 weeks, with the required dosage calculated according to the following formula: Gm iron = (Normal Hgb - pts Hgb) x 0.255. Z-track technique should be used to avoid staining of the skin with IM injection.

(3) IV iron dextran may be given as a single continuous infusion as follows:

(a) Dose (ml) = wt(kg) x (Normal Hgb - observed Hgb) x 0.0429. (Note - concentration of iron dextran is 50mg/ml)

(b) Dilute total dose in normal saline at a 1:20 dilution. Give a test dose, wait one hour. If there is no reaction, infuse the remainder of the solution slowly over several hours. Watch the patient for anaphylaxis. This dose repletes iron stores.

2. Anemia of chronic disease

a. Chronic anemia which may be hypochromic, microcytic or normochromic, normocytic. Hct rarely below 28%, unless an associated iron deficiency is present.

b. Due to chronic inflammation from a variety of causes, including autoimmune disorders, infections and cancer.

c. Improves with treatment of the underlying inflammatory process.

C. Macrocytic anemia (MCV > 100 fl)

1. General

a. Common causes of macrocytosis
   (1) Reticulocytosis
   (2) Alcoholism and liver disease
   (3) Drugs (zidovudine, hydroxyurea, methotrexate)
   (4) Hypothyroidism
   (5) Multiple myeloma

b. Suspect B12 or folate deficiency when the following are present:
   (1) Macrocytosis (even if anemia is not present).
   (2) Other unexplained hematologic abnormalities (neutropenia, thrombocytopenia).
   (3) Neurologic abnormalities (dementia).

2. B12 deficiency

a. General
   (1) Body B12 stores usually last 2-3 years.
   (2) Anemia usually develops slowly, and macrocytosis alone may occur before frank anemia develops.
   (3) Reticulocyte count is not elevated, even when the anemia is severe. Mild neutropenia and thrombocytopenia may be present.
   (4) Peripheral blood smear frequently shows hypersegmented PMNs (> 5% with 5 or more lobes) as well as macrocytosis.

b. Symptoms
   (1) Look for glossitis, stomatitis, GI symptoms, weight loss, orthostatic hypotension.
   (2) B12 deficiency, but not folate deficiency, causes a variety of neuropsychiatric abnormalities. These include impaired vibration and position sense, ataxia and abnormal gait, weakness, decreased muscle strength, spasticity, memory loss, disorientation, depression and acute confusional state. The neuropsychiatric abnormalities can occur early or late in the course of the disease, with or without hematologic abnormalities. They are less responsive to treatment, and may take months to improve, if they improve at all.

c. Diagnosis

(1) Suspect in the appropriate clinical setting.
(2) Review the peripheral smear for macrocytosis and hypersegmentation of WBC.
(3) Evaluate for pernicious anemia if possible (B12 and folate levels, intrinsic factor antibodies, Schilling test).

d. Treatment
(1) Vitamin B12 1000μg IM once a day for one week, then once a week for 4 weeks, then q month for life.
(2) Supplement with iron and folate for the first 4-6 months (phase of reticulocytosis).

3. Folate deficiency
a. Body folate stores usually last 3 months.
b. Causes
(1) Inadequate intake (meatless diet, excessive cooking or lack of green vegetables), gastric resection, pernicious anemia (atrophic gastritis), malabsorption (severe enteritis, *Giardia* infection). It is rarely due to *Diphyllobothrium latum* infection (in Asia).
(2) Increased requirements (sickle cell disease and malaria).
(3) Impaired absorption (tropical sprue, anticonvulsant drugs).

c. Diagnosis and treatment
(1) Suspect in the appropriate clinical setting. A therapeutic trial of replacement is adequate in most settings.
(2) Folic acid 1-2 mg po qd (can give 5mg po qd x 1 week to start).
(3) Treatment with folic acid can improve the anemia of vitamin B12 deficiency, but it has no effect on the neurologic symptoms, which may become irreversible if untreated. Consider treatment with both folate and B12 until a definitive diagnosis can be established.

D. Normocytic anemia
1. General
a. The early stages of most anemias are normocytic, normochromic, so there is considerable overlap in their classification.
b. Normocytic anemias can be further classified into those where there is excessive destruction or loss of RBCs (increased reticulocytosis) or faulty production of RBCs (decreased reticulocytosis).

2. Increased reticulocytosis
a. Blood loss - immediately after an acute major bleed, the hematocrit is normal. After 24 hours, hemodilution occurs, compensating for reduced blood volume, and the hematocrit falls. After 3-5 days, there is a reticulocytosis with accelerated RBC production. At this point, the cause of the anemia may be confused with hemolysis.
b. Hemolysis
(1) Intravascular (transfusion reaction, severe burns or physical trauma, G6PD) or extravascular (autoimmune with positive

    Coombs test, spherocytosis, hypersplenism).

(2) In hemolytic states, the reticulocyte count is very elevated. There is usually hyperbilirubinemia and peripheral smear shows evidence of RBC destruction.

(3) Anemia may occur with malaria due to intravascular lysis and accelerated splenic removal of parasitized RBCs, ineffective erythropoiesis and occasionally autoimmune hemolysis. A malaria smear should be done and splenomegaly looked for. Treatment is to give a curative dose of antimalarials, then prophylaxis for at least 3 months (if massive splenomegaly is present, continue prophylaxis long term). See Chapter 1, section V.

3. Decreased reticulocytosis

a. Bone marrow suppression - aplasia, acute infection, drugs, myelophthisis (leukemia, tumor, fibrosis).

b. Anemia of renal failure - caused by lack of erythropoietin. Degree of anemia is usually proportional to the degree of renal failure.

E. Sickle cell anemia

1. General

a. Produced by a substitution of a valine for glutamic acid in the structure of the hemoglobin S molecule allowing polymerization to occur in areas of low oxygen tension.

b. Sickle cell trait (Hgb AS)

  (1) Heterozygous form.

  (2) Clinical problems are rare.

  (3) The sickle prep is positive, but peripheral smear is normal. Patient is not usually anemic.

c. Sickle cell disease (Hgb SS)

  (1) Homozygous form.

  (2) Laboratory abnormalities

    (a) Sickle prep is positive.

    (b) Peripheral blood smear shows the presence of sickled RBCs. Target cells are common in SC disease.

    (c) Anemia (Hct - high teens to low 30's), leukocytosis and reticulocytosis (10-20%) may be seen.

    (d) Chronic hyperbilirubinemia may be present.

d. Clinical symptoms usually don't appear until 4-6 months of age, due to the protective effect of fetal Hgb.

2. Organs affected

a. Bone - ischemia and infarction, osteomyelitis, aseptic necrosis of the femoral head (especially with SC disease).

b. Pulmonary - thrombosis and embolism are frequent. May lead to pulmonary hypertension and right heart failure.

c. Spleen - splenomegaly disappears by age 8 in patients with SS disease.

d. Liver - hepatomegaly may occur with crises. May have significant intrahepatic cholestasis, which may be difficult to differentiate from cholecystitis (50% of adults have gallstones). Gallstones should not be removed if they are asymptomatic.

e. Cardiac - may develop cardiomegaly secondary to chronic anemia.

f. CNS - cerebral infarction and hematomas are frequent.

g. Leg ulcers - are seen frequently and may be chronic.

3. Common clinical syndromes

a. Musculoskeletal pain - vaso-occlusive crisis causing ischemic infarction of bone. Commonly involves the digits of the hands and feet (hand-foot syndrome). Besides pain, erythema, localized bone or joint tenderness and fever may be present, making it difficult to distinguish from osteomyelitis or septic arthritis. The pain may last for days. Treated with hydration and analgesics.

b. Infection - sickle cell patients have functional asplenia, and are at increased risk of infection with encapsulated organisms (*S. pneumoniae, H. flu*) and *Salmonella*. Febrile children with sickle cell disease should be treated as if they have bacterial infection and hospitalization considered. Treatment with parenteral antibiotics (ampicillin, second or third generation cephalosporin, or chloramphenicol) is often needed initially. If they are not toxic and can be followed closely, treat as outpatients with oral antibiotics (amoxicillin, amoxicillin/clavulanate). Young children should receive prophylactic penicillin from 4 months to 5 years of age: Pen VK 125-250mg bid or benzathine PCN 600,000-1.2 million units IM q 6 weeks.

c. Malaria - consider malaria prophylaxis and early malaria treatment for febrile episodes. Even though children with sickle cell trait are statistically less likely to get malaria, children with sickle cell disease can rapidly become seriously ill with severe malaria and sickling crisis. In malaria-endemic areas, febrile children with sickle cell disease should be treated presumptively for malaria as well as for bacterial infection.

d. Acute chest syndrome - caused by sequestration of RBCs in the lung. Causes chest pain, fever, respiratory distress, rales, decreased breath sounds, infiltrates. Difficult to distinguish between infarction and infection. May progress to respiratory failure and death. Treatment is with antibiotics, hydration and oxygen. If the pO2 is <75mm Hg with oxygen therapy, transfusion is indicated. Major cause of mortality especially in older patients.

e. Stroke - the most devastating form of vaso-occlusive crisis. May be recurrent. Treatment consists of regular transfusions (which are complicated by over-accumulation of iron).

f. Sequestration syndrome (6 months to 2 years of age) is due to trapping of sickled RBCs in the enlarging spleen. It may produce pallor, splenomegaly, respiratory distress, thrombocytopenia. It is treated with transfusion. Elective splenectomy may be done after age 2, if necessary.

g. Aplastic crisis - rapid decrease in Hgb and reticulocytes. Follows parvovirus B19 infection. Treatment is transfusion for Hgb <5gm or if CHF is present (maximum transfusion volume of 10-20cc/kg). May give furosemide at the time of transfusion to prevent volume overload. Rule out infection, which can also cause rapid decrease in Hgb. Supplement with folate 1-5mg/d.

F. Transfusion therapy

1. Because of the risk of transmission of HIV infection, hepatitis B and C, and other infectious agents, transfusion should be used only for life-saving purposes. The high prevalence of HIV infection in many areas, and the possibility of serotypes not identified by screening tests, increases the risk of transfusion. Locally processed blood usually is not screened extensively.

2. Transfusion is indicated if the anemia is acutely life-threatening (cardiovascular decompensation, shock) or contributing significantly to severity of concurrent respiratory infection with hypoxia. Usually not necessary until Hgb<5g.

3. Screen blood for HIV, hepatitis B and C, if possible.

4. Manage chronic anemia as outlined above.

5. Postpone elective surgical procedures until anemia is corrected.

II. EXCESSIVE BLEEDING STATES

A. General

1. Platelet disorders - commonly present with mucosal bleeding (gingival or epistaxis). Spontaneous small superficial ecchymoses occur. Excessive bleeding occurs after minor injury. Petechiae (red, non blanching macules) are present. Heavy, prolonged menstrual bleeding may occur.

2. Coagulation disorders - typically produce large, deep hematomas or hemarthrosis.

B. Coagulation tests

1. Tests commonly available include:

a. Platelet count - can be estimated on peripheral blood smear if an actual count cannot be obtained.

b. Lee White clotting time - gives an estimation of the function of the intrinsic pathway, similar to the aPTT.

c. Bleeding time - measures the time required for bleeding to stop from a shallow, standardized incision. It reflects both platelet and vascular components of coagulation. Normal with coagulation factor deficiencies except Von Willebrand disease. Abnormal in thrombocytopenia, qualitative platelet defects (uremia).

2. Tests less commonly available include:
  a. aPTT - tests the intrinsic coagulation pathway (factors XII, XI, IX, VIII). Elevated with hemophilia, DIC, use of heparin, and Von Willebrand disease.
  b. PT - tests the extrinsic coagulation pathway (factors II, V, VII, IX, X). Elevated by vitamin K deficiency, hepatic dysfunction and warfarin usage.

C. Treatment of bleeding disorders
  1. Discontinue any medication that will interfere with coagulation or platelet function. This includes cephalosporins, dipyridamole, thiazides, alcohol, quinidine, chlorpromazine, sulfonamides, isoniazid, rifampin, methyldopa, phenytoin, barbiturates, NSAIDs, and aspirin.
  2. Administer vitamin K 10mg SQ.
  3. Transfuse fresh, whole blood, if blood products (fresh frozen plasma, platelets) are not available. This will replace some of the coagulation factors and replenish any significant blood losses.

D. Thrombocytopenia - common etiologies
  1. Decreased production due to bone marrow suppression. Common causes are viral infection, alcohol abuse, or following chemotherapy. Treatment is directed at the underlying cause.
  2. Idiopathic thrombocytopenic purpura - Increased destruction of platelets
    a. Criteria for diagnosis: isolated low platelet count without other cell line abnormalities and in the absence of other causes.
    b. Etiology is thought to be antiplatelet antibodies.
    c. Most common in children 2-6 years of age. In adults, most commonly seen in women < age 40.
    d. In children, onset is usually sudden in a previously well child. Symptoms include petechiae and easy bruising. Hemorrhagic bullae of the oral mucosa may be seen.
    e. Often triggered by infection, especially viral.
    f. Platelet count is usually <20,000. Hgb, WBC and differential are usually normal.
    g. 80-90% of children recover spontaneously within 6-8 weeks. Spontaneous recovery in adults is unusual. Patients with stable platelet counts above 30,000 usually do well without treatment. Steroids (prednisone 1mg/kg/d with maximum of 60mg/d tapered over 4-6 weeks after platelet count normalizes) may be used in cases where platelet count is <10,000 or active bleeding is present.
  3. Increased sequestration of platelets occurs in patients with splenomegaly secondary to portal hypertension, or chronic malaria. Bleeding is unusual because overall platelet numbers and function are normal.

CHAPTER 9

ONCOLOGY

I. ONCOLOGY IN DEVELOPING COUNTRIES

A. General

1. Oncology is a particularly confounding problem for doctors in developing countries for the following reasons:
   a. The diagnostic and therapeutic modalities for oncology are often not available, and, if available, are very costly.
   b. There is a tremendous variability among countries and even within countries as to the type of chemotherapeutic agents available and the availability of radiation therapy.
   c. Oncology is heavily dependent on pathology evaluation, which is often unavailable or unreliable in developing countries.
2. If there are local or national standards or regimens available for cancer treatment in a given country, these should be followed as much as possible. Consultation with oncologists who may be practicing in the country could be helpful, as well.

B. Limitations

1. This section will limit itself to therapies that provide either a clear survival advantage or a clear role in palliation, and will assume a situation with either minimal pathologic interpretation or a pathologic interpretation that can be gained with variable quality slides sent back to the US, Canada or Europe.
2. Cost effectiveness of any given treatment will be determined differently than in the US. For example, adjuvant chemotherapy will not be recommended for lymph node negative breast cancer. Aggressiveness of therapy will be reduced, given the greater risk of therapeutic complications in developing countries.

II. TREATMENT OF SPECIFIC MALIGNANCIES

A. Breast cancer

1. Presentation
   a. Most patients present with a breast mass. Examine for lymph nodes in the axilla and supraclavicular area.
   b. Evaluate for enlarged liver, which may indicate metastasis.
   c. Chest x-ray and hepatic ultrasound if nodes are palpable.
2. Localized disease
   a. Primary therapy is modified radical mastectomy and axillary lymph node dissection.
   b. Goal is cure.
3. Lesions which are unresectable or where margins are involved are best treated with radiation therapy.
4. Adjuvant medical therapy is used to achieve a higher cure rate.

    a. Postmenopausal patients - tamoxifen 20mg/d for 5 years. If lymph nodes are positive, chemotherapy (below) can be added.

    b. Premenopausal patients with positive lymph nodes can receive one of the following regimens:

        (1) Cyclophosphamide 600mg/m2 plus doxorubicin 60mg/m2 q 21 days x 4 courses.

        (2) Cyclophosphamide 600mg/m2 plus methotrexate 40mg/m2 plus 5FU 600mg/m2 q 21 days x 8 courses.

        (3) Oophorectomy or tamoxifen 20mg/d x 5 years unless estrogen receptors can be evaluated and are negative or patient insists on further pregnancies at unknown risk.

        (4) Risk benefit ratio does not favor treatment of patients with negative lymph nodes in developing countries with chemotherapy unless tumors are very advanced.

  5. Metastatic disease

    a. Goal is palliation and prolongation of survival.

    b. If disease does not involve liver or lungs, or if chemotherapy is not available, hormonal therapy can be tried first with one of the following:

        (1) Tamoxifen 20mg po daily.

        (2) Progesterone (Megace 40mg po qid).

        (3) Oophorectomy in premenopausal women.

        (4) Aromatase inhibitors, such as letrozole, anastrozole.

        (5) If there is an initial response and then relapse, switch to another of the hormonal regimens.

    c. If visceral disease is present or there is failure to respond to hormonal therapy, try chemotherapy as in 4b above.

    d. Radiation therapy or surgical resection for local recurrence.

    e. Radiation therapy for pain control.

B. Cervical cancer

  1. Presentation - vaginal bleeding, discharge or pelvic pain.

  2. Evaluation

    a. Complete pelvic, rectal and abdominal exam.

    b. Check for supraclavicular lymph nodes.

    c. Chest x-ray, Pap smear and biopsy of the cervix.

  3. Treatment

    a. Goal is cure if disease is confined to the uterine cervix. Otherwise, the goal is palliation.

    b. Microinvasive disease (invasion < 3mm) - simple hysterectomy.

    c. Deeper invasion (>3mm but<4cm in diameter} - radical hysterectomy and pelvic lymphadenectomy.

    d. Diameter > 4 cm (+/- pelvic involvement) can be treated with radiation plus chemotherapy (cisplatin 40mg/m2/week during radiation) or radiation only (external and brachytherapy, if available).

    e. Metastatic disease outside the pelvis is treated with palliative care only.

C. Colorectal cancer

  1. Presentation - blood in stool, change in bowel habits, bowel obstruction with vomiting and/or abdominal pain.

  2. Evaluation

    a. Colonoscopy or barium enema.

    b. Chest x-ray.

    c. Hepatic ultrasound, if available.

  3. Treatment

    a. Primary therapy is surgical resection. Goal is cure.

    b. Adjuvant therapy may be given to achieve a higher rate of cure. It is used for lymph node positive disease, obstructing tumors or perforated tumors. One of the following regimens may be used:

      (1) 5FU 600mg/m2 plus folinic acid 200mg/m2 IV each week for 6 of 8 weeks x 4 cycles.

      (2) 5FU 425mg/m2 plus folinic acid 20mg/m2 IV daily x 5 days, q 28 days x 6 months.

      (3) 5FU 450mg/m2 daily x 5 days, then 4 weeks later 450mg/m2 weekly x 48 weeks, plus levamisole 50mg orally tid x 3 days every 2 weeks x one year.

    c. Localized bowel recurrence is treated with resection.

    d. Unresectable metastatic disease is treated with palliative care. Treat symptomatic disease with b(1) or b(2) above as long as it is effective in controlling disease.

    e. For patients with rectal cancer, radiation therapy with concurrent 5FU is recommended post-operatively in tumors that invade through the bowel wall.

D. Endometrial carcinoma

  1. Presentation - vaginal bleeding, pelvic pain, typically>50 yr old.

  2. Evaluation

    a. Diagnose with D&C, or outpatient endometrial biopsy.

    b. IVP and barium enema should be done, if available.

  3. Treatment

    a. TAH-BSO with lymph node sampling optimal. TAH-BSO alone is acceptable.

    b. Pelvic radiation if disease is outside the uterus.

    c. Palliative radiation if unresectable.

    d. Megace 40mg po qid or other progesterone as trial for palliation in advanced disease.

E. Esophageal cancer

  1. Presentation - dysphagia.

  2. Evaluation

    a. GI endoscopy or barium swallow to diagnose.

    b. Chest x-ray and upper abdominal ultrasound may be done, if available.

  3. Treatment

    a. Goal is cure if disease is confined to the esophagus. Otherwise, preservation of swallowing is the most important.

    b. Treatment measures include:

      (1) Esophagectomy

      (2) Palliative radiation

      (3) Chemotherapy concurrent with radiation. Cisplatin 75mg/m2/day and 5FU 800mg/m2 on days 1-4 by constant infusion IV or 5FU 1000mg/m2 days 1-4 alone if cisplatin not available, repeat days 28-32 of radiation.

F. Gastric carcinoma

  1. Presentation - epigastric pain, blood loss anemia.

  2. Evaluation - GI endoscopy or barium swallow.

  3. Treatment

    a. Primary therapy is resection with attempt at cure, if possible.

    b. Adjuvant therapy after resection, optimal with 5FU and folinic acid and radiation, but probably not best in developing countries given resources and toxicity.

    c. Radiation therapy may be used as palliation for pain or bleeding.

    d. Metastatic disease may be treated with the same regimen as colon cancer.

G. Gestational trophoblastic disease

  1. Presentation - vaginal bleeding in <40 yr old.

  2. Evaluation - D&C in OR; ultrasound and chest x-ray.

  3. Treatment

    a. Suction D&C with methotrexate as below.

    b. If tumor is confined to the uterus, and child bearing is completed, hysterectomy with adjuvant chemotherapy is recommended.

    c. Adjuvant chemotherapy is methotrexate 30-40mg IV weekly or actinomycin D 1.25 mg/m2 or 40 mcg/kg IV q2 wks.

    d. Metastatic disease is treated with above chemotherapy with or without hysterectomy.

H. Lung cancer

  1. Non-small cell cancer

    a. Presentation - lung mass, hemoptysis, chest pain, shortness of breath.

    b. Evaluate with chest x-ray and complete history and physical exam.

    c. Treatment

      (1) If no apparent metastases are present, surgical resection should be done with goal of cure. No adjuvant chemotherapy. Radiation therapy post-operatively if margins positive or mediastinal nodes are positive.

    (2) If disease is unresectable, but confined to the chest, cure is unlikely. Goal of therapy is prolongation of survival and palliation. Radiation therapy is indicated. If chemotherapy is available, treat before radiation with cisplatin 100mg/m2 on day 1, then vinblastine 5mg/m2 weekly x 5 weeks.

    (3) Metastatic disease is treated with palliative care.

2. Small cell cancer

  a. Presentation and evaluation - same as with non-small cell cancer.

  b. Treatment

    (1) Disease limited to the chest

      (a) Cisplatin 75mg/m2 or carboplatin 300mg/m2 (if renal function normal) on day 1 and etoposide 75mg/m2 days 1-3, repeat all every 21 days x 6 courses.

      (b) Cyclophosphamide 1000mg/m2, adriamycin 40mg/m2 and vincristine 2mg IV, repeat every 21 days x 6 courses.

      (c) Irinotecin 60 mg/m2 on day 1 and 8 with cisplatin 60 mg/m2 on day 1.

      (d) If no disease outside of the chest at completion of chemotherapy, radiate the chest and head.

    (2) Metastatic disease - same chemotherapy as above. Radiation as needed for palliation.

I. Lymphoma

1. Presentation - lymphadenopathy, fever, sweats, weight loss, abdominal pain.

2. Evaluation

  a. CBC, bone marrow biopsy to establish the diagnosis.

  b. Chest x-ray, ultrasound of the abdomen and pelvis, if available.

  c. Recommend sending lymph node slides to US, Canada or Europe for review.

3. Treatment

  a. Localized - radiation alone or chemotherapy as below.

  b. Wider spread - for low-grade lymphomas, treat when symptomatic with either chlorambucil 0.1mg/kg/day or cyclophosphamide 2mg/kg/day. Adjust doses every 2 weeks to keep WBC 3-4000 and platelets greater than 100,000.

  c. Aggressive lymphomas, including Burkitt's

    (1) Goal of therapy is cure or prolongation of survival.

    (2) If localized to one or two adjacent lymph node groups, give 3 cycles of chemotherapy 21 days apart followed by radiation therapy to the involved area. Chemotherapy agents: cyclophosphamide 750mg/m2 IV, doxorubicin 50mg/m2 (if normal cardiac function), vincristine 2 mg IV and prednisone 100mg po daily x 5 days.

(3) In cases of more widespread disease (or Burkitt's) or if radiation is unavailable, 6-8 cycles of the same chemotherapy can be given. If there is cardiac enlargement, leave out the doxorubicin.

d. Lymphoma type undetermined, treat as in 3c.

J. Hodgkin's lymphoma

1. Presentation - as with lymphoma.

2. Treatment - unless staging procedures and radiation therapy are sophisticated, it is probably best to treat as advanced disease with 6-8 cycles of one of the following chemotherapy regimens:

a. Doxorubicin 25mg/m2 IV plus bleomycin 10mg/m2 IV plus vinblastine 6 mg/m2 IV plus DTIC (dacarbazine) 375mg/m2 IV. Repeat every 2 weeks x 12 weeks.

b. Nitrogen mustard 6mg/m2 IV on day 1, vincristine 1.4mg/m2 IV on day 1 (maximum of 2 mg), procarbazine 100mg/m2 po on day 1-7 and prednisone 40mg/m2 po on days 1-14. Repeat every 28 days x 6 cycles.

K. Kaposi's sarcoma

1. Presentation - pink to purple or brown lesions on skin, often with edema in lower extremities. In AIDS, may be widely disseminated with oral cavity, lymph node, gastrointestinal or pulmonary involvement. Diagnosis is by biopsy.

2. Treatment

a. Localized lesions - surgery, radiation, cryotherapy or intralesional injection with vinblastine (0.1cc of .1mg/cc).

b. Alpha interferon 5 million units SQ 5 days a week.

c. Liposomal doxorubicin 40mg/m2 q 4 wks.

d. Paclitaxil 100mg/m2 q 3wks.

e. Doxorubicin, bleomycin, and vinblastine in the doses listed under Hodgkin's disease, but q 3 wks.

L. Acute leukemia

Treatment not recommended outside of a major city with trained hematologists.

M. Chronic lymphocytic leukemia

1. Presentation - lymphadenopathy, fatigue, fever, sweats, weight loss.

2. Evaluation - lymphocytosis, anemia, thrombocytopenia.

3. Treatment

a. Goal of therapy is control of symptoms.

b. Treat when symptoms appear, or when hemoglobin is < 10 or platelets < 100,000. Chlorambucil 0.1mg/kg/day or 0.4mg/kg every 2 weeks or cyclophosphamide 2mg/kg/day daily or 1 gram/m2 IV q 3 weeks are given until maximum response, then hold treatment until symptoms recur.

N. Chronic myelocytic leukemia

1. Presentation - fatigue, fever, sweats, splenomegaly.

2. Evaluation - leukocytosis (predominantly neutrophils).

3. Treatment

  a. Goal of therapy is control of symptoms.

  b. One of the following may be given:

    (1) Hydroxyurea 20mg/kg/day in divided doses on an empty stomach. Adjust to keep WBC between 10,000-30,000.

    (2) Busulfan 1mg/kg/day until WBC halves, then use half the dose. Check weekly CBC. Discontinue therapy when WBC < 20,000.

    (3) Interferon alpha 5 million mcg/m2/day SQ. Adjust to WBC of 2,000-3,000.

    (4) STI 571 (Gleevec) 400mg daily is the new preferred treatment, if available.

O. Multiple myeloma

  1. Presentation - bone pain, osteopenia, spontaneous fracture, hypercalcemia, anemia, renal failure.

  2. Evaluation

    a. CBC, creatinine.

    b. Metastatic bone survey with skull films.

    c. X-ray any painful areas.

  3. Treatment

    a. Melphalan 0.25mg/kg/day po x 4 days every 4-6 weeks with prednisone 100mg/day x 4 days every 4-6 weeks, or cyclophosphamide at 2mg/kg/day, continuously, adjusted to white count of 3-4,000.

    b. Dexamethasone 40mg po daily x 4 days every other week.

    c. Radiation therapy to areas of painful, destructive bone lesions.

P. Ovarian cancer

  1. Presentation - pelvic mass, pain, ascites.

  2. Evaluation - abdominal and pelvic ultrasound, chest x-ray, barium enema.

  3. Treatment

    a. TAH-BSO and omentectomy with debulking of all intra-abdominal disease to nodules of <1cm.

    b. If disease is confined to the ovary, then probably should not add adjuvant therapy in developing countries.

    c. If disease has spread outside of the ovary, treat with chemotherapy, after maximum tumor debulking. Use one of the following regimens:

      (1) Carboplatin 300mg/m2 (or AUC of 5 if renal insufficiency) + cyclophosphamide 500mg/m2.

      (2) Cisplatin 75mg/m2 + cyclophosphamide 500mg/m2.

      (3) Paclitaxil 175mg/m2 + carboplatin 300mg/m2 or cisplatin 75mg/m2.

    d. Give for six cycles at 21-28 day intervals depending on blood counts. Do not use cisplatin if creatinine >1.5.

Q. Testicular cancer
1. **Presentation** - testicular mass.
2. **Evaluation**
   a. ß-HCG, alpha fetoprotein, if available.
   b. Abdominal and pelvic ultrasound, ultrasound of the testis.
3. **Treatment**
   a. Goal of therapy is cure.
   b. Seminoma
      (1) Inguinal orchiectomy.
      (2) Lymph node positive disease below the diaphragm is treated with radiation alone if lymph nodes < 5 cm or bleomycin 30 IU/week IV day 1, 8, 15, etoposide 100mg/m2 IV day 1-5, cisplatin 20mg/m2 IV day 1-5. Repeat every 21 days for 3 cycles.
      (3) More advanced disease is treated with the same chemotherapy.
   c. Non-seminomatous
      (1) Inguinal orchiectomy with retroperitoneal lymph node dissection.
      (2) If all positive lymph nodes are resected, either observe frequently with CT scans and tumor markers or treat with 2 cycles of chemotherapy as in b2.
      (3) If residual disease after surgery, 3 cycles of the above chemotherapy may be given. Give 4 cycles of chemotherapy if there is a mediastinal primary or non-pulmonary visceral metastases.

III. OTHER
A. Cancer pain management
1. Treat disease if tumor reduction can reduce pain.
2. Begin stepwise increase in pain medication if pain is not severe:
   a. Step 1 - nonsteroidal anti-inflammatories and paracetamol (acetaminophen).
   b. Step 2 - codeine, hydrocodone, oxycodone.
   c. Step 3 - morphine, hydromorphone, methadone, fentanyl.
3. For severe pain, begin at higher levels to control pain, then reduce dosage to minimize toxicity.
4. For chronic continuous pain, it is best to use a long-acting medication to control most of the pain with short-acting medication as needed for breakthrough pain. Long-acting medication includes preparations of morphine, methadone, fentanyl.
5. Consider potentiating medication such as phenothiazines or tricyclic antidepressants. Carbamazepine or Neurontin can be used for neuropathic pain.
6. Consider ancillary procedures such as nerve blocks.
7. Avoid complications of pain medication such as nausea, constipation, drowsiness, disorientation. Use regular stool softeners. Change medication if nausea or disorientation occurs.

8. Treat underlying depression.

9. Provide hope and mission.

B. Chemotherapeutic drug toxicities

DRUG	TOXICITY
Tamoxifen	Increased risk of venous thrombosis Slight increased risk of uterine cancer Postmenopausal symptoms
Cyclophosphamide	Nausea Minor hair loss Pancytopenia
Doxorubicin and liposomal doxorubicin	Nausea, alopecia Heart damage Pancytopenia
Methotrexate	Stomatitis, pancytopenia Don't use with any renal insufficiency
5-fluorouracil	Stomatitis, diarrhea Pancytopenia
Cisplatin	Nausea Renal damage, pancytopenia
Actinomycin D	Nausea
Vinblastine	Hair loss, muscle pain Neutropenia
Carboplatin	Nausea, pancytopenia Must adjust dose for renal insufficiency
Etoposide	Alopecia Neutropenia
Chlorambucil	Minor nausea Pancytopenia
Vincristine	Neuropathy
Bleomycin	Fever, pulmonary fibrosis
DTIC (Dacarbazine)	Nausea Neutropenia
Nitrogen Mustard	Nausea Pancytopenia
Procarbazine	Nausea, confusion Pancytopenia
Hydroxyurea	Pancytopenia
Busulfan	High risk of pancytopenia, lung damage
Interferon	Fever, malaise, depression Liver damage, pancytopenia
Melphalan	Pancytopenia
Paclitaxil	Allergic reaction on administration, requires steroid premedication. Alopecia and pancytopenia
Alpha interferon	Flu-like symptoms

CHAPTER 10

NEUROLOGY

I. STROKE

A. General

1. Stroke may be defined as a focal neurologic deficit that develops secondary to alterations in cerebral blood flow.
2. Strokes are caused by ischemic infarction (from emboli or thrombi) or hemorrhage (intracerebral or subarachnoid).
3. Risk factors for stroke include hypertension, diabetes, hypercholesterolemia, atherosclerosis and smoking.

B. Embolic stroke

1. Presents with abrupt onset of symptoms that are frequently maximal early in the course. Recovery is frequently rapid.
2. More than one area of the brain may be simultaneously involved.
3. Syndromes
   a. Carotid distribution - transient blindness, transient aphasia, motor and sensory symptoms in a single extremity (upper or lower) or a clumsy hand.
   b. Vertebrobasilar - slurred speech, dizziness, ataxia, syncope, dysphagia, numbness around the lips or face, double vision. Hemiparesis and hemisensory loss do not parallel each other in the individual limb. May be bilateral motor or sensory deficits from a single lesion.

C. Thrombotic stroke

1. Large vessel disease
   a. Deficit develops in a stepwise fashion over hours or days frequently with fluctuating neurologic signs.
   b. May be preceded by warning TIAs (transient ischemic attacks).
   c. Often occurs during sleep or is present on arising in the morning.
   d. Occurs in older patients, commonly from atherosclerosis.
   e. Major syndromes
      (1) Middle cerebral artery syndrome - contralateral hemiparesis, sensory loss worse in the arm and face, expressive aphasia, homonymous hemianopsia.
      (2) Anterior cerebral artery syndrome - contralateral hemiparesis, sensory loss in the leg only, no hemianopsia or aphasia.
      (3) Posterior cerebral artery syndrome - homonymous hemianopsia, little or no paralysis.
2. Small vessel disease - lacunar infarcts
   a. Onset of symptoms is usually over hours.
   b. Common in hypertensive patients.
   c. Affects the midbrain.
   d. Common syndromes
      (1) Pure motor stroke - unilateral face, arm and leg weakness without aphasia or other cortical signs, or sensory changes.

(2) Pure sensory stroke - unilateral numbness of face, arm and leg in the absence of motor or cortical signs.

D. Intracerebral hemorrhage

1. Commonly occurs secondary to hypertension or A-V malformations.
2. Initial symptoms vary with the severity of the hemorrhage; may be catastrophic or gradually increase over minutes to hours without periods of improvement.
3. Common clinical syndromes
   a. Putamen - hemiplegia, eye deviation to side of hemorrhage, away from hemiplegia, cortical deficits, headache and often field defect. Most common.
   b. Thalamus - hemiplegia with marked sensory loss, eyes look at nose, small nonreactive pupils.
   c. Pons - comatose, pinpoint pupils, quadriparesis with up-going toes; usually fatal.
   d. Cerebellar - headache, vomiting, ataxia without paresis or loss of consciousness.

E. Subarachnoid hemorrhage

1. Usually results from rupture of aneurysms or A-V malformations.
2. Onset of symptoms is abrupt and associated with severe headache, vomiting, and loss of consciousness without lateralizing signs.
3. Most common cause of stroke in younger patients.
4. May occur during physical activity (sex).
5. A minority of patients experience a prior "sentinel headache".
6. Bleeding may produce intense vasospasm resulting in ischemic infarction.

F. Risk factors for stroke

1. Hypertension is the most important risk factor in all types of stroke. Treatment substantially reduces the risk.
2. Atherosclerotic risk factors (diabetes, cigarette smoking, hyperlipidemia) increase the likelihood of thrombotic and embolic stroke.
3. Valvular heart disease and atrial fibrillation increase the likelihood of embolic stroke.
4. Sickle cell disease is commonly associated with ischemic stroke.
5. Vasculitis should be considered in younger patents.
6. Bleeding disorders and anticoagulant therapy increase the likelihood of intracranial hemorrhage.

G. Evaluation

1. History and thorough physical exam with detailed neurologic exam. Consider other causes of symptoms, such as hypoglycemia, seizures, migraine, subdural hematoma, tumor.
2. Laboratory tests should include CBC, sed rate, glucose, electrolytes, clotting studies, ECG, chest x-ray. If available, CT scan of the head is helpful. Initially, it will show if a hemorrhage is present. It usually takes a day to become positive after a completed ischemic stroke.

3. Lumbar puncture should be done if subarachnoid hemorrhage is suspected (and CT unavailable or non-diagnostic).

H. Treatment

1. Hypertension - in ischemic stroke, avoid lowering the BP in the first 10 days unless diastolic BP is >120mm Hg. In hemorrhagic strokes, the systolic blood pressure should be maintained at less than 160 mmHg.
2. Vomiting is common and NG suction may be helpful. Patients with facial weakness and impaired gag reflexes should be kept NPO initially.
3. Avoid over-hydration.
4. Anticoagulation is indicated for progressive stroke (stroke in evolution) or frequent, recurrent TIAs only if cerebral hemorrhage can be ruled out with a CT scan. Give heparin 5000-10,000 unit bolus IV, then 1000-2000 units/hr IV to keep the PTT or clotting time 1.5-2.0 x normal.
5. Patients with intracranial hemorrhage may be helped by treatment with calcium channel blockers, especially nimodipine 30mg q6h, if started in the first 12-24h.
6. Observe the patient closely for progression of neurologic defects.
   a. Cerebral edema is maximal at 3-4 days and is more severe with large strokes.
   b. Bleeding into infarcts occurs commonly and may contribute to progression of symptoms.
   c. Watch for headache, nausea and vomiting.
   d. Treat with steroids (dexamethasone 4 mg q 6 hrs) or diuretics (mannitol or furosemide IV).
7. Begin passive range of motion exercises 3-4x/d within 24-48h after the stroke.

I. Prevention

1. Treatment of risk factors (smoking, hypertension, diabetes, hyperlipidemia) has been shown to prevent stroke in patients with underlying hypertension and in those who have already had a stroke.
2. TIA
   a. Aspirin 325mg po qd has been shown to reduce occurrence of subsequent stroke.
   b. Ticlopidine 250mg bid is better than aspirin.
   c. Carotid endarterectomy is superior to medical therapy for reducing subsequent stroke in patients with TIA or mild stroke in the hemisphere supplied by a carotid artery with 70-99% stenosis. No benefit of endarterectomy in patients with vertebrobasilar ischemia or infarction.
3. Anticoagulation with low dose warfarin should be considered in patients with non-valvular as well as valvular atrial fibrillation, if possible.
4. Asymptomatic carotid artery stenosis (asymptomatic carotid bruits) - control risk factors. Aspirin 325mg po qd may be of benefit.

II. SEIZURES
A. General
1. Seizures result from excessive electrical activity in the cerebral cortex.
2. Primary epilepsy - recurrent seizures without known etiology.
3. Consider the following secondary causes of seizures:
   a. Cerebral malaria
   b. Meningitis
   c. Hypoxia
   d. Hypoglycemia
   e. Head trauma
   f. Alcohol or drug withdrawal
4. Febrile seizures (see Chapter 14, section III, B, 3, e)
   a. Are most common at 12-18 months of age, and are rare after age six.
   b. Occur when the temperature is greater than 38° C., frequently when the temperature is increasing rapidly.
   c. Are usually benign, and do not require anticonvulsant medication.
   d. In children with a history of febrile seizures, treat any temperature elevation promptly with antipyretics.

Seizures		
Type	**Characteristics**	**Treatment**
Grand-mal (tonic/clonic)	Tonic-clonic activity with LOC Patient falls, becomes rigid, rhythmic jerking of extremities	Phenytoin Carbamazepine Phenobarbital Valproic acid
Petit-mal (absence)	Brief LOC without loss of postural tone School-age children	Valproic acid Ethosuximide
Partial - simple	No alteration in consciousness Affects motor, sensory, visual or olfactory areas	Carbamazepine Phenytoin Valproic acid Phenobarbital in children
Partial - complex (temporal lobe)	Consciousness or mentation affected May have automatic behaviors, psychiatric features	Carbamazepine Phenytoin Valproic acid Phenobarbital in children

B. Classification
1. **Generalized seizures** (begin with loss of consciousness)
   a. Grand mal (tonic-clonic) - abrupt loss of consciousness, patient becomes rigid and falls. May become apneic and have urinary or fecal incontinence. Rigid (tonic) phase is followed by rhythmic (clonic) jerking of all extremities. Consciousness returns gradually with postictal confusion and fatigue.
   b. Petit mal (absence) - brief (few second) loss of consciousness without loss of postural tone or incontinence. Patients may stare, have

twitching of the eyelids, not respond to stimulation. Cease abruptly with no postictal symptoms. May occur multiple times daily. Usually occur only in school-age children.

2. Partial (focal) seizures

    a. Simple - no alteration of consciousness. Seizure pattern is determined by the site of the electrical discharge (motor, sensory, visual, olfactory).

    b. Complex (psychomotor or temporal lobe) - focal seizure in which consciousness or mentation is affected. Often occur in the temporal lobe causing bizarre symptoms with psychiatric features (hallucinations, memory disturbances, automatisms, dream-like states).

C. Evaluation

    1. History - determine if a seizure has occurred (LOC, tonic-clonic activity, loss of control of bowel or bladder, post-ictal state), type of seizure, prior history of seizures.

    2. Physical exam - look for injuries occurring as a result of the seizure and for any secondary causes of the seizure. Include a thorough neurologic exam. Check vital signs, especially blood pressure. Seizure may be the presenting symptom in acute hypertension.

    3. Laboratory - CBC, electrolytes, glucose, creatinine, and calcium should be checked at the time of a first seizure. Laboratory studies (except drug levels) are usually not necessary in patients with a history of seizures and no signs of intercurrent illness. CT scan and EEG should be done at the time of initial evaluation, if available. Lumbar puncture is indicated in cases of suspected meningitis. Malaria smear should be done in febrile patients with seizure.

D. Acute treatment of seizures

    1. Avoid trauma - lay patient on side, on the ground or a bed, away from walls.

    2. Maintain airway by turning face to side and downward. It is not necessary to put a tongue blade or other object in the mouth. Suction secretions, if possible. Administer oxygen, if available.

    3. Give medication (diazepam or paraldehyde) if seizure lasts longer than 10 minutes.

    4. Obtain laboratory studies, if indicated.

    5. Patients with status epilepticus (seizure activity lasting longer than 30 minutes or in which there is incomplete recovery between recurrent seizures) should be treated with diazepam or paraldehyde, as above, as well as another anticonvulsant (loading dose of phenobarbital or phenytoin). If seizures continue, a second dose of phenobarbital 10mg/kg may be given after 20 minutes. Phenobarbital may be given IM, if venous access is not possible.

    6. Status epilepticus may occur with any primary or secondary cause of seizures listed above.

Anticonvulsant Drugs		
Drug	**Dosage**	**Comments**
Diazepam**	Acute seizure: 0.3 mg/kg slow IV (not to exceed 2 mg/min) Rectal dose: 0.5 mg/kg	Repeated doses may cause respiratory depression.
Carbamazepine	Children: 5-10 mg/kg/d up to 20-30mg/kg/d div. 2-4x/d Adults: 200mg bid up to 400-1200mg/d div. 2-4x/d	May cause drowsiness, dizziness, nausea, vomiting
Paraldehyde*	0.2 ml/kg deep IM Rectal dose 0.4 ml/kg	Dosed in ml/kg not mg.
Phenobarbital	Children - loading dose: 10-20mg/kg/dose IV or IM (1mg/kg/min). Maintenance: 5-8 mg/kg/d in 1-2 doses. Adults - loading dose: 300-800mg IV (1mg/kg/min) Maintenance: 120-150mg/d Do not use for seizure prophylaxis in cerebral malaria (see note)	May cause drowsiness, respiratory depression, rash
Phenytoin	Children - loading: 15-20mg/kg (not to exceed 1 mg/kg/min) Maintenance dose: 5 mg/kg Adults - loading: 10-15 mg/kg (usual dose - 1gm IV) (max rate of administration - 50mg/min). Maintenance: 5 mg/kg/d (3-400 mg/d)	May cause nystagmus, ataxia, gingival hyperplasia, hepatotoxicity, pancytopenia
Valproic acid	Children > 10 yrs, adults: 10-15mg/kg/d div. 3x/d up to 30-60mg/kg/d div. 3x/d. Usual adult dose: 1000-2500 mg/day	May cause nausea, drowsiness, hepatotoxicity, bone marrow suppression

* Note paraldehyde is dosed in ml, not mg. Paraldehyde will cause deterioration of plastic, however plastic syringes can be used for administration if the drug is drawn up and used immediately. The syringe must be discarded after use. Paraldehyde causes less respiratory depression than diazepam and is safer if repeated doses are required.
** Intramuscular administration of diazepam and phenytoin is not recommended because of unreliable/delayed absorption.

E. Long-term management of seizures
1. Family education.
2. Avoidance of activities which increase risk of injury with convulsion (tree-climbing, swimming, driving, operating machinery).
3. Chronic anticonvulsant medication is indicated if seizures are frequent or severe or if they significantly impair normal activity and development.
4. Start with a single drug. If it is not effective in controlling seizures, switch to a second drug. If seizures still uncontrolled, give two drugs together. Measure serum drug levels, if available.
5. Consider discontinuing anticonvulsants only after at least a 2 year seizure-free period.

F. Management of seizures in severe malaria

1. Check for and treat hypoglycemia.
2. Control hyperpyrexia. If the rectal temperature is > 39°C. specific measures to reduce body temperature are indicated (oral or rectal paracetamol or acetaminophen and cooling).
3. A single brief seizure does not require anticonvulsant therapy. For prolonged or recurrent seizures, diazepam and paraldehyde are the initial drugs of choice.
4. Prevention of seizures - phenobarbital has been used prophylactically in children with cerebral malaria. However, recent studies raise concerns about efficacy and increased mortality in children receiving prophylactic phenobarbital. Until further studies clarify the role of prophylactic phenobarbital, it can no longer be recommended for routine use. Since the manifestations of seizure activity can be subtle and covert status epilepticus has been demonstrated in children with cerebral malaria, vigilance and a low threshold for initiating anticonvulsant therapy is essential. Children with persistent minor twitching (even if restricted to a single muscle or muscle group), nystagmus and salivation should be treated for seizures according to the same protocols as those with full blown tonic-clonic convulsions.

III. HEADACHE

A. Types

1. **Migraine** - unilateral, throbbing headache, aggravated by physical activity. May be accompanied by nausea, vomiting, photophobia. Scotomata, focal transient sensory changes may precede development of headache by minutes to hours (aura). Fatigue and changes in the weather may provoke a migraine headache.
2. **Tension** - pressing/tightness quality of pain with mild or moderate intensity (doesn't prohibit activities), bilateral location, not aggravated by physical activity. Nausea and vomiting are usually absent.
3. **Cluster** - severe, unilateral, penetrating, non-throbbing pain, usually felt behind the eye. Pain has maximal intensity 2-15 min. after onset, waning over 30-60 minutes. Regular recurrence 1-2x/d for 4-8 weeks. Usually associated with ipsilateral Horner syndrome, lacrimation, nasal stuffiness and rhinorrhea. Alcohol may trigger an attack. Uncommon type of headache.
4. **Post lumbar puncture** - usually bilateral, pulsatile, worse in the upright position. Usually occipital or cervical location.
5. **Other** - headaches may be secondary to sinus infection, allergic disease (frontal headache), dental disease, ear infection (facial pain), fatigue, stress, meningitis, malaria, hypertension, trauma (generalized headache) or intracranial disease (frontal or occipital headache present with arising in the morning, associated with neurologic deficits).

B. Evaluation

1. **History** - ask about the following:
   a. Age at onset
   b. Frequency, pattern
   c. Location, character
   d. Duration and course
   e. Auras and associated symptoms
   f. Neurologic symptoms
   g. Precipitating factors
   h. Family history

2. **Physical exam**
   a. Check BP.
   b. Funduscopic exam.
   c. Facial tenderness (sinuses, temporal arteries).
   d. Neck stiffness.
   e. Screening neurologic exam - check for asymmetry in the following: cranial nerves, heel and toe walking, squatting, Romberg, gait, finger-to-nose, reflexes.

3. **Laboratory**
   a. No tests are needed if the diagnosis is clear after the history and physical.
   b. CBC, sed rate if meningitis or temporal arteritis are suspected.
   c. LP to rule out meningitis or subarachnoid hemorrhage.
   d. CT scan, if available, is helpful in evaluating patients with headache which is either very severe, or "the worst headache" the patient has ever had. These patients have a higher chance of having a subarachnoid hemorrhage.

C. Treatment

1. **Migraine headache**
   a. Abortive therapy - any of the following may be tried: NSAIDs, prochlorperazine or chlorpromazine, metoclopramide, sumatriptan, narcotic analgesics.
   b. Prophylaxis - propranolol, amitriptyline, verapamil may be effective. Treat for at least three months to determine effectiveness.

2. **Tension-type**
   a. Nonnarcotic analgesics - paracetamol (acetaminophen), NSAIDs.
   b. Amitriptyline, if the headache is chronic.

3. **Cluster headache.**
   a. Acute - oxygen at 5-8L/min for 10 minutes may resolve the headache. Treatment as for migraines may be tried if oxygen is unsuccessful.
   b. Prophylaxis - verapamil 120mg tid, prednisone 80mg/d x 7d, then taper over 7d. If headache persists >48h, discontinue. If it recurs while tapering, increase the dose.

IV. DIZZINESS
A. Definitions
1. **Dizziness** - nonspecific, subjective term used to indicate a sensation of weakness, unsteadiness, instability, or faintness.
2. **Vertigo** - illusion of motion where no motion exists. Occurs due to peripheral or brainstem dysfunction.
3. **Disequilibrium** - feeling of imbalance or unsteadiness while walking. May be produced by decreased sensory input (decreased vision, peripheral neuropathy) associated with aging.
4. **Syncope and near syncope** - "gray out" feeling which may progress to loss of consciousness. Common causes are vasovagal syncope, orthostatic hypotension, or arrhythmias.

B. Evaluation
1. **History**
   a. Establish which of the above symptoms best describes the patient's feeling.
   b. Determine relationship to movement, head position, lying, standing.
   c. Ask about duration of symptoms, history of trauma and medications.
   d. Note any associated symptoms such as nausea, vomiting, visual changes, tinnitus, weakness, numbness, palpitations, or loss of consciousness.
2. **Physical examination** - should include attention to the following:
   a. Ears and hearing acuity (whispered voice).
   b. Eye movement (testing for spontaneous and positional nystagmus).
   c. Cranial nerve testing.
   d. Coordination (Romberg, finger-to-nose).
   e. Gait
   f. Heart rhythm and murmurs.
3. **Laboratory testing** - should be based on the history and physical exam.

C. Differential diagnosis
1. **Vertigo**
   a. Peripheral vertigo (vestibular nerve or inner ear) - characterized by intense whirling feeling, often associated with nausea, vomiting, sweating, and diarrhea. Usually abrupt in onset, affected by movement or changes in position. Symptoms are transient. There may be tinnitus or hearing loss. Nystagmus testing shows fatigable, unidirectional nystagmus, which is inhibited by ocular fixation.
   (1) Benign positional vertigo - most common. Episodes are brief in duration, but are usually recurrent. Symptoms are associated with head movement, or change in body position. Symptoms are usually brief. Drug treatment is usually not indicated.
   (2) Viral labyrinthitis - acute onset of vertigo with nausea, vomiting, bilateral tinnitus and decreased hearing. Usually follows a viral URI. Lasts 1-4 days. Treat symptomatically with meclizine.

(3) Ménière's disease - recurrent episodes of severe vertigo, nausea, vomiting, unilateral tinnitus and progressive hearing loss. Low-sodium diet and thiazide diuretics may be helpful.

   b. Central vertigo - much less intense vertigo, not exacerbated by motion or position. Usually has little or no associated nausea, vomiting, or diaphoresis. There is non-fatigable, multi-directional nystagmus, not inhibited by ocular fixation. Caused by conditions affecting the cerebellum and brain stem. May have other neurologic signs associated with the vertigo. Causes of central vertigo include:

     (1) Cerebellar infarction or hemorrhage.

     (2) Vertebrobasilar insufficiency.

     (3) Acoustic neuroma (cerebellopontine angle tumor) - slow, steady increase in vertigo associated with unilateral neurosensory hearing loss.

     (4) Multiple sclerosis.

2. Other causes of dizziness

   a. Disequilibrium syndrome - usually occurs in elderly patients with diminished vision, hearing or peripheral neurologic function. Exacerbated by unfamiliar surroundings.

   b. Near syncope - should be evaluated as in patients with syncope. Consider hypoglycemia, orthostatic hypotension, vasovagal and drug effects, cardiac arrhythmias, peripheral neuropathy.

   c. Hyperventilation - patient may be able to reproduce their symptoms with directed hyperventilation.

V. ALTERED MENTAL STATUS

A. Delirium

1. General

   a. Alteration in the ability to think with customary speed and clarity.

   b. Principle features include an alteration in level of consciousness, change in cognition, onset over short period of time, and fluctuation in mental functioning over the course of day.

   c. Commonly occurs in older patients in response to stress of major illness (especially common in the post-operative period), sensory deprivation, or use of multiple drugs (especially psychoactive agents).

2. Etiology

   a. CNS origin - trauma, seizures, infections, nutritional problems, mass lesions, dementing diseases.

   b. Toxic-metabolic disorders - disorders of fluids and electrolytes (volume depletion, hypo or hypernatremia, hypo- or hypercalcemia), drug intoxication and withdrawal, and metabolic encephalopathies.

3. Evaluation

   a. Do a thorough history and physical examination. Evaluate the patient's orientation to time, place and person and knowledge of generally available information. Neurologic exam is usually unremarkable. Presence of asterixis is suggestive of metabolic encephalopathy.

   b. Laboratory studies: CBC, glucose, electrolytes, urinalysis, malaria smear, lumbar puncture, chest x-ray.

4. Treatment - treat according to likely cause.

   a. Correct underlying metabolic abnormalities.

   b. Discontinue medication whenever possible, since medication is frequently a cause of confusional states.

   c. Treat infection, if present.

   d. Antipsychotics (haloperidol 0.5-1mg) are effective in treating acute confusional states. Sedative-hypnotic agents (such as benzodiazepines, barbiturates, or chloral hydrate) should not be used as they may exacerbate the confusion.

B. Coma

1. General

   a. Definition - lack of responsiveness to stimulation or to the surrounding environment.

   b. Most common causes of obtundation are endogenous or exogenous toxins.

2. Differential diagnosis

   a. No focal neurologic signs

     (1) Metabolic - hypoglycemia, uremia, DKA, hyperosmolar hyperglycemic nonketotic syndrome, hepatic coma, hypothyroidism (myxedema coma).

     (2) Respiratory - hypoxia.

     (3) Intoxication

     (4) Infectious - malaria, sepsis, pneumonia, typhoid fever.

     (5) Shock

     (6) Seizure disorder.

     (7) Hypertensive encephalopathy.

   b. Meningeal irritation with no focal neurologic signs

     (1) Meningitis

     (2) Subarachnoid hemorrhage.

   c. Focal signs

     (1) CVA

     (2) Subdural/epidural hemorrhage.

     (3) Brain abscess.

3. Evaluation

   a. Examine patient for evidence of trauma.

   b. The anatomic level of neurologic impairment can be assessed by evaluating state of consciousness, pupils, eye movements, respirations, and motor function. Deterioration in neurologic function follows a rostral-caudal progression (cerebral cortex, diencephalon, midbrain, pons and medulla).

	Motor response to pain	Pupils	Extraocular movement	Respirations
Diencephalon	Spontaneous movements to loud clap; limb withdrawal to deep pain; decorticate posturing	Small, reactive	Doll's eye reflexes	Normal or Cheyne-Stokes
Mesencephalon	Decerebrate posturing	Unresponsive	Need cold-calories to elicit Doll's eye reflexes	Hyperventilation
Pons	Flaccid tone	Unresponsive	No response	Apneustic respiratory rhythm
Medulla	Flaccid tone	Unresponsive	No response	Ataxic/irregular respirations, respiratory arrest

    c. Laboratory - CBC, electrolytes, BUN, creatinine, glucose, calcium, magnesium, liver enzymes. Drug screen, ABGs, if available.

    d. Lumbar puncture if meningitis or subarachnoid hemorrhage suspected.

    e. Assess using the Glasgow Coma Scale (See Chapter 20, page 428). Useful especially in trauma cases.

  4. Immediate treatment

    a. Assess airway, breathing and circulation. Intubate the patient to protect the airway if no gag reflex is present.

    b. Position the patient to prevent aspiration. Protect the cervical spine in cases where trauma is involved.

    c. Check fingerstick glucose, if possible.

    d. Rapidly administer the following medication, if the cause of the coma is not readily obvious:

      (1) Thiamine 100mg IV.

      (2) Glucose 25-50gm IV (D50W).

      (3) Naloxone 2mg IV (0.1mg/kg), if narcotic ingestion is suspected. Repeat with 4 mg if there is no response.

  5. Treat the underlying cause when identified.

C. Dementia

  1. Definition

    a. Nonspecific, progressive deterioration in intellectual and cognitive functioning. Usually an irreversible process. Involves memory, abstract thinking, judgment, personality, and language.

    b. Differentiate from delirium, which is an acute deterioration in mental status from a previously stable baseline.

  2. Evaluation

    a. Mini-mental status exam - establish if cognitive function is impaired.

b. Physical exam may show frontal release signs (grasp, snout, suck), loss of inhibitions, depression.

c. Laboratory (to look for treatable causes) - CBC, electrolytes, BUN, calcium, thyroid tests. Others to consider are B12, VDRL, liver function tests, sed rate, ECG, chest x-ray, head CT, lumbar puncture.

3. Differential diagnosis (DEMENTIA)

    a. D epression

    b. E ndocrine (T3, T4, TSH)

    c. M etabolic (electrolytes, Ca, phosphorus, Mg, BUN, creatinine, LFTs)

    d. E tOH (+ meds + drugs)

    e. N utritional (B12, folate), normal pressure hydrocephalus (CT)

    f. T rauma, tumor (CT)

    g. I nfections (VDRL)

    h. A lzheimer's (psychologic testing, EEG)

4. Treatment

    a. Supportive care.

    b. Rule out other causes of altered mental status.

VI. PARKINSON'S DISEASE

A. Clinical

1. Progressive, chronic disorder resulting from atrophy or destruction of areas within the basal ganglia.

2. May be secondary to neuroleptic drugs (usually reversible), but most cases are idiopathic.

3. Manifestations

    a. Gait disturbance - slow, shuffling gait, with rapid propulsion forward and an inability to stop.

    b. Tremor - fine, resting tremor (pill-rolling).

    c. Rigidity of the musculature (cog wheeling on passive movement).

    d. Dementia

    e. Depressed affect.

4. Laboratory - no specific tests are helpful. Diagnosis is made clinically.

B. Treatment

1. Discontinue neuroleptic agents.

2. Selegiline (Eldepryl) 5mg po bid seems to slow progression of the disease and should be given to all patients initially, if available.

3. Begin antiparkinsonian agents when the patient is symptomatic (will develop tolerance over time). Purpose of treatment is to enhance dopaminergic transmission or inhibit cholinergic transmission.

4. Anticholinergic drugs (useful for mild disease; control tremor and reduce rigidity).

    a. Biperiden 1mg PO tid-qid, max 16mg/day.

    b. Trihexyphenidyl (Artane) 2mg po tid up to 5mg tid.

    c. Benztropine (Cogentin) 1mg/d up to 5mg/d.

d. Diphenhydramine (Benadryl) - weak agent.

5. Amantadine (Symmetrel) 100mg bid-tid. May be used alone in early disease.

6. Levodopa + carbidopa (Sinemet) 25/250 tid-qid. Can start with 10/100mg tab tid, increase q2d until improved or side effects occur. Maximum dose 50/500 qid. Sinemet is the most potent drug available for advanced Parkinson's disease. Clinical fluctuations, "wearing off" and/or dyskinesia may benefit from the addition of amantadine or anti-cholinergic drugs.

7. Bromocriptine 1.25mg bid up to 10 - 20mg/d with increases q 2 weeks.

8. Special considerations:

a. Tricyclic antidepressants can be used for patients with depression who are on L-dopa. MAO inhibitors not recommended.

b. Phenothiazines, haloperidol, reserpine aggravate Parkinsonian syndrome.

c. Pyridoxine antagonizes the effect of L-dopa, but not Sinemet.

d. Methyldopa (Aldomet) may potentiate or antagonize the effects of L-dopa.

VII. NEUROPATHIES

A. Mononeuropathy

1. Involves a single peripheral nerve.

2. Commonly due to trauma (eg: pressure injury as in radial, or common peroneal nerve compression).

3. Entrapment syndromes include:

a. Carpal tunnel syndrome

(1) From median nerve entrapment (C6-T1).

(2) Symptoms - pain in wrist and arm, especially at night, paresthesias in thumb and first three fingers, weakness and atrophy of thenar muscles.

(3) Treatment- wrist splints or steroid injections may be helpful.

(4) Surgery with medial nerve release may be required in severe cases.

b. Ulnar nerve entrapment (C8-T1)

(1) Paresthesias over fourth and fifth fingers. Later, may produce claw hand deformity.

(2) Treatment is difficult and surgery is not always helpful.

c. Lateral femoral cutaneous nerve (L2-L3)

(1) Produces paresthesias and numbness over the lateral thigh associated with obesity, wearing tight clothing or heavy tool belts.

(2) Treatment is mainly eliminating aggravating factors.

B. Mononeuropathy multiplex

1. Random involvement of multiple nerves, sensory or motor.

2. Occurs secondary to other medical diseases - diabetes, vasculitis or infection (HIV, leprosy).
3. Treatment depends on the underlying cause.

C. Polyneuropathy

1. Bilateral, symmetrical involvement of the peripheral nerves, usually affecting legs more than arms, and distal segments earlier and more severely than proximal ones (stocking-glove pattern). May produce changes in reflexes, vibratory sense and proprioception.
2. Commonly associated with diabetes, B-vitamin deficiencies, and HIV disease.
3. Treatment consists of adequate vitamin replacement. Symptomatic improvement may be obtained with tricyclic antidepressants (amitriptyline) or anticonvulsants (carbamazepine).

D. Radiculopathy

1. Symptoms are due to compression of spinal nerve roots.
2. Commonly due to herniation of intervertebral disc.
3. Less frequently associated with degenerative disease of spine (osteoarthritis), epidural abscess or tumor.
4. Treatment depends on the underlying cause.

CHAPTER 11

RHEUMATOLOGY

I. MONOARTICULAR ARTHRITIS
A. Etiology
1. Definition - pain localized in a single joint.
2. Most common etiologies include trauma, infection, or crystal disease (gout or pseudogout). The differential diagnosis is broad and includes the causes of polyarticular disease. See below.
3. The presence of synovitis (inflammation of the lining of the joint) indicates an inflammatory process and is characterized by swelling, pain, erythema, warmth, and decreased range of motion of the joint. Joint effusion may be present.
4. It is critical to rule out infectious arthritis.

Differential Diagnosis of Acute Arthritis Syndromes			
Etiology	Acute Monoarticular	Chronic Monoarticular	Polyarticular Arthritis
Infectious Causes	*Staphylococcus aureus* *Strep. pneumoniae* Group A Streptococcus Other Streptococci *Neisseria gonorrheae* *Salmonella* Other Gram negative bacilli	Mycobacterial tuberculous Non-tuberculous Fungal *Sporothrix* *Cryptococcus* *Blastomycosis* Bacterial *Nocardia* *Brucella* *Treponema pallidum* *Borrelia*	Bacterial *Neisseria meningitidis* *Neisseria gonorrhea* Viral Hepatitis B HIV Rubella Parvovirus B19
Non-infectious causes	Gout Pseudogout Fracture Hemarthrosis	Osteoarthritis	Reactive arthritis Serum sickness Rheumatic fever Rheumatoid arthritis Systemic lupus Sickle cell flare and others......

B. Infectious arthritis
1. Septic arthritis (bacterial)
   a. Infectious arthritis usually follows hematogenous inoculation of organisms into the joint, or extension of a focus of osteomyelitis into the joint space.

(1) In children less than one year of age and adults, osteomyelitis can extend across the epiphysis into the joint. In children older than one year, until closure of the epiphysis, the epiphysis acts as a barrier to the extension of osteomyelitis and secondary septic arthritis occurs only in those joints where a portion of the metaphysis is inside the joint capsule (elbow, shoulder, hip).

(2) Less commonly, septic arthritis is caused by penetrating trauma (particularly bite wounds of the hand). Intra-articular steroid injections can introduce bacteria into joints if there is a break in sterile technique.

b. Clinical presentation

(1) Pain, swelling, and limited range of motion due to joint effusion are key signs of septic arthritis. Detection of effusion in the shoulders and hips is difficult due to the deep location of these joints.

(2) Systemic features of infection are frequently present.

(3) Pyogenic bacteria typically cause acute onset of symptoms while arthritis due to mycobacteria or fungi (most commonly *Sporothrix*) have a more indolent presentation.

(4) Disseminated gonorrhea infection causes an immune mediated polyarticular arthritis accompanied by tenosynovitis and hemorrhagic skin lesions. Cultures of the joint fluid are negative. True septic gonococcal arthritis can follow unrecognized disseminated gonococcemia and typically involves a single large joint. Gram-negative diplococci are only occasionally detectable in joint fluid on Gram stain. In a sexually active young adult, *Neisseria gonorrheae* is the most common cause of acute monoarticular arthritis.

(5) The knee is the most commonly affected joint in both adults and children, in both acute pyogenic and mycobacterial arthritis.

(6) Infection of small joints of the hands suggests *Neisseria gonorrhea*, mycobacteria or septic arthritis secondary to bite wound.

(7) The sacroiliac joint is a common site for pyogenic arthritis due to *Brucella* but is also commonly infected by *Staphylococcus aureus* and streptococci.

(8) In cultures where young children are carried on the back, there is a high incidence of septic shoulder if children are picked up and transferred to the mother's back by holding the child's upper arm.

(9) *Salmonella* arthritis is common in children (particularly in Africa) and, unlike osteomyelitis, is not related to sickle cell anemia.

c. Diagnosis

(1) Joint aspiration and examination of synovial fluid is essential in diagnosis.

Synovial Fluid Analysis				
	Normal	**Bacterial Infections**	**Inflammatory Arthritis**	**Traumatic**
Appearance	Clear, pale yellow Viscous	Cloudy, purulent Serosanguinous (20%) Low viscosity	Translucent or opaque, yellow Low viscosity	Pink-red, opaque, low viscosity
WBC	< 200/mm³ < 25% neutrophils	> 50,000/mm³ > 75% neutrophils	2,000-75,000/mm³ 50-100 neutrophils	<200/mm³
Glucose (fluid to serum ratio)	90-100%	< 50% (poor sensitivity & specificity)	40-90%	100%
Gram stain	Negative	50% positive	Negative	Negative
Culture	Negative	90% positive (*N. gonorrhea*: 50%)	Negative	Negative

d. Treatment

  (1) Drainage - acute bacterial infection of the joint space causes rapid destruction of the articular cartilage due to direct invasion by bacteria, the presence of enzymes and inflammatory substances released from neutrophils, and increased intra-articular pressure. Drainage is an essential component of management of septic joints to remove bacteria and inflammatory mediators and reduce intra-articular pressure. In most cases needle aspiration will suffice. Repeated aspiration is needed if the fluid re-accumulates. Surgical arthrotomy is usually necessary for septic arthritis of the hip and for those joints where repeated needle aspirations fail to control the effusion.

  (2) Antibiotics - empiric antibiotic choices should follow those used in hematogenous osteomyelitis.

    (a) Results of the Gram stain of joint fluid can be used to guide the initial antibiotic choices. Initial treatment should be with parenteral antibiotics. The duration of therapy varies depending on the organism:

      Staphylococcus aureus and Gram negative bacilli - 4 wk.

      Hemophilus Streptococci - 2 wk.

      Neisseria - 1 wk.

    (b) Intra-articular injection of antibiotics is unnecessary and not recommended.

    (c) Arthritis due to *Neisseria gonorrheae* will need to take into consideration local resistance patterns; where available, ceftriaxone or cefotaxime are recommended until local and systemic signs are resolving. Therapy can be completed with oral ciprofloxacin or cefixime.

2. Septic bursitis

a. Most commonly affects the olecranon and pre-patellar bursas.

b. Patients present with a painful, erythematous swelling overlying the bursa, often mistaken for cellulitis. Since the infection does not involve the joint space, range of motion is well preserved and relatively painless. Fluid may be detectable within the bursa on examination. Aspiration of the bursa yields pus.

c. Etiology

(1) *Staphylococcus aureus* causes 95% of acute cases.

(2) Chronic cases may be caused by atypical mycobacteria or fungi.

d. Treatment - drainage is important and may need to be repeated. Repeated needle aspiration is preferable to placement of a drain, which may promote secondary infection. Anti-staphylococcal antibiotics should be given in acute cases (cloxacillin, cefazolin, clindamycin, TMP/SMX). Treatment duration is 3 weeks.

3. Viral synovitis

a. Viral infections commonly cause arthralgias but true joint inflammation is much less frequent.

b. Viral arthritis can occur as a major clinical manifestation of infection as in Chikungunya (East Africa, India), O'nyong-nyong (East Africa), Barmah Forest Virus and Ross River virus (Australia), as a common but not characteristic feature (rubella, mumps, hepatitis B) or as an unusual manifestation of infection (varicella, measles).

c. Joint aspiration will show normal glucose and lymphocyte predominance in the synovial fluid.

C. Gout

1. Definition

a. An acute arthritis resulting from the deposition of crystals of sodium urate in the joints and tendons.

b. Symptoms are usually recurrent and can become chronic with development of deformities over time.

2. Acute gout

a. Usually presents with a monoarticular arthritis involving the first MTP joint (podagra), knee or wrist. Other joints may be involved. The patient rarely has associated systemic symptoms and is usually afebrile.

b. The acute attack lasts 3-10 days without treatment.

c. Examination shows an acute synovitis of the affected joint. The joint is hot, erythematous and exquisitely tender to palpation. Inflammation may extend beyond the joint and resemble cellulitis.

d. Definitive diagnosis is made by joint aspiration with identification of sodium mono-urate crystals on polarizing microscopy (yellow, needle-like, with negative birefringence). Synovial fluid usually shows 2000-100,000 WBCs and should be differentiated from a septic arthritis by Gram stain, culture, etc.

e. Serum uric acid levels are usually normal in an acute attack, and do not help with management.

f. X-rays are not necessary unless trauma or osteomyelitis are suspected.

g. Treatment

    (1) Colchicine is specific treatment for gout, and can be used as a diagnostic trial. If relief occurs, the diagnosis of gout is established. Side effects limit its usefulness as a first-line drug, however. Dosage is 0.6mg q 1-2 hours for a total of 8-10 doses, or until GI side effects occur (nausea, vomiting, diarrhea). If the patient responds, then colchicine is given 0.6mg po bid for 4-6 weeks.

    (2) Any NSAID in appropriate dosage may be used to treat acute gout. Indomethacin 50mg po tid or ibuprofen 600mg po qid are effective. Narcotic analgesics may need to be given concomitantly for the first few days of treatment due to the severity of the pain.

    (3) Glucocorticoids (prednisone 40-60mg/d) may be given to those unable to take colchicine or NSAIDs or those who are unresponsive to these medications. Intraarticular steroids may also be used.

    (4) Patients with recurrent attacks of gout, uric acid nephrolithiasis or tophaceous gout should receive long-term treatment with allopurinol or probenecid.

3. Chronic (tophaceous) gout

  a. Joints may show evidence of destruction.

  b. Tophi can be found in subcutaneous tissues along tendons and in small joints. They may also be found along the pinna of the ear.

  c. X-rays may show periarticular or intraarticular bony erosions with a sclerotic margin.

  d. Chronic gout usually develops over 10-20 years.

  e. Treatment

    (1) Probenecid (blocks tubular reabsorption of uric acid) 250mg-500mg 1-2x/d.

    (2) Allopurinol (blocks formation of uric acid) 100-300mg/d.

    (3) Concurrent colchicine 0.6mg po bid should be given during the first 6-12 months of therapy with these agents. It should be started 1-2 weeks before these meds, to prevent an acute gouty attack.

D. Pseudogout (chondrocalcinosis)

  1. Caused by the accumulation of calcium pyrophosphate dihydrate (CPPD) crystals in joints and adjacent tendons.

  2. Knees, wrists, second and third MCP joints are most commonly involved.

  3. May complicate osteoarthritis.

4. Acute attacks mimic gout and combined disease may occur. The two are differentiated by examination of the synovial fluid under a polarizing microscope. CPPD crystals are blue, rhomboid shaped, and positively birefringent. Synovial fluid may have up to 100,000 WBCs.

5. X-rays may show calcium deposition in the joints or articular cartilage.

6. Treat with NSAIDs. Colchicine is less effective than in gout. Joint aspiration with intra-articular steroid injection is effective.

II. POLYARTICULAR ARTHRITIS

A. General

1. See the discussion under monoarticular arthritis.

2. Important historical characteristics of polyarticular disease include the following:

   a. Number of joints involved
   - (1) Pauciarticular - involvement of 2-4 joints.
   - (2) Polyarticular - involvement of more than 4 joints.

   b. Degree of symmetric joint involvement.

   c. Size of the joints involved.

   d. Systemic manifestations
   - (1) Inflammatory arthritides, such as rheumatoid arthritis often have systemic findings such as malaise, fever, morning stiffness.
   - (2) Noninflammatory processes, such as osteoarthritis, cause painful joints without systemic findings.

3. Consider infection with fever, inflamed joints.

4. Differential diagnosis - overlaps with monoarticular disease.

   a. Post-infectious (rheumatic fever, viral, Reiter's syndrome)

   b. Gout, pseudogout

   c. Rheumatologic disease (rheumatoid arthritis, systemic lupus, vasculitis)

   d. Ankylosing spondylitis

   e. Osteoarthritis

5. Other medical problems may present with joint complaints

   a. Hypothyroidism

   b. Depression

   c. Fibromyalgia

   d. Metabolic bone disease

6. Laboratory - check CBC, sed rate, antibody tests (RF, ANA), if available and synovial fluid analysis.

B. Osteoarthritis (DJD)

1. Clinical

   a. Chronic arthropathy characterized by degeneration of cartilage and bony hypertrophy at the articular margins.

   b. Most commonly involved are the knees, hips, spine and hands.

   c. Distribution may be symmetric or asymmetric.

d. Deep aching joint pain associated with stiffness after periods of inactivity is an early symptom. Pain is aggravated by activity and relieved with rest. With more severe disease, pain may be persistent, interfering with sleep and normal activities. Systemic symptoms are usually absent, even with severe disease.

e. Examination frequently shows crepitus of the joints and limited range of motion. Bouchard's nodes (non-tender nodules at the PIP joints) and Heberden's nodes (non-tender nodules at the DIP joints) are common. The foot may show hallux valgus of the great toe (bunion). With destruction of the cartilage of the knees, valgus (knock-knee) deformity develops.

2. Laboratory

a. Synovial fluid shows minimal abnormalities (noninflammatory pattern).

b. X-rays show joint space narrowing, marginal osteophyte formation and subchondral sclerosis and cysts (with advanced disease). X-ray findings may not correlate with symptoms. Severe abnormalities on x-ray may be asymptomatic.

3. Treatment

a. Paracetamol (acetaminophen) up to 4 gm/day is as effective as NSAIDs in treating pain in patients with osteoarthritis.

b. Occasionally, narcotics may be necessary for severe pain. Long-term narcotics should be avoided.

c. Treatment with heat or cold application and range of motion exercises are helpful in treating joint stiffness and maintaining mobility.

d. Intraarticular steroids are helpful in acute flares, but should not be given more frequently than 3-4x/year in any one joint.

e. With severe disease, joint replacement may be considered.

C. Rheumatoid arthritis (RA)

1. General

a. RA is a chronic, inflammatory disorder primarily affecting joints but occasionally with systemic manifestations.

b. Female to male ratio of 2-3 to 1. Affects 1% of whites, but less than 0.1% of Africans.

c. Criteria for diagnosis includes at least four of the following:

(1) Morning stiffness persisting for > one hour of more than six weeks duration.

(2) Swelling involving three or more joints of more than six weeks duration.

(3) Swelling of the metacarpophalangeal or PIP joints of at least six weeks duration.

(4) Symmetric joint swelling.

(5) X-ray changes of the hands typical of RA (erosions or bony decalcification).

(6) Subcutaneous rheumatoid nodules.

(7) Positive rheumatoid factor.

2. Clinical

a. Early manifestations

(1) Insidious onset of swelling, pain, and stiffness, initially involving the small joints (esp. MCP, PIP, MTP). It usually starts with symmetric involvement of the hands, wrists, knees and feet. With time, it may affect the elbows, shoulders, sternoclavicular joints, hips and ankles. Spinal involvement is limited to the upper cervical spine. It does not cause disease in the lumbar or thoracic spine.

(2) One third may present more acutely with fatigue, morning stiffness, arthralgias and myalgias, and occasionally low grade fever.

(3) Morning stiffness lasting greater than one hour is unusual in other conditions. The duration of morning stiffness is often used as a guide to the activity of the inflammatory process.

(4) Non-tender rheumatoid nodules may develop over the extensor tendon surfaces.

b. Late manifestations

(1) Hand - usually involves MCP and PIP joints, with sparing of the DIP joints (distinguishes it from osteoarthritis). Later effects include ulnar deviation of the fingers at the MCP joints, swan-neck deformities (hyperextension of the PIP joints with flexion of the DIP joints) and Boutonniere deformities (flexion contractures of the PIP joints with hyperextension of the DIP joints).

(2) Wrist - loss of motion at the wrist, and carpal tunnel syndrome are frequent.

(3) Knee - synovial proliferation and effusion are common. Quadriceps atrophy may occur and a flexion contracture of the knee may develop. Baker's (popliteal) cysts may form and can sometimes rupture into the calf, causing acute pain.

(4) Feet - MTP joints are commonly involved. Deformities of the toes may cause painful walking. Fibular deviation of the toes is common.

(5) Neck - pain and stiffness are common. Subluxation of C1 on C2 may occur, and can be seen radiographically. It is often asymptomatic.

(6) Shoulder - advanced disease may cause limitation of motion.

3. Laboratory

a. A chronic normocytic, normochromic anemia is common.

b. Sed rate (ESR) is elevated in most patients but does not indicate severity of the disease.

c. Rheumatoid factor is positive in 80% of patients. ANA may be positive in one third of patients.

   d. Synovial fluid analysis shows an inflammatory arthritis with poor mucin clot, WBC 5000-20,000 (50-70% polys), normal or low glucose.

   e. X-rays show decalcification, surface erosions and subsequent joint space narrowing. May progress to destruction of the joint.

4. Management

   a. Rest - significantly decreases the inflammatory response. During acute attacks, longer periods of rest, and sometimes complete bed rest are required to treat the inflammation.

   b. Maintain joint motion - during acute attacks, passive range of motion exercises should be done to maintain joint function. Once the acute inflammation has subsided, heat treatments (showers, baths, hot packs) are used to loosen the joints and relieve stiffness. This should be followed by mild exercise to maintain joint function and prevent atrophy. Over-activity will increase inflammation, and should be avoided.

   c. Anti-inflammatory therapy

   (1) Salicylates may be used, due to their efficacy and low expense, and low side effect profile. Usual dose is 3-6 gm of aspirin/day. If salicylate levels cannot be followed, the patient should be advised to be aware of signs of toxicity, such as tinnitus.

   (2) NSAIDs are effective analgesics and antiinflammatory agents, but more expensive than aspirin.

   (3) These drugs improve symptoms but do not affect disease outcome.

   d. Corticosteroids

   (1) Try to limit use to treating flares of disease.

   (2) In unresponsive or severe cases where chronic administration is necessary, use the smallest dose possible (5-10 mg/day) or use alternate day therapy.

   (3) Calcium (1000 mg/day) and Vitamin D (400-800 IU/day) will decrease the incidence of steroid induced osteoporosis.

   e. Disease-modifying therapy. These drugs improve outcomes in RA and should be used early, if possible. They do have significant toxicities which need to be followed closely.

   (1) Hydroxychloroquine 200mg 1-2x/d.

   (2) Oral gold salts (auranofin) 3 mg 2-3x/d.

   (3) Sulfasalazine 2-3 gm/d.

   (4) Methotrexate 7.5-15mg once/week.

   (5) Penicillamine 125-250mg/d up to 750mg/d max.

III. LOW BACK PAIN

A. Evaluation

1. History

    a. Determine duration of symptoms, initiating event (e.g. trauma), quality and intensity of the pain, radiation pattern.

    b. Look for symptoms suggesting serious disease

      (1) Cauda equina syndrome - leg weakness and bowel or bladder dysfunction.

      (2) Infection - fever, pain unrelieved by lying down, night pain.

      (3) Cancer - age >50 yrs, history of cancer, weight loss, or prolonged pain greater than 6 weeks duration.

2. Physical exam

    a. Palpate the spine and paraspinal muscles for tenderness or muscle spasm.

    b. Assess range of motion (flexion, extension, lateral bending, rotation).

    c. Test for radicular involvement

      (1) Motor strength can be tested with toe walking (S1), heel walking (L5), leg extension at the knee or squatting (L4).

      (2) Straight leg raising - assess for pain by passively flexing each leg at the hip. It is significant if pain is present at <60° of flexion, especially if the pain radiates into the posterior thigh and leg.

      (3) Examine for sensory deficits in the lower extremity (L4 - medial border of the foot, L5 - base of the middle toes on the dorsum of the foot, S1 - lateral margin of the foot and distal calf).

3. Diagnostic tests

    a. Check the following:

      (1) CBC may be helpful if fever is present.

      (2) Sed rate (ESR)

    b. LS spine X-rays are indicated in the following conditions: recent trauma, recurrent or prolonged pain, radicular symptoms, compression fracture suspected, malignancy suspected, or back pain with fever.

    c. Mantoux test if TB suspected (see Chapter 1, VIII, C, 3)

B. Differential diagnosis

    1. Acute musculoskeletal or ligamentous sprain or strain (mechanical LBP)

    a. Usually associated with an acute injury or strain (i.e. lifting a heavy object, MVA).

    b. Spasm and tenderness of the back muscles is present.

    c. No radicular findings and no neurologic deficits (pain may radiate into buttocks).

    d. X-rays not usually needed.

    e. Treatment

      (1) Local heat, activity as tolerated.

      (2) Scheduled analgesics (NSAID and/or muscle relaxants) for 4-7 days. Narcotic analgesics are usually not necessary.

      (3) Advise patient to sleep on the side with knees flexed and a pillow between the legs.

(4) Flexion exercises after the acute pain has resolved.

2. Sciatica (pain secondary to nerve root involvement)

  a. Pain characteristics

    (1) Radiates down one or both lower extremities.

    (2) May increase with coughing or straining.

    (3) May increase with sitting or standing, relieved by lying.

    (4) With time, there may be associated weakness and/or numbness of the leg.

  b. Exam may show weakness on motor testing (heel and toe walking) or depressed knee or ankle reflexes. Sensory changes may be present.

  c. Treatment

    (1) Consider hospital admission for intractable pain, loss of function, or symptoms indicating serious disease.

    (2) LS spine X-rays should be obtained.

    (3) Bedrest until pain begins to improve, then activity as tolerated. Application of ice or heat may help pain.

    (4) Provide adequate analgesia (NSAIDs, narcotic analgesics, and muscle relaxants).

    (5) Follow closely, especially if symptoms of serious disease are present.

3. Tuberculosis of the spine (Pott's disease) (see Chapter 1, section VIII, B, 3)

  a. Common cause of back pain and neurologic dysfunction in countries with a high prevalence of TB.

  b. Neurologic dysfunction may occur as the vertebral bodies collapse. At this stage, adequate antitubercular therapy can reverse the neurologic abnormalities. Once gibbus formation has occurred, the spine is sclerosed and stable, and any neurologic abnormalities present will probably remain, even with treatment.

  c. Treatment (see Chapter 1, VIII, D)

    (1) In patients with uncomplicated Pott's disease (especially those without neurologic findings), standard anti-tubercular therapy is adequate for treatment. Continue treatment for one year.

    (2) Patients with unstable-appearing spine X-rays (vertebral collapse without gibbus formation) or those with acute neurologic dysfunction should be placed at strict bedrest for 4-6 weeks, in addition to receiving standard chemotherapy. Some of these patients might benefit from treatment with a body cast, if they are still unstable when beginning to ambulate.

    (3) Patients in whom gibbus formation has already occurred do not need to be at bedrest, unless they have new neurologic symptoms (which is unusual). They may be treated with standard chemotherapy.

4. Vertebral compression fractures

   a. Usually present with acute onset of sharp pain at the level of the fracture. May or may not be associated with a fall (most commonly a jump or fall onto the feet). Occur frequently in patients with osteoporosis.

   b. Physical exam shows tenderness over the affected vertebra.

   c. X-ray shows loss of height of the vertebral body. In osteoporosis, the thoracic vertebrae are usually involved. In neoplastic or infectious processes, the lumbar vertebrae are more commonly affected.

   d. Treatment

   (1) Bed rest for 1-2 weeks.

   (2) NSAIDs or narcotic analgesics for pain, which is usually severe.

   (3) Consider biopsy if neoplasm is suspected.

   (4) Antibiotics or anti-tubercular agents if an infectious process is identified.

5. Facet disease (spondylolisthesis)

   a. Usually causes chronic low back pain with recurrent acute exacerbations. Rarely are there radicular symptoms.

   b. Physical exam is usually unremarkable.

   c. Caused by an acquired anterior subluxation of a vertebral body upon an adjacent vertebral body (spondylolisthesis). This occurs due to degenerative disease of the facet joints.

   d. Treatment - bedrest, NSAIDs and narcotic analgesics.

6. Consider non-orthopedic causes of back pain

   a. Acute pyelonephritis

   b. Renal colic

   c. Dissecting aneurysm

   d. Pneumonia

CHAPTER 12

DERMATOLOGY

I. PRINCIPLES OF DERMATOLOGY

A. Diagnosis

1. History should include information about the following:
   a. Earliest lesion, duration, associated symptoms (itching, pain, systemic symptoms).
   b. Distribution of lesions (location, symmetry or asymmetry, relationship to outside influences, i.e. sun exposed, under clothing, where patient can reach, where bites are apt to occur, where chemical exposure has occurred at home or work etc.).
   c. Therapy and response to therapy thus far.
2. Examination principles
   a. The skin must be exposed and examined with adequate lighting.
   b. Description should include color, size, elevated or not elevated, texture (firm, soft, compressible), description of border (poorly demarcated, well demarcated, elevated, depressed) depth, tender or non-tender, temperature, distribution, location, and secondary changes (excoriation, infection).

B. Terminology

1. Macule-flat skin lesion <0.5cm with color different from the surrounding skin.
2. Patch-flat skin lesion >0.5cm with color different from the surrounding skin.
3. Papule-elevated skin lesion <0.5 cm.
4. Plaque-elevated skin lesion >0.5 cm.
5. Nodule-lesion with depth <0.5 cm.
6. Tumor-lesion with depth >0.5 cm.
7. Vesicle-blister filled with clear fluid <0.5 cm.
8. Bullae-blister filled with clear fluid > 0.5 cm.
9. Wheal (hive)-papule or plaque than is evanescent (moves, changes or disappears within 24 hours).
10. Crust-liquid serum, pus or blood that has dried on the skin.
11. Scale-visibly thickened stratum corneum that is at least partially unattached to the skin. Usually dry but can be greasy as in seborrheic dermatitis.
12. Induration-sensation of firmness or hardness to the skin.
13. Erosion-superficial, not full thickness, loss of skin.
14. Ulcer-deep full thickness loss of skin replaced by a scar.
15. Lichenification-accentuation of the normal markings of the skin usually due to rubbing.
16. Excoriation-lesion left on the skin as a result of scratching.
17. Pustule-blister filled with cloudy fluid.
18. Cyst-sac-like lesion filled with semisolid material.

19. Atrophy-thinning of the skin. Can be deep with a definite indentation or superficial with a fine wrinkling of the skin (cigarette paper atrophy) as seen in mycosis fungoides or steroid induced skin atrophy.
20. Hypertrophy-thickening of the skin.
21. Verrucous-rough and warty.
22. Arciform-with a curved edge.
23. Erythematous-red.
24. Diascopy-fading or disappearance of a lesion upon pressure such as in a spider nevus (nevus araneus).
25. Reticulate-lace-like or net-like.
26. Keratotic-rough.
27. Eczematous-oozing or crusted.
28. Id Reaction (auto-eczematous reaction)-generalized symmetrical papular or eczematous reaction resulting from a severe long-standing localized inflammatory condition. In children, most often associated with a kerion due to a fungal infection in the scalp and in adults, most often due to stasis dermatitis.
29. Koebner Phenomena (isomorphic response)-reproduction of a previously existing skin disease at a site of trauma of the skin. Seen most characteristically in psoriasis, lichen planus, and flat warts.

C. Principles of topical therapy
1. Vehicles
   a. Cream - water-based preparation that disappears when rubbed into the skin and tends to be hydrophilic (picks up extra water from the skin and leaves the skin drier). Use it when you want to dry the skin.
   b. Ointment or oil - oil-based preparation that is greasy and does not rub well into the skin. It is hydrophobic (holds moisture in the skin). Use it when you want to lubricate or moisturize the skin. Allows better penetration of the skin and thus makes a topical steroid in an ointment more potent. Examples: Vaseline, zinc oxide, Aquaphor, olive oil, peanut oil, cooking oil, vegetable oil.
   c. Lotion - may be a moisturizing lotion with properties similar to an ointment or a drying (shake) lotion with properties similar to a cream. Drying lotions are powders suspended in water/alcohol, which evaporate and leave the active ingredient on the skin. This type of lotion is even more drying than a cream and is useful in hairy areas. Examples of this type of lotion are calamine or a nonalcoholic shake lotion (24 parts zinc oxide, 24 parts talc, 12 parts glycerin and add water to make 120) or an alcoholic shake lotion (zinc oxide 24, talc 24, glycerin 12 and isopropyl alcohol to make 120).
   d. Gel - clear, colorless emulsion that liquefies when applied to the skin. May be useful in hairy areas.
2. Application
   a. With the exception of sunscreens, a thin coat is always preferred. This

saves medicine, works well, and allows for full visualization of the disease process.

b. Creams should be rubbed in until they disappear.

c. Ointments spread easily and can cover large areas with one application.

3. Topical steroids

a. Use the smallest quantity and weakest preparation that is effective.

b. Use low potency on the face and intertriginous regions. Avoid long-term use of medium and high potency topical steroids to avoid skin atrophy.

c. Occlusion with gauze, plastic wrap, tape, gloves, socks, etc. increases potency greatly.

d. Relative potency - see Appendix I, Formulary.

e. Frequency of application and not thickness of application increases benefit.

f. Ointments are more potent the creams.

g. Super high potency topical steroids should not be used longer than 2 weeks unless a systemic corticosteroid effect is desired. Every other day or Monday-Wednesday-Friday usage or 2 out of 3 weeks usage will help with this problem.

h. To increase the strength of the steroid, 5-20% urea, 5-10% salicylic acid, or 5-12% alpha hydroxy acid (citric acid, glycolic acid, or lactic acid) can be added.

4. If the skin is too dry

a. Use an ointment, oil or moisturizing lotion to seal water in the skin.

b. Application immediately after bathing or hand washing is important to keep the skin from drying out.

c. Oil (bath oil, liquid cooking oil) in water soaks in a tub of water for the whole body or a basin of water for a hand or foot will allow the oil to cover the skin as it is removed from the water and hold the water in. 5-10 minutes of soaking is all that is needed several times a day. Gauze can be dipped into this oil in water emulsion and then the gauze can be applied directly on the dry skin for 5-10 minutes.

d. 5-20% urea will allow the skin to retain moisture.

e. 5-12% of an alpha hydroxy acid will be moisturizing.

f. Simply soaking for a few minutes with water or wrapping the skin with wet gauze or cotton fabric and immediately applying an ointment, oil or moisturizing lotion is helpful.

g. Limit frequent water exposure.

5. If the skin is oozing or too wet

a. Water compresses with gauze or cotton fabric for 5-10 minutes several times a day will dry the skin.

b. Water can be made more drying by adding one or two packets or tablets of aluminum acetate (Domeboro) to one pint of water. Water with or without the Domeboro can be used to soak the affected skin. Aveeno in the amount of one to two tablespoons can be used in the same way. The Aveeno solution may be substituted with one half cup of white vinegar to 1 quart of water or 1 tablespoon of salt to one quart of water.

    c. Frequent exposure to water and gauze or cotton fabric wraps without adding an ointment or oil to the skin will dry the skin.

    d. Gels and drying lotion vehicles will dry the skin.

  6. Control of pruritus (itching)

    a. Local measures include cooling lotions such as calamine, emollient lotions, alpha- hydroxy products and urea products. 0.25 % menthol is also effective.

    b. Local, low potency steroid therapy can be used if there is inflammation.

    c. Systemic antihistaminic agents are useful.

II. SKIN LESIONS

  A. Common papules, plaques, nodules, and tumors

    1. Warts

      a. General

        (1) Papules, or more rarely, tumors caused by the human papilloma group of viruses.

        (2) Common in children, especially on the hands and feet. Plantar warts, (on the bottom of the feet), are particularly difficult to treat due to the thick epidermis.

        (3) Warts are contagious but transmission is more dependent on susceptibility rather than exposure.

        (4) Diagnosis can usually be made clinically but biopsy may be used in difficult cases. Warts have a rough, verrucous surface and will often show tiny black dots representing clotted capillaries. This differentiates them from corns, which are more painful and have a central keratotic core without the black dots. Flat warts are small (1to 4 mm), more common on the extremities and may spread by skin abrasion.

      b. Genital warts

        (1) Caused by human papilloma virus (HPV). Very difficult to cure.

        (2) The virus is sexually transmitted.

        (3) HPV virus infection is strongly associated with development of cancer of the cervix. Cancer of the rectum is associated with HPV, especially in male homosexual patients with AIDS. Anogenital warts greater than 0.5cm should be biopsied to check for transformation into a squamous cell cancer.

        (4) Delivery of a newborn through an infected birth canal can result in wart transmission and vocal cord papillomas.

c. Warts on the nail bed
  (1) Especially on the thumbs, warts can mimic and rarely be associated with squamous cell cancer.
  (2) Caution in therapy at the base of the nail is warranted if a dystrophic nail is to be avoided.
d. Treatment
  (1) Warts often disappear spontaneously and, if asymptomatic and not increasing in size or number, they can be left alone (except in the anogenital area). Many folk remedies are successful when strongly believed in by the patient. If harmless, they should not be discouraged.
  (2) For areas of thick skin, such as palms, soles and flexor digits, use the following:
    (a) 40% salicylic acid plaster each night with weekly paring of the skin with a scalpel blade for several months is the most conservative form of therapy.
    (b) Chemical therapy with 20% podophyllum or 1% cantharidin under tape overnight isn't painful at the time of application, but will form a painful blood blister.
    (c) Excision may be effective, but requires local anesthesia.
    (d) If available, freezing with liquid nitrogen or dry ice, electrodessication or laser therapy also may be effective.
  (3) For areas of thinner skin, such as anogenital, face, backs of hands and tops of feet, freezing with liquid nitrogen or dry ice to give a 1mm white halo, scissor excision under local anesthesia, topical imiquimod (Aldara) overnight 3 times a week on Monday-Wednesday- Friday for several months, and topical retinoic acid under tape each night for months can be used.
2. Molluscum contagiosum
  a. General
    (1) Molluscum contagiosum lesions are caused by the molluscum virus and are very contagious.
    (2) They are common in children and consist of 2-4 mm white umbilicated papules that, upon scraping with a scalpel blade and spreading on a glass slide, reveal tiny white, round, firm molluscum bodies.
    (3) They are also common in HIV patients, where they may be very numerous, larger, and erosive. They are most commonly seen on the face.
  b. Treatment
    (1) Most molluscum contagiosum lesions in children will resolve spontaneously without treatment. Parents usually want therapy instituted, however. In HIV positive patients, the lesions will probably not resolve without therapy unless the patient's immune status improves.

(2) The lesions may be lightly scraped with a scalpel blade, curette or pin to remove the molluscum bodies. Light liquid nitrogen or dry ice application, or toothpick application with 25% trichloroacetic acid or 1% cantharidin is also effective.

3. Skin tags
a. General
   (1) Usually tiny (2-4mm) fleshy and most often pedunculated tumors that are flesh-colored or hyperpigmented. They are very common and are found most often on the sides of the neck, axillae, and in the groin.
   (2) They are more common during pregnancy.
   (3) Occasionally they are much larger (1-2 cm).
   (4) Other names include fibroepithelial polyps and acrochordon.

b. Treatment
   (1) Removal is unnecessary if they are not bothersome to the patient. If they are rubbed by clothing or jewelry they can twist and be painful. If they twist enough they may become black and hemorrhagic and fall off by themselves.
   (2) They can be snipped off with surgical scissors with or without local anesthetic. Bleeding is usually minimal for the small tags.

4. Seborrheic keratosis
a. General
   (1) Very common verrucous tumor that may be white to brown or black. It may have tiny pin head sized dots of white, brown or black.
   (2) Always benign, very common.
   (3) In dark skinned people these lesions are often small, multiple and symmetrical on the face (dermatosis papulosa nigra).

b. Treatment
   (1) None necessary but can be treated by cryosurgery, scissor excision or shave excision.
   (2) Reassurance may be important because they can be black, come up quickly, itch and mimic a malignant melanoma.

5. Malignant melanoma
a. General
   (1) Multi-colored or black malignant tumor with an irregular border that is fatal 20% of the time due to distant metastasis.
   (2) Melanoma is rare in dark skinned patients. It most frequently occurs as a very aggressive form of melanoma called an acrolentiginous melanoma. These lesions are usually located around the mouth, hands, feet, under nails or in the genital area.

b. Treatment
   (1) Early and aggressive surgery with 1-3 cm margins is life saving if done early.

(2) Radiation and chemotherapy are minimally successful once metastasis has occurred.

6. Keloid

a. General

    (1) Firm, elevated scar that extends beyond the border of the wound that caused it. These are common in blacks and occur frequently at the site of body piercing for jewelry. They can become large, grotesque, and painful.

    (2) Certain patients have a tendency to develop keloids. If a patient has a keloid already, elective surgery should be avoided.

b. Treatment

    (1) Treatment is often inadequate. Intra-lesional injection with triamcinolone 8-20 mg/cc may be beneficial. Injections may be repeated as necessary.

    (2) Excision with intra-lesional triamcinolone the day of surgery, then monthly as needed can be tried.

    (3) Massaging the keloid for 60 seconds daily, immediately after bathing, with ointment (any type, but preferably a high potency corticosteroid ointment) may be beneficial.

    (4) When keloids are removed, they may recur, often larger than before treatment.

7. Kaposi's sarcoma

a. General

    (1) May present as papules, plaques, nodules or tumors that are purple in color and arise not only in the skin but also in vascular tissue throughout the body.

    (2) The skin is the most common location followed by the mucous membranes, gastrointestinal tract, and lungs.

b. Types

    (1) The endemic form seen in Africa is a common tumor that has a strong association with underlying reticuloendothelial malignancies such as leukemia and lymphoma.

    (2) There is a form mainly in people of Mediterranean ancestry that is seen in the elderly on the lower extremities and is not usually associated with underlying cancer.

    (3) There is an iatrogenic form associated with immunosuppressive therapy for cancer or in transplant patients. It usually improves with a decrease in immunosuppression.

    (4) The most recently described form is in HIV positive patients. This is the most aggressive form, can occur at any site, and be widespread and life threatening. Improvement in HIV status results in improvement of Kaposi's. This form can also be seen in male homosexuals that are not HIV positive.

c. Treatment

      (1) Cryosurgery with liquid nitrogen or dry ice for mild disease.
      (2) Intralesional adriamycin 0.2 to 0.5 cc can also be used.
      (3) Various forms of chemotherapy can be of benefit.
      (4) Radiation may be helpful but rarely causes dramatic worsening.

8. Squamous cell cancer
  a. General
      (1) A firm tumor that may be ulcerated or hyperkeratotic.
      (2) In fair skinned patients this is seen in sun-exposed areas.
      (3) In all races this malignancy is seen at the site of chronic draining ulcers, non-healing wounds, burn scars, and in the mouth of people who abuse tobacco products and ethanol.
  b. Treatment - excision with a clear border on histopathology is the treatment of choice and is usually curative.

9. Dermatofibroma
  a. General
      (1) Common, perfectly round nodule seen most often on the extremities. It is rock-hard and indents upon squeezing; hyperpigmented brownish or reddish.
      (2) Always benign.
  b. Treatment - no treatment is necessary unless the nodule is painful or felt to possibly be a squamous cell cancer. Simple excision with a small margin is all that is necessary.

B. Eczematous rashes
  1. Atopic dermatitis (eczema)
    a. General
      (1) Common eruption that usually begins in childhood and disappears in 60-70% of patients by puberty.
      (2) The hallmarks of the disease are lichenification, severe pruritus, generalized dry skin, dermographism (scratch causing a welt), signs of scratching (excoriations), and a family or personal history of asthma, allergic rhinitis (hay fever), penicillin allergy, hives (urticaria), or eczema.
      (3) The disease tends to involve extensor surfaces (malar areas, fronts of legs, outer arms) in younger children and flexor surfaces (antecubital fossae, popliteal fossae, around the neck) in older children. It tends to be localized in adults, seen commonly on the hands, genital area, back of neck, and lower extremities, especially around the ankles.
      (4) It can be a generalized eruption or form dramatic, oozing, yellow-crusted circles called nummular eczema in all age groups.
      (5) Common associated findings include:
        (a) Keratosis pilaris - very common tiny keratotic papules located on the upper outer arms and upper legs and sometimes malar areas. This is seen as part of the atopic dermatitis.

(b) Pityriasis alba - poorly demarcated, slightly hypopigmented patches see mainly on the cheeks but sometimes the upper outer arms in eczema patients. A fine, dry scale may be present.

(c) Nail pits - tiny pits seen in fingernails and toenails in eczema patients. Also occur in psoriasis.

(d) Lichen simplex chronicus - very pruritic, localized plaques of hyperkeratotic, lichenified eczema seen most often on the lower extremities and genital areas.

b. Treatment

(1) First-line treatment is with topical corticosteroid ointments using the mildest potency that is effective.

(2) Patients with eczema should use mild soaps and avoid hot water for bathing or hand washing. Cool to lukewarm water is preferable. Adding an oil to bath water can help decrease dryness. Dry skin can be treated with any kind of an ointment, especially after water exposure. Keeping the patient as cool as possible is beneficial.

(3) Antihistamines help to decrease itching.

(4) Secondary infection with *Staphylococcus aureus* is not uncommon and should be treated with systemic antibiotics.

(5) When severe and crusted, cool wet towels can be applied for 10 to 15 minutes, followed by a lubricant.

(6) Topical tacrolimus is quite safe and effective for eczema, when available. When very severe, systemic corticosteroids, methotrexate, and oral cyclosporine may be used.

2. Stasis dermatitis

a. General

(1) Chronic skin changes of the lower extremities due to venous stasis.

(2) The rash is located mainly in the area of the medial malleolus. In addition to oozing and crusting there is brown discoloration of the skin and varicosities are present. Secondary infection may occur.

(3) When severe and long lasting a generalized eczematous skin eruption may occur called an auto-eczematous or Id reaction. This is very pruritic and excoriation to the point of lichenification and bleeding may occur.

b. Treatment

(1) Diuretics may help reduce swelling of the extremity. Pressure with support stockings or firm elastic bandages can improve venous return.

(2) Prolonged standing or sitting with the legs dangling is to be avoided. When sitting, the legs should be slightly elevated and straight.

     (3) Cool wet compresses may be helpful. Infection should be treated with systemic antibiotics. A corticosteroid ointment or cream will help reduce itching and inflammation.

3. Contact dermatitis

  a. General

     (1) A delayed hypersensitivity reaction occurring 1-7 days after exposure to a substance contacting the skin. Caused by either a primary irritant (such as a strong chemical or soap) or a specific allergen to which an individual is sensitized.

     (2) Usually presents with redness, peeling and fissuring of the skin. Occasionally, blisters will be present.

     (3) Chemicals used to clean the skin are the commonest offenders. Plants are common causes, producing reactions that are typically linear, asymmetrical, and often blistered. The reaction does not spread from ruptured blister fluid but will spread from repeated exposure from the offending plant or from objects that have the oil from the offending plant on them.

  b. Treatment

     (1) Identify and avoid the irritant or allergen.

     (2) Topical corticosteroids are the mainstay of therapy. Systemic steroids may be used in severe cases.

     (3) Topical lotions with 0.5-2% phenol, 0.25% menthol, 1-2% camphor, or pramoxine may relieve the itching. Oral antihistamines may also be used for pruritus.

C. Papulosquamous rashes (elevated rashes with scaling or peeling of the skin)

  1. Psoriasis and related conditions

    a. General

     (1) Considered by some authors to be rare in dark skinned races but not in this author's experience.

     (2) Elevated, well-demarcated, red plaques covered with a dry, thick, and characteristic silvery-white adherent scale. Prefer extensor locations on knees and elbows. Common also on pretibial areas, in the external auditory canals, scalp, palms, and soles. Koebnerization does occur. Not rare in the genital area, including the glans of the penis.

     (3) 7% of patients develop psoriatic arthritis, especially in the spine and the distal joints in the fingers.

    b. Types

     (1) Guttate psoriasis - sudden onset of widespread, symmetrical, drop-shaped psoriasis often associated with a streptococcal throat infection. The only form of psoriasis that may spontaneously disappear over several months only to reappear with another streptococcal sore throat.

(2) Pustular psoriasis - a relatively rare form of the disease with multiple tiny sterile pustules that can be localized to the palms and soles (acropustulosis) or form a generalized life-threatening pustular rash.

(3) Exfoliative erythroderma - generalized redness and desquamation of the skin due to many underlying skin diseases, the most common of which is psoriasis. It can also be associated with underlying illness, most often a drug allergy or lymphoma, or rarely, it can be idiopathic.

c. Topical treatment

(1) Topical corticosteroids are the treatment of choice for localized disease. If the plaques are thick, occlusion with gloves or socks, gauze or plastic wrap overnight may be beneficial. 2-5% salicylic acid can be added to increase penetration of the corticosteroid and decrease scaling. 5-10% urea will accomplish the same thing.

(2) 5-10% coal tar (LCD) can be added to any ointment.

(3) 1% crude coal tar in vaseline nightly is effective and safe but smells and stains skin and clothes.

(4) For the scalp, corticosteroid solutions can be used. Using shampoos containing salicylic acid, tar, corticosteroids, and selenium sulfide will help. They should be scrubbed in aggressively, used daily, let set for as long as possible, and, after being rinsed out, they should be lathered in a second time.

(5) Sunlight or artificial light sources are helpful. Use PUVA therapy, if available.

d. Systemic treatment

(1) Systemic corticosteroids are contraindicated due to rebound that may occur when they are stopped. The psoriasis may be transformed into a more severe, pustular phase.

(2) Methotrexate is helpful but limited by liver toxicity. Liver function tests alone are not accurate for such monitoring. Liver biopsies need to be done after 1500mg total dose and, depending on the result, at other dosage intervals after that.

(3) Retinoids (Accutane or Soriatane) are slowly effective over several months, but can't be given if pregnancy is a possibility. They may cause muscle aches, dryness, elevated triglycerides, and other side effects.

(4) Cyclosporine is very helpful for severe disease, if available, but blood pressure and creatinine must be carefully monitored.

2. Pityriasis rosea

a. General

(1) A common rash seen mainly in older children and young adults but may occur at any age. It resolves in 6 to 8 weeks without sequelae. Itching is usually absent or mild. Recurrences may uncommonly occur.

(2) Initial presentation is with a "herald patch" that is larger than the rest of the spots and comes 2 days to 2 weeks before the rest of the rash. The rash consists of oval, pink, barely elevated plaques with a collar of fine, adherent scale forming a ring that begins just inside the oval. The long axis of the ovals is parallel to the normal folds in the skin. This gives a pine tree-like distribution on the back.

(3) The rash is not contagious. Some drug eruptions can mimic pityriasis rosea.

b. Treatment - reassurance and mild antipruritics.

3. Secondary syphilis (see Chapter 1, section VI, C, b)

a. General

(1) A rash which can mimic pityriasis rosea, however it often affects the palms and soles and can be papular. Lesions do not necessarily line up along the lines of cleavage of the skin.

(2) The rash may be accompanied by mild, moth-eaten scalp hair loss. White plaques in the mouth or genital area called mucous patches may occur. Pruritus is usually absent. Lymphadenopathy is common and hepatosplenomegaly can occur.

(3) The serologic blood test for syphilis is positive.

b. Treatment - responds rapidly to appropriate antibiotic therapy.

4. Lichen planus

a. General

(1) Rash consisting of pruritic, purplish, polygonal papules occurring most commonly on the flexor surface of the wrists. It may be symmetrical and widespread.

(2) When occurring in the scalp it causes a scarring hair loss. It commonly forms reticulate, milky-white confluent papules on mucous membranes. Ulcers may occur in the mouth and, rarely, on vaginal mucous membranes. It exhibits Koebnerization.

(3) Some drug eruptions mimic lichen planus.

b. Treatment -topical corticosteroids are the treatment of choice. Systemic steroids may be used in severe disease. Up to 20% of patients may have hepatitis C.

5. Seborrheic dermatitis

a. General

(1) Erythematous, dry, scaling, crusting lesions with or without greasy, yellow appearance. Common in the scalp, external auditory canals, eyebrows, nasolabial areas, and intergluteal area. It responds readily to therapy but always recurs.

(2) It can occur as a generalized eruption in the newborn but this form usually dissipates by 6 months of age.

(3) HIV positive patients may develop severe, recalcitrant, generalized disease.

b. Treatment

(1) Usually responds easily to low strength topical corticosteroids. Adding 2-5% sulfur is helpful.

(2) Shampoos containing ketoconazole, selenium sulfide, tar, and salicylic acid are helpful.

(3) Topical miconazole, clotrimazole, and ketoconazole may help, especially when combined with a corticosteroid cream.

(4) Oral ketoconazole or fluconazole is often beneficial, especially in HIV positive patients.

D. Pustules

1. Acne

a. General

(1) This disease may be divided into 3 main types. All 3 types are caused by obstruction of the duct of the oil gland. Epidermal debris gets stuck in the duct of the oil gland, as in comedones, ruptures through the duct superficially, as in papules and pustules, or deeply through the duct or oil gland as in cystic acne.

(2) Acne begins at puberty and may last for years. It is especially long lasting in women and often flares the week before their menstrual period.

(3) Common locations are the face, back, and upper chest.

b. Types

(1) Comedonal acne

    (a) This consists of open comedones or blackheads and closed comedones or whiteheads.

    (b) It does not respond well to oral medications. It responds best to topical retinoids (vitamin A derivatives), which are effective but take 4 to 6 months of application every night. Nighttime application is important since these products may cause sun sensitivity. Initial irritation occurs from these products but over several weeks this usually subsides.

    (c) Adding a product containing a benzoyl peroxide in the morning is synergistic with the retinoids. It is available from 3 to 10 %.

(2) Pustular and papular acne

    (a) This type of acne consists of red bumps and pustules usually less than 0.5 cm.

    (b) The mainstay of therapy is oral antibiotics which often must be given for many months or years. The most commonly used are tetracycline 250-500mg twice a day (avoid giving with food, dairy products, and vitamins with calcium or iron), doxycycline 50-100mg twice a day, minocycline 50-100mg twice a day, clindamycin 150-300mg twice a day, erythromycin 250-500mg twice a day, and trimethoprim 100-200mg twice a day.

    (c) Topical therapy, such as topical erythromycin and clindamycin 1-2% may be helpful. In women who flare before their periods, spironolactone 25-50mg twice a day may be used.

(3) Cystic acne

    (a) Topical agents are usually not very effective.

    (b) Oral antibiotics are usually tried first for at least 2 months and at least two or three different drugs should be tried if the first is not effective.

    (c) If scarring occurs, the disease is severe, and is not responding to therapy, then oral Accutane (13 cis-retinoic acid) 40mg twice a day with food for 5 months should be given. After this course of therapy, approximately 75% of patients will stay clear for 10 years. The other 25% who recur are usually not as severe as before Accutane and conservative therapy causes a better response. Repeat courses are occasionally used. There are many side effects from Accutane, the most significant of which is birth defects. A negative pregnancy test should be done on the first visit and again a few days after the patient's menstrual period begins and monthly during therapy. Two forms of contraception should be used during therapy. Pregnancy should be avoided for at least 3 menstrual cycles after the drug is stopped. Other side effects include depression, severely chapped lips, muscle pain (especially of the back and ankles), sun sensitivity, very dry skin, headaches, night blindness, mild hair loss, blurred vision, epistaxis, and elevated serum triglycerides.

    (d) Intralesional corticosteroids (Celestone 2mg/cc or triamcinolone 4mg/cc) are helpful for treating individual cysts.

2. Folliculitis

a. General

(1) Folliculitis is a common condition, especially in hot humid environments.

(2) It consists of multiple and often symmetrical, usually small (2-4mm) pustules surrounding a hair.

(3) The trunk, groin, scalp, and proximal extremities are common locations.

(4) Itching is a significant problem.

b. Types

(1) Chronic noninfectious folliculitis

    (a) This is the commonest type, frequently causing scalp lesions in men. Oily hair care products as well as body oils will often make this worse in men and women.

    (b) Treatment is similar to acne with the exception that Accutane is usually not used. Treatments that cool the skin such as cool baths, wiping with alcohol, and cool compresses that are drying such as Domeboro and Aveeno are helpful. Shampoos containing salicylic acid (2 to 5%) may be helpful.

(2) Eosinophilic pustular folliculitis
  (a) This is usually seen in HIV positive patients and has severe disabling pruritus. If unsure of the diagnosis a biopsy can be done.
  (b) It is difficult to treat. Sometimes potent topical corticosteroids or short courses of systemic corticosteroids are beneficial.

(3) Staphylococcal folliculitis
  (a) These lesions are purulent and can progress to boils or occasionally cellulitis.
  (b) Bacterial culture is positive for *Staphylococcus aureus*. Remember that *Staphylococcus epidermidis* is a normal inhabitant of the skin and culture showing this organism is not significant. *S. aureus* is quite contagious and can be harbored in the external nares.
  (c) Neosporin, Polysporin, triple antibiotic ointment or especially mupirocin (Bactroban) ointment in the nose of all family members twice a day for 1 week should help eliminate family carriers. Appropriate oral doses of antibiotics that are anti-staph should be given to the patient. Recurrence is common.

III. INFECTIONS
A. Bacterial
1. Impetigo
a. General
(1) Superficial bacterial infection of the skin. Consists of scalloped, oozing, honey-colored crusted circles that may begin with a central pustule. Spreads rapidly and is very contagious.
(2) Common in children. Favors hot, humid climates.
(3) Due to *Staphylococcus aureus* or *group A beta hemolytic streptococcus*. Some streptococcal strains may cause glomerulonephritis.
b. Therapy
(1) Localized disease may be treated with Neosporin, bacitracin, Polysporin or triple antibiotic ointment.
(2) More widespread disease will respond to oral antibiotics such as penicillin and erythromycin. Staph. resistance to these two drugs can be treated with cloxacillin, dicloxacillin or cephalexin. Methicillin-resistant staph is treated with mupirocin (Bactroban) topically or Zyvox systemically.
2. Ecthyma

a. This is a deeper infection than impetigo, with oozing and honey-colored crusts or pus on the surface of the skin, and red, indurated surrounding tissue. Usually due to staph or strep. May progress to form a cellulitis.

b. Therapy - the same as systemic therapy for impetigo.

3. Cellulitis

a. General

(1) This is an infection of the deeper tissues underlying the skin. Signs of impetigo or ecthyma may be seen over the surface. It is characterized by pain, redness, tenderness, swelling. It is most often seen on the lower extremity.

(2) Bacteria that are causative of impetigo are the usual culprits. The site of entry of the bacteria may be apparent (scratch, insect bite or chronic interdigital fissured tinea between the toes), or the site of entry may not be apparent.

(3) The patient is often febrile and may have signs of systemic sepsis.

b. Treatment

(1) Rapid institution of systemic antibiotics is mandatory. Depending on the severity of illness, intravenous therapy may be indicated for the first 3 to 5 days or longer.

(2) Antibiotics which are effective against strep and staph should be given (cephalexin, cloxacillin, dicloxacillin, or clindamycin). For severe infections, IV nafcillin, cephalosporins or, if resistant organism, vancomycin are indicated. Blood cultures are helpful, if available.

4. Erysipelas

a. General

(1) This is a rapidly spreading form of cellulitis due to *group A beta hemolytic streptococci*. The patient is febrile and toxic.

(2) It is seen most commonly on the face. Recurrences may occur.

b. Therapy - oral or intravenous anti-strep antibiotics are mandatory.

5. Staphylococcal scalded skin syndrome (toxic epidermal necrolysis)

a. General

(1) Rare, life threatening sepsis due to certain specific strains of *Staphylococcus aureus*. More common in young children.

(2) The patient develops sudden onset of generalized red skin that may be easily wiped off with light pressure in thin sheets (Nikolsky's sign). The patient is febrile and very ill.

(3) Survival depends on early use of intravenous antibiotics.

(4) Blood cultures are usually positive. Cultures taken from a nidus of infection may be positive, as well.

(5) Adult toxic epidermal necrolysis is usually due to drugs and is fatal in 50% of patients. Intravenous IgG may be life saving.

b. Treatment

(1) IV anti-staphylococcal antibiotics.
(2) Cool water compresses may be soothing.
(3) Complete recovery with therapy is common.
B. Mycobacterial
1. Leprosy (Hansen's Disease)
a. General
(1) This disease is caused by *Mycobacterium leprae*. It is contracted mainly through household contacts.
(2) Types
  (a) Lepromatous leprosy - shows indurated, red to purple lesions with ill defined borders. Lesions are numerous and may be symmetric. Thickening of the face leads to leonine facies. Lateral loss of eyebrows may occur. Diffuse nerve involvement occurs. These patients have low resistance and severe disease with a negative lepromin skin test. The bacilli may be seen on biopsy or in smears obtained from the skin exposed through a small incision made through the lesion into the dermis.
  (b) Tuberculoid leprosy - erythematous plaques with elevated borders and central dry, anesthetic, hairless atrophy. These result in scarring. Decreased sensation is a characteristic finding. These patients have high resistance to the organism and are not as sick. Their lepromin skin test is positive. Organisms are usually not found on tissue biopsy or smear.
  (c) Borderline disease is an overlap between the above two types.
b. Treatment
(1) Lepromatous disease is treated with dapsone 50-100mg q day plus clofazimine 50-200mg q day plus rifampin 450-600mg q day. If cost is an issue, rifampin may be used once a week or once a month. Treatment is given for a minimum of 2 years.
(2) Tuberculoid disease is treated with rifampin 600mg q month for 6 months plus dapsone 100mg q day for 6 months. Systemic corticosteroids may be used for disease complications.
2. Buruli ulcer (Seorl's ulcer)
a. Caused by *mycobacterium ulcerans*. The organism may be seen on histology or in smears with Ziehl-Neelsen or Fite-Faraco stains. It may be cultured with difficulty.
b. The diagnosis is usually made clinically in areas of tropical rain forests where it usually occurs. It evolves from painless solitary hard nodules to progressive skin necrosis and ulceration over weeks. Morbidity is related to scarring and amputation. Gangrenous changes may be deep and mutilating. Most commonly seen in children and young adults in central Africa.
c. Therapy - aggressive surgical debridement is the treatment of choice. Appropriate antibiotics, local heat (40°C.), and hyperbaric oxygenation have been used. (See Chapter 1, section VII, E)

DERMATOLOGY

3. Tuberculosis
a. General
   (1) Primary tuberculosis occurring in previously unexposed patients may produce a chancre at the site of infection. Multiple symmetrical erythematous papules are seen in miliary tuberculosis secondary to seeding via the blood stream. Tubercle bacilli are present in tissue and the tuberculin skin test is negative.
   (2) Secondary tuberculosis has scant bacilli in tissue and a positive tuberculin skin test indicating prior exposure. Lupus vulgaris is the commonest form and exhibits nodules, ulcers, and plaques in every possible configuration. Scarring, atrophy, and contracture can lead to mutilating changes. Facial involvement is most common. HIV positive patients may have severe drug resistant disease.
b. Treatment - surgery and anti-tuberculous drugs are indicated. Treatment follows guidelines for extra-pulmonary TB. See Chapter1, section VIII.

C. Fungal
1. Tinea capitis
a. General
   (1) Scalp infection caused by dermatophyte fungi transmitted from person to person or animal to person or sometimes by fomites. Most often seen in children.
   (2) The inflammatory type shows much scaling, hair loss, and may appear as a boggy, pustular, erythematous mass called a kerion. A less common non-inflammatory type called "black dot" tinea occurs. Black stubs of broken off hairs are seen. There may be slight or no scaling. A high index of suspicion is needed for diagnosis.
b. Treatment
   (1) Griseofulvin in a dose of 15mg/kg per day for 1 to 3 months is the treatment of choice. Systemic fluconazole, itraconazole or terbinafine have also been used.
   (2) Shampooing with a selenium sulfide shampoo or ketoconazole (Nizoral) shampoo may help treat and decrease transmission.
2. Tinea corporis ("ringworm")
a. General
   (1) Dermatophyte infection of the body that produces a characteristic erythematous ring with an elevated border and central clearing. It is contagious and can be acquired from infected humans, infected animals or the soil. It is pruritic and common especially in hot, humid climates. If it occurs on the hand there is usually a fine, white adherent scale in the folds of the skin mimicking dry skin but usually only one hand is involved.

(2) Diagnosis can be made by examining a KOH mount. Skin scrapings from the lesion show distinctive branching hyphae under low power on a microscope. The scraping is acquired using a scalpel blade scraping just deep enough to cause slight bleeding. The scraping is spread on a slide and covered with 10% potassium or sodium hydroxide solution and a cover slip. It is then heated lightly.

b. Treatment

(1) Topical therapy is often successful with imidazoles (miconazole, econazole, clotrimazole) or allylamines (naftifine, butenafine, terfenadine) twice a day for 2 to 4 weeks.

(2) Oral agents as for tinea capitis may be necessary, if there is no response to topical therapy.

3. Tinea cruris

a. This groin dermatophyte infection is seen mainly in men who are involved in activities that increase moisture and heat in the groin area (hot working conditions, athletic activities or exercise). It may be very pruritic.

b. Treatment - usually treated topically the same as tinea corporis.

4. Tinea pedis

a. General - dermatophyte infection of the feet with three distinct forms

(1) Interdigital disease is seen most often between the 4th and 5th toes as macerated skin with a central fissure. Treatment is important since this can be a portal of entry for bacteria leading to cellulitis, especially in diabetics.

(2) The dry or "moccasin" type mimics dry skin with fine adherent scale in the lines of the skin. It usually involves both feet. A similar eruption of the hands may occur, but it usually involves only one hand.

(3) The vesicular form consists of small vesicles and is very pruritic. The organism can be observed by removing the top of the blister and examining the underside of the skin under low power on the microscope in a KOH mount. All three forms of tinea pedis have a positive scraping.

b. Treatment

(1) Topical therapy is usually adequate as explained for tinea corporis. This is a very chronic recurrent infection and long term daily use of topical anti-fungals may be necessary.

(2) Powdering of socks with talcum powder or a powder with an antifungal may be a helpful prophylactic measure.

5. Tinea versicolor

a. General

(1) A common infection caused by a yeast-like organism. A KOH mount will show very tiny round spores and tiny short hyphae ("spaghetti and meatballs").

(2) The rash is most common on the trunk and will show areas of non-tanning hypopigmentation with a very fine, dry, adherent scale upon scratching the skin. These areas may be confluent or form small well-defined circles. There is no elevated border. In areas of skin where the patient has not tanned the areas may be light brown or light pink-hence the name versicolor (varied color). In areas where the skin has tanned, the skin is white since the fungus inhibits formation of melanin.

(3) This is a common, incurable, non-contagious disease. Lesions are usually not pruritic. When extensive, however, itching may be significant.

b. Treatment

(1) Any of the topical imidazoles twice a day for 2 weeks will cause a temporary remission. Treatment with a selenium sulfide shampoo daily for 2 weeks is often effective (lathering up for five minutes and then rinsing).

(2) For severe disease, oral ketoconazole 200mg twice a day for 5 days may be used.

6. Onychomycosis

a. General

(1) Dermatophyte infection of the toenails. Treatment may be indicated when the infection causes ingrowing of the nail especially in diabetics and patients with significant neuropathy or compromise of circulation to the lower extremities.

(2) It is very common in elderly patients, primarily in the toenails. It is not curable and treatment is not easy.

b. Treatment

(1) Topical agents may be helpful (ciclopirox solution, gel or nail lacquer twice a day for 12 to 18 months). Debridement of the nail may decrease disability.

(2) Oral agents such as itraconazole 200mg twice a day for 1 out of 4 weeks for 3 months, or terfenadine 250mg a day for 3 months are effective if topical agents are not helping. Liver enzyme elevation may rarely occur with both of these oral agents.

(3) Griseofulvin may be used, but is less effective and must be taken for 12 to 18 months.

7. Candidiasis

a. General

(1) Opportunistic infection caused by a normal inhabitant of the mouth, rectum, and vaginal tract.

(2) Diabetes, systemic antibiotics, any activity that increases heat and sweat, or immunosuppressive drugs and conditions predispose to this infection. It is common in the vaginal tract in women and the groin in men.

(3) It causes an erythematous dermatitis without an elevated border and surrounding satellite papules or pustules. An overhanging whitish fringe of epidermis may be present around the periphery. It causes dramatic itching and burning.

(4) In the mouth white plaques are formed that may be thick and wiped off with a tongue blade. This oral form of the disease is often very severe in HIV positive patients.

b. Treatment

(1) Topical imidazoles or nystatin twice a day for 1 week is usually effective.

(2) Oral mucous membrane disease may be treated with nystatin liquid one half hour after each meal to swish and swallow, or clotrimazole troches to suck on one half hour after meals and at night for 1 week.

(3) HIV patients may require oral ketoconazole, fluconazole or itraconazole.

D. Viral

1. Herpes simplex

a. General

(1) DNA virus which occurs as 2 types. Type I usually causes oral lesions and type II usually causes genital lesions. Both can occur at any site, however.

(2) Herpes simplex is an acute painful viral eruption of grouped vesicles on a red base seen most often around the mouth or genitalia. The lesions are associated with pain, fever and malaise. They rapidly ulcerate and may produce an exudate. They heal in 5-7 days.

(3) Primary infection may be subclinical. The viral DNA may remain in the ganglion of the anatomic region of initial infection, however, and subsequently be reactivated, resulting in recurrent infection.

(4) Herpes simplex has also been associated with cutaneous erythema multiforme.

(5) The diagnosis can be made by cultures or a Tzanck smear (Wright-Giemsa stain of smear taken from the ulcer shows multinucleated giant cells).

b. Treatment is with oral acyclovir, valacyclovir, and famciclovir. Topical acyclovir or valacyclovir is less effective but helpful.

2. Varicella Zoster (shingles)

a. General

(1) This is a common viral disease characterized by the appearance of several groups of vesicles along the distribution of a cutaneous nerve (dermatome). Zoster and chicken pox are caused by the same virus. Zoster results from reactivation of the virus that has remained latent in dorsal root ganglion after an earlier exposure to chickenpox. It is usually unilateral and occurs in the thoracic region, face and, less frequently, in the lumbosacral region. Any site may be involved. Eye involvement may cause corneal scaring and can be very serious.

(2) New crops of vesicles appear for 3-5 days, then dry up and form crusts. They usually heal in 3 weeks. The lesions can be secondarily infected with bacteria. Severe neuropathic pain may precede the rash. Some patients develop persistent pain (post herpetic neuralgia), which can persist for months to years. This occurs in up to half of patients over the age of 50. The disease is more severe in immunocompromised patients.

(3) Diagnosis is generally made clinically. It can be confirmed by culture or Tzanck smear.

b. Treatment

(1) Acyclovir 800 mg five times a day. Famciclovir and valacyclovir can also be used. They must be started within 48 hours of onset for maximum benefit.

(2) Analgesics for pain, amitriptyline, phenytoin, and carbamazepine can be tried for post herpetic neuralgia.

(3) Systemic antibiotics if secondary infection is present.

(4) Zoster cannot be caught from someone with zoster, but chickenpox can be caught by a susceptible person by touching zoster lesions.

IV. BITES AND INFESTATIONS
A. Scabies
1. General

a. Common contagious infestation caused by a mite, *Sarcoptes scabei*. The organism cannot be seen with the naked eye but may be demonstrated on skin scraping.

b. Examination of a wet mount prepared by scraping the lesion with a scalpel blade just enough to cause bleeding, then examining the scrapings under low power microscopy will reveal the mite. Oval eggs and small brown oval feces may also be seen.

c. Papules, pustules, and occasionally vesicles are seen most often on the flexor surfaces of the wrists, between fingers, axillae, elbows, girdle areas, genital area, ankles, palms, and soles. The major complaint is pruritus. Excoriations may be numerous and dramatic, as itching is often intolerable.

d. The most diagnostic skin finding is a thread-like burrow several mm in length which is tiny and difficult to see. The adult mite is often present in the burrow.

e. The mite is transmitted mainly by prolonged skin to skin contact. It can be sexually transmitted. It is very common in children.

f. A non-infectious form called nodular scabies may persist many months after the mite has been exterminated. It consists of extremely pruritic red nodules. No mites are found in nodular scabies.

2. Treatment

a. Kwell (lindane, gamma benzene hexachloride) should be applied from the neck down in adults and children over one year of age. In children under one year of age the scalp and face must also be treated. All areas of skin should be treated. This is left on overnight and repeated in 24 hours.

b. Sulfur ointment (10 % in petrolatum) can be applied overnight for 3 consecutive nights in all age groups and during pregnancy.

c. Elimite (permethrin) is the preferred treatment in infants where the cream is applied above the neck. It may also be used in pregnant women. Application regimen is similar to that described above for Kwell.

d. Oral ivermectin (Stromectol) 200 mg/kg in a single oral dose repeated in 10 days can be used in non- pregnant adults.

e. All bedding and clothing should be laundered in hot soapy water.

f. All family members and household contacts should be treated regardless of signs of the disease. This is essential to clearing up an outbreak of scabies.

g. The itching may be worse the first week after therapy and, if persistent, potent topical corticosteroids or a short course (ten to fourteen days) of systemic corticosteroids is very helpful. Antihistamines may help, as well.

B. Lice (pediculosis)

1. Types

a. Head lice are the largest organisms and can easily be seen with the naked eye. Shared fomites such a hats, combs, and hair decorations can transmit the disease. Nits are 2 to 3 mm white concretions that adhere firmly to the hair. Examining clipped hairs on low power microscopy can easily identify them. The egg is flask shaped and eccentrically attached to the hair with an outline of the organism within.

b. Body lice are slightly smaller and are often transmitted in bedding materials.

c. Pubic lice are the smallest and are difficult to see with the naked eye. They are present mainly in the pubic area but can also be seen on abdominal areas and eyelashes. The organism is usually sexually transmitted.

2. Treatment

a. Head lice are treated by discarding all fomites or storing them for 30 days in a plastic bag.

  (1) Kwell (lindane, gamma benzene hexachloride) shampoo is lathered in and left for 3 to 4 minutes before rinsing. Treatment is repeated in 3 days.

  (2) Nix (permethrin) cream rinse is left on for 10 minutes after shampooing and repeated in 3 days.

  (3) Mayonnaise (not low fat) can be left in overnight under a shower cap. Treatment is repeated in 3 days.

  (4) Attempts should be made to remove all nits by trimming hair, or by using a fine toothed comb to remove them.

  (5) Step Two (formic acid) rinse, or shampoos containing salicylic acid may be helpful.

  (6) All family members should be treated. All fomites should be discarded or stored for 30 days in a plastic bag to prevent recurrent infestation after treatment. Secondary infection should be treated, if present.

b. Body lice

  (1) May be treated with 10 % sulfur in petrolatum applied to involved skin and left overnight for 3 nights.

  (2) Topical Kwell (lindane, gamma benzene hexachloride) is applied and left over night. Treatment is repeated in 3 days.

  (3) Ivermectin may be used as for scabies in non-pregnant adults.

c. Pubic lice are treated in the same manner as head lice. Sexual contacts should be treated.

d. Lice on the eyelashes can be treated with sulfacetamide ophthalmic ointment 4 times a day for 5 days. Petrolatum may also be used in the same way.

C. Chiggers

1. General

a. Seen worldwide and common in tropical areas, these mites are red-orange and 0.25-0.4 mm in size.

b. Red very pruritic papules are seen in areas under socks and waistbands, and also on exposed skin. Infection is acquired by sitting or walking through infested vegetation. Rarely vesicular.

2. Treatment

a. Topical corticosteroids or, when severe, 10 to 14 days of systemic corticosteroids are used for therapy.

b. Antihistamines and topical anti-pruritics are helpful to ameliorate the itching. Insect repellants containing diethyltoluamide or sulfur may help prevent the bites.

D. Spider bites

1. General

a. Several species of spiders throughout the world, such as the brown recluse spider, can cause acute cutaneous necrosis within hours after the bite. The lesion is painful and can be severe. The spider is usually not seen.

b. Bites are single and most common on the extremities.

2. **Treatment**

a. No therapy has been shown to be reliably beneficial. Dapsone 100 mg a day for 5 days, short-course high-dose systemic corticosteroids, ice compresses, elevation of the affected limb are all therapies advocated by some.

b. Debridement and treatment of secondary infection is appropriate follow-up therapy.

V. MISCELLANEOUS
A. Urticaria (hives)
1. General

a. Urticaria are erythematous or white plaques and occasionally papules that are evanescent. They disappear and reappear in less than 24 hours and often in minutes or hours.

b. This is a Type I or anaphylactic hypersensitivity reaction. It can be life-threatening if bronchospasm or laryngeal edema occurs.

c. Angioedema is a large hive involving a body region such as a hand, lip, side of face, etc. The cause is often not ascertained. The commonest causes are drugs (especially aspirin, sulfa-derived medications, penicillins, anti-convulsants, and non-steroidal anti-inflammatory drugs), foods (most notably shellfish, nuts, chocolate, fresh berries, melons), emotional upset, and physical agents (cold, heat, pressure).

d. Dermatographism (a hive produced by scratching the skin) is more common in these patients or may be present as a separate condition.

e. Asthma, hayfever, marked reactions to insect bites, and eczema are also more common in patients with urticaria.

2. Treatment

a. Antihistamines are the mainstay of therapy. Sedating antihistamines include chlorpheniramine, diphenhydramine, hydroxyzine, and cyproheptadine. Non-sedating antihistamines include cetirizine, loratadine, fexofenadine and clemastine.

b. Combination of these medications may be very helpful. Adding an H-2 blocker such as ranitidine or cimetidine may be helpful. Doxepin can be very beneficial alone or in combination with the antihistamines already mentioned. It can be very sedating.

c. Systemic corticosteroids may be necessary if antihistamines fail. Short courses are preferable due to side effects.

d. Subcutaneous epinephrine is used when the condition is life threatening such as in an anaphylactic reaction.

B. Drug eruptions

1. General

a. There are many different types of reactions to drugs. The most common variant is morbilliform or maculopapular which consists of symmetrical red macules and papules that are usually very pruritic.

b. All patterns of drug eruptions are most common with antibiotics, non-steroidal anti-inflammatory drugs, anti-seizure medications, thiazide diuretics, sulfonylureas, and allopurinol. Drug eruptions can mimic lichen planus and pityriasis rosea and be manifested as pruritus or hives.

c. The drug reactions can cause a vasculitis that can affect the skin and other organs, especially the joints and kidneys.

d. A fixed drug eruption occurs as a localized severe inflammatory or bullous eruption leaving marked hyperpigmentation. The lesions recur at the same sites if the same drug is re-introduced. The penis is the most common location in men for a fixed drug eruption. Phenolphthalein, non-steroidal anti-inflammatory drugs, and antibiotics (especially tetracycline derivatives) are common offenders.

e. Photosensitivity drug eruptions and hives (see urticaria) are other types of drug eruptions.

2. Treatment

a. Discontinue the offending drug, if possible. If the drug is too important to stop and the reaction is not life threatening, sometimes the drug can be continued and the drug reaction will resolve with or without treatment.

b. A short course of high dose systemic corticosteroids is the treatment of choice.

c. Topical antipruritics or antihistamines can be used to control symptoms.

C. Toxic epidermal necrolysis (TEN)

1. General

a. This is a life-threatening blistering disease that is usually due to drugs in adults and staphylococcal infection in children (see Chapter 1, section I).

b. Anti-seizure medications and sulfa derivatives are the most common offenders.

c. The skin next to large flaccid blisters can be wiped off with gentle pressure with the finger (Nikolsky's sign).

d. Patients with TEN appear very ill, with fever and generalized skin rash. It is fatal 50% of the time when drug induced in adults.

2. Treatment

a. Supportive therapy is the most important with electrolyte and fluid replacement.

    b. Cool wet compresses with saline, water, Aveeno or Domeboro may be soothing. Topical antibiotics (Silvadene, Polysporin, mupirocin) and, when indicated, systemic antibiotics are helpful.

    c. Systemic high-dose corticosteroids are a very controversial therapy but may be helpful if given early in the course of the disease. Intravenous immunoglobulin is felt to be very beneficial in some cases.

D. Erythema multiforme (minor)

1. General

    a. In its minor form painful oral erosions are accompanied by skin lesions with concentric rings of white and red circles and, at times, a central blister. This is called a "target" lesion.

    b. Lesions are symmetric and are common on the palms and soles.

    c. Herpes simplex is the most common cause of erythema multiforme. Drugs and other infections may also be causative.

    d. In its most severe form, it is called Stevens-Johnson syndrome.

2. Treatment

    a. Short course, high dose systemic corticosteroids are usually effective.

    b. Acyclovir, famciclovir, and valacyclovir can be used prophylactically when herpes simplex is recurrent and is the cause.

E. Stevens-Johnson syndrome (erythema multiforme major)

1. General

    a. Some experts consider this a variant of TEN with severe mucous membrane disease (eyes, oral, genital). Blindness may occur.

    b. Circular "bulls-eye" or "target" iris lesions can occur with a central blister.

    c. Drugs are usually the cause (eg. as anti-seizure medications and antibiotics).

2. Treatment

    a. Supportive care as for TEN.

    b. Early in the course of the disease high-dose systemic corticosteroids may be beneficial.

    c. Intravenous IgG immunoglobulin may be life saving, if available.

VI. How to Improvise Topical Medications

1. Creams - whenever a cream is needed, water can be mixed with equal parts of vaseline, lard, shortening, lanolin, zinc oxide or any other solid plant or animal oil.

2. Ointments - whenever an ointment is needed and Aquaphor is unavailable, vaseline, lard, cold cream, petrolatum, shortening, liquid oils such as olive oil, palm oil, coconut oil, olive oil, safflower oil, canola oil, mineral oil or any other plant or animal-derived oil can be used as a substitute.

3. Compresses to dry the skin - include the following (substitute for Domeboro or Aveeno):

a. Luke-warm water.

b. Equal parts of water and white vinegar (adds antibacterial properties).

c. Camomile or other teas.

d. Salt or epsom salts (2 tablespoons of salt to one pint of water).

4. **Compresses to moisturize the skin** - these include any of the liquid oils above mixing 2 capfuls of oil per pint of water.

5. **Compresses in general** - should be applied to the affected area for 10-15 minutes 2 to 3 times a day and kept moist during the entire compress period.

6. **Shake lotions** - can be made as follows:

   a. For a drying and antipruritic lotion, mix 24 parts zinc oxide, 24 parts talc, 12 parts glycerin and enough distilled water to make a total of 120.

   b. For more drying and more antibacterial properties, mix 24 parts zinc oxide, 24 parts talc, 12 parts glycerin and enough 70% isopropyl alcohol to make 120. This lotion will sting at first if open areas are present, then it cools.

7. **Baths** (soak for 10-15 minutes)

   a. Coal tar solution (LCD) baths - add 2 tablespoons of coal tar to 6-8 inches of lukewarm water. This is antipruritic, anti-eczematous.

   b. Starch baths (alternative for Aveeno or Domeboro) - small box of starch to 6-8 inches of cool water. This is soothing, drying, and antipruritic.

   c. Oil baths - add 2-3 tablespoons or capfuls of oil to 6-8 inches of water. This is moisturizing for dry skin.

   d. Oatmeal baths (alternative to Aveeno or Domeboro) - add 2-4 tablespoons of oatmeal to tub of water. This is antipruritic and drying.

   e. Clorox baths - add one half cup of Clorox or bleach to tub of water. Use for impetigo, folliculitis or other infections.

8. **Psoriasis** - can be treated using 1% coal tar in any ointment. It is malodorous and stains clothing, but is safe and effective. Apply overnight 3-5 times a week.

9. **Eczema** - any of the ointments applied immediately after water exposure (such as hand washing or bathing) will help to keep the skin moist. Bag balm or udder cream are also effective.

10. **Acne**

   a. Clindamycin topical solution may be made by adding 600 mg of clindamycin (powder contents of two 300mg or four 150mg capsules) dissolved in 2 ounces or 4 parts isopropyl alcohol with 1 part propylene glycol.

   b. Erythromycin topical solution can be made by substituting 1000mg of erythromycin in place of clindamycin.

   c. 2% to 5% sulfur can be mixed in the above mixtures or added to any of the creams bid. (Salicylic acid can be added to this or substituted for the sulfur, also at 2% to 5%)

CHAPTER 13

NEONATOLOGY

I. BASICS

A. Definitions of maturity
1. **Pre-term** - < 37 weeks
2. **Term** - 37-42 weeks
3. **Post-term** - > 42 weeks

B. Classification of size
1. **Large for gestational age (LGA)**
   a. > 4000gm at term.
   b. Could be a sign of maternal diabetes.
   c. Associated with risk of difficult delivery, hypoglycemia.
2. **Appropriate for gestational age (AGA)**
3. **Small for gestational age (SGA)**
   a. <2500gm at term.
   b. Might suggest poor prenatal nutrition, placental insufficiency or gestational infection, such as malaria.
   c. At risk for hypoglycemia.

C. Classification of heart rate
1. **Bradycardia**
   a. < 100/minute
   b. May be due to inadequate ventilation, sepsis or, rarely, heart block (seen with maternal digoxin use, maternal lupus).
2. **Tachycardia**
   a. > 180/minute
   b. May suggest pain, hypovolemia, fever.

D. Understanding of temperature
1. **Technique** - only rectal temperatures are reliable in newborns.
2. **Low temperature** (< 36° C.)
   a. Might need more covers/hat/clothes or external warmth.
   b. May be sign of sepsis.
3. **High temperature** (> 38° C.)
   a. Suggestive of infection, such as bacterial sepsis, or malaria in endemic areas, even in newborns.
   b. Needs further investigation. See Section VI below.

E. Output
1. **Urine**
   a. First urine usually passed within 24 hours after birth. Subsequent voiding should then occur at least every six hours.
   b. Delayed urine passage raises concern of obstruction (posterior urethral valves).
2. **Stool**
   a. First stool is usually passed within 24-48 hours after birth. Tarry, green/black "meconium" is passed for the first 1-3 days.

    b. Brownish, runny "transition stool" passes for 1-2 days.

    c. Then, yellow pasty or seedy "normal" infant stool is passed.

    d. Frequency varies with method of feeding. Breastfed infants pass stool more frequently than formula-fed. May vary from once every few days to many stools each day.

    e. Delayed initiation of stool suggests possibility of intestinal atresia or Hirschsprung's disease.

F. Weight changes

  1. Initial weight loss during the first week

    a. Breastfed infant loses 6%, on average.

    b. Formula-fed infant loses 3%, on average.

  2. Then weight regained, usually back to birth weight by 10-14 days.

  3. Weight gain is about 15-30 gm per day during early months of life.

  4. Excessive weight loss or delayed weight gain

    a. Usually suggestive of inadequate intake

      (1) Poor feeding technique.

      (2) Inadequate supply.

    b. Sometimes due to excessive losses

      (1) Emesis

      (2) Intestinal malabsorption.

    c. Rarely due to hypermetabolic state

      (1) Infection

      (2) Endocrine

      (3) Intoxication

II. INITIAL CARE OF NEWBORN INFANT

A. "Resuscitation" for all newborns

  1. Clear airway (oral and nasal suctioning).

  2. Stimulate (rub back, stimulate cry).

  3. Maintain warmth

    a. Dry wet skin.

    b. Provide external warmth.

    c. Cover skin (especially head) to maintain temperature.

B. Resuscitation for struggling newborns

  1. **Apgar score** - can be used to evaluate need for resuscitative efforts. Assess at 1 minute and 5 minutes after birth:

Apgar Score			
Sign	**0**	**1**	**2**
Heart Rate	Absent	<100/min	>100/min
Respirations	Absent	Weak Cry	Vigorous Cry
Muscle Tone	Limp	Decreased	Normal
Response (to nasal stimulation)	None	Grimace	Cough, Sneeze
Color	Blue	Pink/Blue	Entirely Pink

a. Low 1 minute Apgar suggests need for more aggressive immediate resuscitative care.

b. Low 5 minute Apgar suggests guarded neurological prognosis.

2. Score 7-10

a. Continue usual care.

b. No special resuscitative efforts needed.

3. Score 5-6

a. Increasingly stimulate the infant.

b. Consider oxygen supplementation.

4. Score 0-4

a. Maintain airway patency.

b. Ensure adequate warmth of infant.

c. Oxygen supplementation, if possible.

d. Increase ventilation (bag/mask vs. intubation, depending on resources).

e. Cardiac massage if heart rate < 60/minute despite good ventilation.

f. Medications to consider, if available:

(1) Epinephrine 1:10,000, 0.1cc/kg IV or SQ, repeat q 15 min prn if bradycardia despite good ventilation.

(2) Volume (normal saline, albumin or blood) at 10cc/kg if persistently poor perfusion.

(3) Naloxone 0.1 mg/kg IV, IM or SQ, repeat q 5 min prn if poor inspiratory effort and maternal narcotic.

(4) Bicarbonate 1 mEq/kg IV if prolonged resuscitation (>10 minutes) and poor perfusion.

C. Initiation of feeding

1. Selection

a. Breast milk is usually the best choice.

(1) If mother is able, this should be strongly encouraged.

(2) There is a risk to the infant if the mother is HIV +. The parent(s) and health care provider(s) need to balance the nutritional and psychosocial values of breastfeeding and the following risks:

(a) Real risk of mother to child HIV transmission through breast-milk. This accounts for perhaps one third of all mother to child transmission, mostly in the first few months of nursing.

(b) Risk of combined breast-milk and formula feedings (perhaps more risk of transmission of HIV than for children who receive only breast-milk or formula).

(c) Risk of formula feeding - cost, water-born diseases in areas of unhygienic water supplies.

(3) Personal, local and cultural situations will contribute to the decision about whether to have a mother breastfeed or not.

b. Formula

          (1) Difficulty in obtaining clean water and correctly preparing the formula makes this a less ideal choice in developing countries.

          (2) Lactose-free formulas may be of help in the uncommon situation where an infant is unable to tolerate lactose-based formula.

     c. Cows' milk

          (1) Risk of intestinal irritation and blood loss during first 6-12 months of life.

          (2) Not recommended until infant is 12 months old.

   2. Timing

     a. Best to start feeding during first two hours after birth.

          (1) Maximizes maternal milk supply.

          (2) Initial breast milk (colostrum) is very nutritious and anti-infective.

     b. Feed frequently - usually every 2 to 4 hours, on demand.

D. Routine neonatal cares

   1. Ophthalmic prophylaxis

     a. Done to prevent neonatal infection with *N. gonorrhea* or *Chlamydia*, which can cause blindness in the infant. These infections may be inapparent in the mother. Routine prophylaxis of all newborns is recommended.

     b. Treat with topical therapy, once during early minutes/hour of life. One of the following should be used: silver nitrate drops, erythromycin ointment or tetracycline ointment.

   2. Prevention of hemorrhagic disease of the newborn

     a. Vitamin K, 1 mg IM or SQ, if available, especially if traumatic delivery.

     b. Should be given during early hours of life.

   3. Vaccination

     a. Follow local schedules.

     b. Hepatitis B

          (1) Immune serum globulin, if available, if mother HBsAg+.

          (2) Vaccination reasonable for all newborns, if available (first of three doses may be given during first days of life).

     c. BCG

          (1) Limited benefit if good access to medical care.

          (2) Routinely given in many countries.

III. CARE OF PRETERM INFANTS

A. Determination of gestational age

   1. Useful for some legal-social situations (paternity issues, especially). Accurate determination may be made using standard texts.

   2. Useful to determine some post-natal management

     a. Abbreviated scoring scale:

Modified Gestational Age Assessment

Points	0	1	2	3	4
Plantar Creases	No creases	Faint red marks	Ant. transverse crease only	Creases anterior 2/3	Creases cover entire sole
Breast	Barely perceptible	Flat areola, no bud	Stippled areola, 1-2mm bud	Raised areola, 3-4mm bud	Full areola, 5-10mm bud
Ear	Pinna flat, stays folded	Sl. curved pinna, soft with slow recoil	Well curved pinna, ready recoil	Formed, firm pinna, instant recoil	Thick cartilage, ear stiff
Genitals (Male)	-	Scrotum empty, no rugae	Testes descended, few rugae	Testes down, good rugae	Testes pendulous, deep rugae
Genitals (Female)	-	Prominent clitoris and labia	Majora, minora equally prominent	Majora large, minora small	Clitoris and minora completely covered

Score	2	3	5	7	9	10	12	14	16
Age (Weeks)	26	28	30	32	34	36	38	40	42

   b. Consider nasogastric feeding if < 36 weeks
     (1) Pre-term infants have increased risk of aspiration due to poor suck or uncoordinated suck-swallow.
     (2) Use intermittently placed tube (remove after each feeding).
     (3) Oral feedings when able clinically.
   c. Consider respiratory stimulant if < 34 weeks
     (1) Monitor closely and initiate treatment if apnea > 20 seconds and bradycardia episodes noted. If monitor not available, treat pre-emptively.
     (2) Aminophylline 6mg/kg IV or PO x1, then 1.5mg/kg q8 hours or caffeine 10mg/kg IV or PO x1, then 2.5mg/kg daily.
     (3) Treat until > 36 weeks corrected gestational age (add number of weeks since birthday to number of weeks of pregnancy at time of birth, stop treatment when this total is more than 36 weeks).

B. Routine pre-term cares

  1. Feeding
   a. Route
     (1) Usually from breast (or bottle or spoon/cup if not breastfeeding).
     (2) Consider nasogastric feeding if:
       (a) < 36 weeks gestational age.
       (b) Neonatal asphyxia.
       (c) Difficulty with initial attempts at oral feeding.
   b. Solution

      (1) Colostrum and/or breast milk, if available.
      (2) Sugar water (5% dextrose) first day if no colostrum available.
      (3) Formula only if no breast milk available. Needs careful preparation.

  c. Quantity
      (1) Ad lib if breastfeeding (monitor weight if concerns about adequacy of volume).
      (2) Ad lib if bottle feeding.
      (3) Nasogastric feeding:

          Day 1   80 cc/kg/day (9cc/kg every 3 hours)
          Day 2   100 cc/kg/day (12cc/kg every 3 hours)
          Day 3   120 cc/kg/day (15cc/kg every 3 hours)
          Day 4+ 150-180 cc/kg/day (18-24cc/kg every 3 hours)

  d. Cautions
      (1) If formula is being used, careful attention must be paid to preparation, using pure water, appropriate concentration.
      (2) Premature infants need to have right side down, head up for feedings. Supine/side position for sleep is okay after feeding.

2. Warmth
  a. Ensure adequate environmental warmth (often about 31-32° C. for small premature babies).
  b. Cover skin and scalp to prevent loss of body warmth.
  c. Keep baby dry to prevent evaporative heat losses.
  d. Monitor temperature closely to help keep it normal.

3. Oxygen therapy
  a. In premature infants with respiratory distress, keep oxygen concentration as low as possible to keep infant pink or O2 saturation 89-95%.
  b. In term infants with meconium aspiration or at risk for pulmonary hypertension, keep the oxygen as high as possible.

IV. CARDIO-RESPIRATORY PROBLEMS

  A. Clinical signs of respiratory distress
    1. Tachypnea (respiratory rate > 60/minute at rest).
    2. Retractions (indrawing, prominent chest muscle use).
    3. Nasal flaring.
    4. Grunting (moaning expiration).
    5. Cyanosis (central, especially).

  B. Central cyanosis
    1. General
      a. Involves the trunk as well as the extremities.
      b. Can result from pulmonary insufficiency, congenital heart disease or hypoventilation from a central nervous system lesion.

   c. Differentiate from peripheral cyanosis, which is often a normal variation. Most often occurs when the baby is undressed and exposed to a cool environment. Peripheral cyanosis does not usually indicate serious disease, unless it persists after the baby is warmed up. Usually involves the hands, feet and circumoral area.

2. Congenital heart disease

   a. Early central cyanosis, without respiratory distress, is usually caused by congenital heart disease. These patients need referral to a cardiovascular center where surgery is available. Echocardiography and cardiac catheterization can help localize the specific diagnosis if these modalities are available. A PaO2 that does not rise about 100mm Hg with the administration of 100% oxygen (hyperoxia test) suggests cyanotic heart disease, with a right-to-left shunt.

   b. Tetralogy of Fallot

      (1) Sometimes mild cyanosis. A right-to-left shunt is present.

      (2) Murmur after first day (ventriculoseptal defect, systolic murmur along left sternal border and to apex).

      (3) Sometimes able to live without intervention.

   c. Transposition of great vessels

      (1) Most patients present with cyanosis and tachypnea. Hypoxemia can be severe. Heart failure is not usually present.

      (2) Usually requires surgical intervention in first 5 days.

   d. Truncus arteriosus

      (1) Most patients develop heart failure due to increased pulmonary blood flow. Cyanosis is not usually clinically significant.

      (2) Precordium is hyperactive and there is a systolic ejection murmur.

      (3) Medical management until surgical correction can be done.

   e. Total anomalous pulmonary venous return

      (1) Often requires surgical intervention in first 5 days.

      (2) Might not present until second month or so of life.

   f. Tricuspid atresia

      (1) Usually requires surgical intervention in first 5 days.

C. Respiratory distress with or without cyanosis

  1. Congenital cardiac malformation with heart failure

   a. Coarctation of the aorta

      (1) Can be diagnosed anytime in childhood. In neonates, acute congestive heart failure is the most common presentation.

      (2) A systolic murmur is usually present, heard best in the back. Hepatomegaly may be present also.

      (3) Femoral pulses are decreased compared with those in the upper extremity and there is a discrepancy in blood pressure between the arms and legs.

(4) Since patent ductus arteriosus is often associated, infusion of prostaglandin E1 may improve blood flow to the extremities. Diuretics may relieve symptoms of heart failure. Immediate surgical repair may be necessary.

b. Hypoplastic left heart
    (1) Presents in first 5 days of life, sometimes with a systolic flow murmur. Heart failure develops quickly.
    (2) Complex surgical procedures might help, but the condition is usually fatal in developing countries.

c. Patent ductus arteriosus (PDA)
    (1) Presents around second week of life.
    (2) Systolic/diastolic murmur near left clavicle.
    (3) Bounding pulses, palmar pulses notable.
    (4) Short term fluid restriction and indomethacin sometimes effective 0.1-0.2 mg/kg IV over 30 minutes, repeat q 12-24 hours up to 3 doses prn.
    (5) Surgical ligation helpful when medical interventions not successful.

d. Ventriculoseptal defect (VSD)
    (1) Manifestations depend on size. Small defects may be audible early but remain asymptomatic. Large VSDs can be silent at birth and then develop signs of congestive heart failure in the first few postnatal weeks.
    (2) A systolic murmur in the apical area, often with a thrill is characteristic. Pulses are normal.
    (3) Heart failure can be treated with digoxin 5mcg/kg/dose bid and a diuretic such as furosemide 1mg/kg/dose 1-2 times a day.
    (4) Spontaneous closure may occur during the first 18 months of life. If it doesn't, surgery is necessary.

2. High output failure with anatomically normal heart
  a. Anemia
  b. Vascular malformation
    (1) Bruit over fontanelle, eyes, abdomen.
    (2) Ultrasound to image head, abdomen.
    (3) Complex surgery might be needed.

3. Pulmonary disease
  a. Tracheomalacia - usually causes inspiratory stridor, due to the abnormally weak airway. Stridor may get worse during feeding or when the baby cries. Infants usually do not experience respiratory distress and do well with no treatment.
  b. Tracheoesophageal fistula - usually diagnosed within the first 24 hours after birth. Infants may present with choking, gagging or cyanotic episodes during feeding. Aspiration pneumonia can occur. Diagnosis is made with bronchoscopy or contrast x-rays.

c. Pneumonia - see G below.

4. Infection

  a. Sepsis and pneumonia are both possible causes of cyanosis with respiratory distress.

  b. Diagnose pneumonia with elevated white blood count, positive chest x-ray. Blood cultures, if available, often positive in sepsis.

  c. Antibiotics to treat.

D. Respiratory distress syndrome (hyaline membrane disease)

  1. Usually with premature birth (<34 weeks).

  2. Progressive over first 3 days, then stable until death or resolution.

  3. Treat with oxygenation, possible continuous positive airway pressure, or intubation.

  4. Intra-tracheal surfactant helpful, when available.

E. Meconium aspiration

  1. Usually occurs with stressful delivery, asphyxia.

  2. May cause a necrotizing pneumonitis.

  3. Antibiotics are indicated if bacterial superinfection seems likely.

  4. Oxygenation and ventilation as needed.

F. Transient tachypnea of the newborn

  1. Most common if operative (Cesarean) delivery.

  2. Up to 48 hours of tachypnea, rarely cyanosis.

  3. Hazy appearance on chest x-ray, fluid in fissure.

G. Pneumonia

  1. Often *group B streptococci* or gram-negative enteric pathogens.

    a. Infant may have associated fever.

    b. X-ray with diffuse and/or focal infiltrates.

    c. Antibiotics helpful (see under "Fever" below).

    d. Supportive care (oxygen, ventilation) as needed.

  2. *Chlamydia* pneumonia

    a. Afebrile pneumonia between 4 and 8 weeks of age.

    b. May or may not have had earlier conjunctivitis.

    c. Cough is usually staccato in nature.

    d. Treatment is with erythromycin 50mg/g/d po for 14 days.

    e. Mother and her partners might also benefit from treatment.

V. VOMITING

A. General

  1. Vomiting (forceful expulsion of stomach contents) must be distinguished from regurgitation, which is common in all babies. Regurgitation can be managed by reducing the volume of each feeding and increasing the frequency with which the baby is "burped".

  2. True vomiting is characterized as bilious (never normal, signifies an obstructive lesion) or non-bilious.

B. Green emesis (bilious)

   1. **Possible ileal atresia** - if there is no stool and no distal intestinal gas on x-ray, consider exploratory surgery and ileostomy (versus re-anastomosis).

   2. **Possible mid-gut malrotation with volvulus** - if acutely ill, give nothing by mouth and perform emergent surgery. If not acutely ill, do contrast x-ray (upper GI study shows abnormal small intestine with proximal dilatation and, often, gasless area distally).

C. Non-bilious emesis

   1. **Imperforate anus** - diagnosed on physical exam.

   2. **Intestinal atresia**

      a. No significant stool output.

      b. Abdominal distension often present.

      c. Abdominal x-ray may show the following:

         (1) "Double bubble" representing air in the stomach and proximal duodenum if duodenal atresia.

         (2) No gastric/intestinal air if esophageal atresia.

      d. Surgical intervention needed if atresia is present.

   3. **Systemic infection**

      a. Vomiting is a common finding in neonates with sepsis or meningitis.

      b. Management as under "Fever", Section VI below.

   4. **Pyloric stenosis**

      a. Presents around 4 weeks of age (rarely before). Infant typically has projectile vomiting.

      b. Healthy-seeming child, good appetite.

      c. Often in first-born males.

      d. Delayed emptying of contrast on stomach x-ray.

      e. Treatment by surgical pyloromyotomy.

   5. **Gastroesophageal reflux** - helped with head-up positioning during and after feedings.

VI. FEVER

A. General

   1. Ensure absence of extrinsic temperature source.

   2. Always consider infectious etiology.

   3. Rectal temperature >38° C., 100.4° F. is considered significant.

B. Congenital malaria

   1. Possible in endemic areas.

   2. Malaria smear usually positive.

   3. Treat as in older child with malaria, with age-adjusted dosing.

C. Serious bacterial infection

   1. **Presentation**

      a. The general appearance of the infant is important in determining extent of illness. Irritability is a cause of concern. Lethargy, apnea or cyanosis are ominous signs, indicating grave illness. Mottled extremities, decreased peripheral pulses or delayed capillary refill are signs of cardiovascular instability, indicating the need for aggressive fluid resuscitation. Serious bacterial infection can be generalized with sepsis and bacteremia or present with localized infection, as below.

b. Meningitis
    (1) Full fontanelle.
    (2) Irritability.
    (3) Spinal fluid (CSF) with white cells, organisms.

c. Pneumonia
    (1) Sometimes with respiratory distress.
    (2) Chest x-ray with infiltrates.
    (3) Might benefit from oxygen.

d. Osteomyelitis, septic arthritis
    (1) Sometimes with decreased use of involved part.
    (2) X-rays not usually helpful until late in course.

e. Urinary tract infection
    (1) Usually hematogenous in first 2 days.
    (2) Possibly ascending later.
    (3) Urinalysis with white cells, organisms.

2. Evaluation
  a. All newborns with fevers >38° C. (100.4° F.) should have a sepsis workup done, and be admitted to the hospital for parenteral antibiotic therapy.
  b. Recommended laboratory studies include CBC, urinalysis, chest x-ray and spinal tap. Blood, urine and CSF cultures should be done, if available.
  c. CBC may show elevated WBC's with neutrophilic predominance and left shift. Sometimes, neutropenia may be present or the WBC may be normal. Low platelet count suggests severe disease.

3. Treatment (for proven or possible "sepsis")
  a. Supportive care
    (1) Feeding
    (2) Temperature control
  b. Antibiotics
    (1) Most common bacterial pathogens include *Group B streptococci* (GBS), Gram negative enteric organisms and, rarely, *Listeria*.
    (2) Broad coverage with ampicillin 100mg/kg/dose IV q12h and gentamicin 2.5mg/kg/dose IV q12h the first week, then q8h should be given.
    (3) Alternative regimen is ampicillin as above and cefotaxime 50mg/kg/dose IV or IM.
    (4) If cultures are available, antibiotic therapy can be adjusted according to results of the susceptibility testing.

    c. Duration of treatment
      (1) 7-10 days if bacteremia, pneumonia.
      (2) 10 days if urinary tract infection.
      (3) 10 days if Group B strep meningitis.
      (4) 14 days if gram negative meningitis.

VII. Seizures
A. General
1. Seizures in the first two days of life often result from neonatal asphyxia but do not necessarily imply a poor prognosis for ongoing seizures.
2. Seizures during the neonatal period, but after 48 hours of age suggest ongoing CNS pathology (infection, intracranial hemorrhage).
3. Neonatal seizures are often subtle with eye and/or mouth movements with or without "swimming movements" or frank tonic-clonic movements of the extremities. They may be focal, involving one extremity or the muscles of the face. They may be accompanied by apnea, bradycardia or cyanosis.
4. As with older children, attention to airway protection, injury prevention and aspiration avoidance are important.

B. Evaluation
1. Careful attention to the skin exam (neurocutaneous syndromes), temperature, signs of infection (sepsis or meningitis), anemia, electrolyte imbalance and hypoglycemia can often identify causative or aggravating factors.
2. EEG testing, if available, can help determine if a seizure disorder is present and if there is a localized CNS process.
3. Intracranial ultrasonography or CT may be helpful, if available.

C. Treatment
1. Attention to airway, breathing and circulation.
2. Phenobarbital and phenytoin are often useful (for dosing see Appendix I, Formulary), but higher cumulative loading doses of phenobarbital are sometimes needed in newborns.

VIII. Jaundice
A. Physiologic jaundice
1. Occurs in first 3-10 days. Bilirubin usually less than 10-12mg/dL.
2. Due to relative hepatic immaturity, hemoglobin "recycling" as physiologic polycythemia resolves and birth-related hematomas resolve.
3. May be brought on by limited oral intake, especially if breastfeeding.
4. The infant is usually mildly icteric, feeds well and has normal stools.

B. Pathologic jaundice
1. Suspect in infants with visible jaundice during the first 24 hours of life and with associated anemia.
2. Causes

a. Blood incompatibility (Rh, ABO).

b. Other hemolytic disease, such as spherocytosis.

c. Metabolic disease (hypothyroidism, galactosemia).

d. Sepsis or other infections (especially urinary tract).

e. Biliary obstruction
   (1) Biliary atresia - high direct bilirubin, pale color to stool. Requires surgical intervention. Poor prognosis.
   (2) Choledochal cyst - high direct bilirubin. Diagnose by ultrasound. Surgical correction is curative.

f. Neonatal hepatitis - elevated liver enzymes. Treat with supportive care.

3. Evaluation
   a. CBC - to see if anemia is associated (suggesting hemolytic origin of jaundice).
   b. Coombs and blood type for mother and infant to evaluate for antibody-mediated hemolysis.
   c. Blood smear to look for spherocytosis (rare).
   d. Reticulocyte count - elevated in hemolytic states.
   e. Evaluation for infection, if clinically indicated.

4. Treatment
   a. Clinical estimates of the degree of hyperbilirubinemia are possible based on the level at which blanched skin appears yellow.
   b. Phototherapy is indicated if the indirect bilirubin is >25mg/dL. This correlates with jaundice visible on or below the level of the thighs. Visible jaundice in the first 24 hours of life usually implies a need for phototherapy and, perhaps, exchange transfusion. Jaundice on the second day of life or in small preemies will benefit from phototherapy at a level of 15mg/dL.
   c. Consider exchange transfusion if the indirect bilirubin is >30mg/dL. This correlates with jaundice which is visible below the knees. Kernicterus is rare with bilirubin <20-25mg/dL.
   d. May need to exchange transfuse earlier in areas where G6PD deficiency is prevalent and kernicterus more common (such as Nigeria).
   e. Maximize enteral feedings.
   f. Treat associated problems such as sepsis.
   g. Phenobarbital is not of proven effectiveness for treatment of jaundice.

IX. BUMPS AND BULGES

A. Head: cephalhematoma

1. Description
   a. Hematoma between skull and its periosteum.
   b. Seen in newborns, related to minor trauma during delivery.
   c. Palpable, soft swelling on head.
   d. Does not cross suture lines.

    2. Diagnosis - clinical. No x-ray or aspiration is indicated.

    3. Treatment

      a. No treatment needed.

      b. Gradual resolution over several weeks.

B. Neck/Chest: fractured clavicle

    1. Description

      a. Frequently seen after difficult delivery of large baby.

      b. Initial pain with movement/palpation of clavicle.

      c. Sometimes not noticed until palpable callus present.

    2. Diagnosis - clinical. Confirmation possible by x-ray, if desired.

    3. Treatment

      a. Full resolution expected without residual deformity.

      b. No splinting or wrapping necessary.

C. Umbilicus: granuloma

    1. Description - Pink swelling at base of umbilical stump.

    2. Diagnosis - clinical. Should not be confused with patent urachus, which has serous drainage without granulomatous material.

    3. Treatment

      a. Silver nitrate topically to cauterize.

      b. May need to be repeated in several days.

D. Abdomen/Groin: hernia

    1. Description

      a. Soft protrusion due to muscle wall defect allowing abdominal contents to bulge.

      b. Inguinal hernia most common in boys.

      c. Femoral hernia possible in boys and girls.

      d. Umbilical hernia more common in boys and in children with more darkly pigmented skin.

      e. Incarceration

        (1) Firm, non-reducible tender swelling, often with overlying bluish discoloration. Untreated incarceration will lead to vomiting.

        (2) Extremely rare with umbilical hernias.

    2. Diagnosis - usually clinical. Ultrasound is possible to confirm difference between hernia and hydrocele (fluid-filled sac around the testicle or along the spermatic cord). Waxing and waning size suggests communicating hydrocele or associated hernia with need for surgical repair.

    3. Treatment

      a. Surgical repair of inguinal and femoral hernias.

      b. Emergent repair if incarcerated (risk of necrosis of incarcerated bowel).

      c. Elective, cosmetic repair of umbilical hernia if still present after age 4 years.

X. RASH

A. Congenital rubella infection
1. Causes petechial/purpuric rash.
2. Follows first trimester maternal infection.
3. May be associated with congenital heart disease, poor hearing, cataracts and low birthweight.
4. No specific therapy.

B. Herpes
1. Vesicular rash, skin or mucosal surfaces. Hepatitis and encephalitis possible. Sometimes with fever.
2. Diagnose with viral culture and/or PCR tests, if possible.
3. Therapy with acyclovir, 20 mg/kg/dose q8h IV x 14-21 days.

C. Milia
1. White 1mm "pustules" on nose and face.
2. Benign condition, self-limited, no treatment needed.

D. Impetigo
1. Causes bullae, usually due to *Staphylococcus aureus*.
2. Usually occur in the periumbilical and diaper areas at 7-10 days of age.
3. Diagnosis is clinical, although Gram stain and culture may be done to confirm.
4. Treat with oral antibiotic (penicillin if staphylococci generally susceptible, otherwise cephalexin, cloxacillin or amoxicillin/clavulanate) for a 10 day course.

E. Congenital syphilis.
1. Consider with rash involving palms and soles.
2. Lumbar puncture should be done and treponemal antibodies evaluated, if available.
3. Treat with aqueous crystalline penicillin G 50,000 units/kg IV q8-12 hours for 10-14 days or procaine penicillin G 50,000 units IM daily for 10-14 days.

F. Erythema toxicum
1. Causes transient, migratory maculopapular 5-10 mm blotches on face, chest, trunk, and extremities between 24 and 72 hours after birth.
2. Self-limited course, resolving over 3-5 days.
3. No treatment needed.

XI. ANOMALIES

A. Trisomy 21 (Down Syndrome)
1. Presentation
   a. Flat face with broad nasal bridge.
   b. Small, low-set, posteriorly rotated ears.
   c. Often single transverse palmar creases.
   d. Widely spaced 1st and 2nd toes.
   e. Hypotonia

    2. Associated features
      a. >30% with cardiac malformation.
      b. Most all with neurodevelopmental delay.
    3. Diagnosis
      a. Clinical suspicion.
      b. Karyotype, if possible.
      c. Echocardiogram to rule out treatable heart anomaly.

B. Myelomeningocele
  1. Description
    a. Sac-like midline protuberance from spinal column.
    b. Contains CSF and/or spinal cord (or brain).
    c. Associated hydrocephalus in 90% (progresses rapidly after surgical closure of the defect).
  2. Diagnosis - made by physical examination. Ultrasound or CT scan can be done to look for associated hydrocephalus.
  3. Treatment
    a. Immediate treatment if leaking CSF is to apply sterile dressings, treat as for meningitis and refer for urgent surgical closure.
    b. At 1-2 weeks of age, a ventriculo-peritoneal shunt can be placed if hydrocephalus is present, with repair of the defect as elective surgery later.

C. Cleft lip and/or palate
  1. Developmental defect with opening(s) of palate and/or lip.
  2. Risk of brain and/or pituitary anomaly if central cleft.
  3. May develop feeding problems, respiratory infections. Allow to breastfeed. If unable, use NG.
  4. Treat with staged operative repairs, beginning after 1-2 months of age.

D. Externalized abdominal contents (omphalocele, gastroschisis)
  1. Moist, sterile dressings around defect.
  2. Antibiotics to cover presumed peritonitis.
  3. Nothing by mouth. Give IV fluids until emergent surgical closure can be done.

E. Polydactyly
  1. Ligation if no bone present in extra digit.
  2. Surgical excision if bone present in extra digit.

F. Undescended testes
  1. Karyotype and endocrine testing (congenital adrenal hyperplasia) if ambiguous genitalia.
  2. Surgical exploration and descent if still not descended by 1-2 years of age.

G. Club foot
  1. If able to passively obtain neutral position, physical therapy to maintain mobility.
  2. If unable to reach neutral position, orthopedic referral for possible serial casting and/or surgical repair.

XII. OTHER NEONATAL PROBLEMS

A. Poor feeding/lethargy

1. Hypoglycemia (especially if associated jitteriness)
   a. More common in premature, SGA or LGA infants, and infants of diabetic mothers.
   b. Symptoms include jitteriness, irritability, lethargy, cyanosis or convulsions.
   c. Treatment
      (1) If blood sugar < 40, feed infant.
      (2) If blood sugar < 30, feed infant or give intravenous dextrose (2.5 - 5.0ml/kg 10% glucose IV, followed by an infusion).
   d. Follow blood glucose carefully before feedings until problem is resolved.
2. Infection (consider especially if fever present).
3. Neurologic injury or anomaly. Examine the skull for evidence of trauma, microcephaly or craniosynostosis. Palpate the fontanel for size, check pupillary response and evaluate reflexes.
4. In premature infants, consider NG feeding if infant not feeding well on its own.
5. Environmentally induced hypothermia - ensure normothermia.

B. Apnea

1. Try to distinguish between true apnea and normal periodic breathing.
2. Pathologic apnea (>20 seconds) is always cause for concern, especially if associated with pallor, mottling of the skin, cyanosis, oxygen desaturation or bradycardia.
3. Possible causes include serious bacterial infection (especially meningitis), metabolic abnormalities (hypoglycemia), seizures, severe anemia, hypothermia.
4. Treatment is directed at the underlying cause.

C. Diarrhea with bleeding

1. **Hemorrhagic disease of the newborn** - occurs in the second week of life. Treated with Vitamin K 5-10mg IM x 1, supportive care and transfusion, if needed.
2. **Bacterial enteritis** - treatment as for serious bacterial infection pending stool culture, if available.
3. **Milk protein intolerance** - blood and mucus mixed in the stool, otherwise the child is well. Diagnosis of exclusion after considering infectious and hematologic processes. Treat by limiting cow milk protein in formula or, for breastfed babies, in mothers' diet.

D. Thrush

1. White coating on the tongue and/or buccal mucosa, which doesn't easily scrape off. Rarely are there feeding problems or fussiness.
2. Treat with Gentian Violet or nystatin.

E. Blocked nasolacrimal (tear) duct

1. Usually unilateral obstruction at the distal end of the duct.
2. Occurs at 2-3 weeks of life.
3. Presents with constant tearing, accumulation of dried mucoid material at the inner canthus or secondary conjunctivitis.
4. The duct usually opens spontaneously by 6-9 months. If persistent after 9 months, refer to an ophthalmologist.

F. **Breast engorgement**
1. Secondary to transfer of maternal hormones and is physiologic.
2. Usually bilateral.
3. Peak enlargement may take 4-6 weeks and persist for several months.
4. No treatment is needed.

G. **Vaginal discharge/bleeding**
1. Usually occurs in the first week of life (milky-white vaginal discharge or bleeding),
2. Due to estrogen withdrawal.
3. No treatment is necessary.

CHAPTER 14

PEDIATRICS

I. GENERAL CARE AND MONITORING
A. Development
1. Knowledge of the average timing of developmental milestones can help one recognize delays and deviations from the normal pattern. These abnormalities may signal the presence of a chronic illness or mental retardation which could benefit from further evaluation and intervention.
2. General developmental milestones:

Birth	Alerts to sound
6 weeks	Smiles responsively, coos
4-5 months	Rolls over
6 months	Sits without support
9 months	Pincer grasp Crawls
12 months	Stands independently, takes first steps First specific words with meaning
18 months 2 years	Runs Combines words in phrases

B. Nutrition and growth
1. General
   a. Both genetic and environmental factors determine the growth of an individual from the intrauterine period to adulthood. Growth is especially sensitive to environmental or external factors, such as nutrition and disease.
   b. Measurement of growth, if accurately done, is a simple and useful way of monitoring the health of children. Malnutrition can be detected by means of growth monitoring before clinical signs and symptoms become apparent. Metabolic and genetic disorders are usually associated with failure of statural growth, but acute malnutrition may occur before statural delay can be detected.
   c. Measurement of both weight and length provides the most accurate assessment of the nutritional status of the child, however length is difficult to measure accurately. The most commonly used method for monitoring the health progress of an individual child is weight for age.
2. Growth charts
   a. The public health department of most countries should have a standard growth chart for that particular country. WHO has produced a prototype growth chart that may be used as a reference (see Appendix I). The upper reference curve represents the 50th percentile for boys (slightly higher than that for girls) and the lower curve represents the 3rd percentile for girls (slightly lower than that for boys). It can be used for both sexes and measures weight-for-age, which is the most common parameter measured on growth charts.

    b. A growth chart is designed for longitudinal follow-up of a child, so that changes in weight over time can be evaluated. A single measurement is difficult to interpret. Longitudinal data allows one to act when 10 percentile lines have been crossed.

    c. Periodic weighing is recommended by WHO as follows:

      (1) Obtain the first weight at birth or as soon as possible afterwards.

      (2) Children should be weighed once every month during the first year, every two months during the second year and every three months up to the age of five.

      (3) Every child should also be weighed each time he or she is brought to the health service for any reason.

    d. The growth chart should include other information, such as immunizations, vitamin A administration, dietary changes, illnesses, etc.

    e. Children growing normally will follow curves running parallel to the reference curves. If the growth curve of a child drops, something is wrong with his health. Health workers should be trained to interpret the growth chart and to explain its significance to mothers. It is especially important to emphasize that it is the direction of growth which is important, rather than the position of the growth curve in relation to the reference curves. A rising growth curve means a healthy child. A flat curve is a warning signal. A growth curve that turns downward calls for immediate action (may indicate nutritional inadequacy, hypermetabolic state from infection or chronic disease or intestinal malabsorption).

3. Neonatal growth

    a. Weight drops during first week (breastfed baby loses 6%, formula-fed baby loses 3%, on average). Weight loss more than 10% of birthweight suggests a significant problem is present (illness, poor feeding technique) and that further evaluation and care is needed.

    b. After the first week, weight is regained, usually back to birth weight by 10-14 days.

    c. Thereafter, weight is gained at about 15-30 gm per day during the early months of life.

4. Subsequent growth

    a. Birth weight doubles by 4-5 months.

    b. Birth weight triples by 12 months.

    c. Six times birth weight around age 4-5 years.

C. Immunization

  1. General

    a. Immunization is a cost-effective, generally feasible means of dramatically saving lives and reducing suffering and disability.

    b. Curative health services should be organized within a system that includes good coverage of preventive health services (hygiene, nutrition, growth monitoring, and immunization).

c. Schedules of immunization vary in relation to individual patient situations, regional and local disease epidemiology, availability of vaccines, and extent of resources. In general, the national or regional immunization schedule should be followed. Specific individuals, however, might need varied schedules and/or additional vaccines because of their own specific medical conditions or travel plans.

d. A commonly used guideline is the EPI Immunization Recommendations chart produced by WHO:

EPI Immunization Recommendations				
Contact No.	Age in Weeks	Vaccine	Option I	Option II
1	Birth	BCG, OPV-0	HBV-1	-
2	6	DTP-1, OPV-1	HBV-2	HBV-1
3	10	DTP-2, OPV-2	HBV-3*	HBV-2
4	14	DTP-3, OPV-3	-	HBV-3
5	26-52	Measles, yellow fever**	-	-

* Some countries give HBV-3 with measles
** Yellow fever

2. Diphtheria, Tetanus, and Pertussis (DTP)
a. Combined vaccine which includes three agents.
b. No live agents; incapable of causing disease. Safe for HIV + children.
c. Side effects are common. ~20% of recipients will develop fever, swelling and discomfort at the injection site. This usually resolves in 48 hours.
d. Newer acellular pertussis vaccine has equal efficacy with fewer side effects.
e. DTP is often given at 6, 10, and 14 weeks of age in developing countries (2,4,6,15 and 60 months in the US).
f. Tetanus "boosters" (more effective with diphtheria included as Td)
   (1) Every 10 years throughout life to boost waning immunity.
   (2) Three injections (0, 1, 6 months) provides primary series for unimmunized older children and adults.
g. Adequate vaccination of pregnant women protects against neonatal tetanus.
h. Tetanus illness does not provide future protection from disease. Therefore, tetanus vaccine should be given at the time of treatment of tetanus illness.

3. Polio
a. Trivalent vaccine, covers all three strains.
b. Generally given at same time as DTP.
c. Oral form
   (1) Live virus vaccine. Potentially dangerous for HIV + individuals.
   (2) Inexpensive and very effective.
   (3) Polio can rarely be caused by the vaccine itself:

          (a) 1 of 750,000 after first dose.

          (b) 1 of 2,400,000 after subsequent dose.

          (c) Half of such cases in immunocompetent individuals.

      (4) Generally preferred in developing countries.

    d. Inactivated form

      (1) Non-infectious vaccine given by injection. Safe for HIV+ individuals.

      (2) Somewhat expensive, very effective.

      (3) Cost and injection risks are only disadvantages. Safe without adverse reactions.

4. Tuberculosis (BCG)

  a. Long history of safety. Some risk for HIV+ children.

  b. Questionable effectiveness

    (1) Minimal protection against pulmonary TB.

    (2) Some protection against TB meningitis and miliary TB.

  c. Use

    (1) Generally used in developing countries and Europe.

    (2) Not routinely recommended in US.

  d. Dosing

    (1) Usually a single intradermal dose at birth in developing countries.

    (2) Single dose later in first year in some countries.

    (3) "Boosters" used in some countries.

5. Measles, Mumps, and Rubella (MMR)

  a. Three separate live virus vaccines. Safe in HIV + individuals, if signs of severe AIDS are not yet present.

  b. Effectiveness

    (1) 95% effective if given after 12 months of age.

    (2) Second dose 1+ month(s) later increases to 98+% effective.

    (3) 60% effective when given at 6-9 months (limited due to maternally-acquired antibody).

  c. Side effects

    (1) Very rare serious complications.

    (2) 10% with fever, rash, aches/pains 6-10 days following injection.

  d. Dosing

    (1) Usually at 6-9 months in developing countries.

    (2) Two doses after 12 months of age in areas with low incidence of measles.

6. Hepatitis A

  a. Non-live vaccine, sometimes available in combination with Hepatitis B vaccine.

  b. Young children are usually asymptomatic with hepatitis A infection but can transmit infection to adults.

  c. Vaccine effective in seronegative individuals (after 12-15 months of age if born to seropositive mother); some immune priming effect earlier.

d. May be given to non-immune travelers.

e. Now recommended for all children in several western US states to decrease some childhood illness and, mostly, to decrease spread to adults.

f. Possible for children in developing countries.

g. One dose gives ~2 years of protection; booster extends protection for 10+ years.

7. Hepatitis B

a. Very safe, even in HIV + individuals.

b. Very effective at any age (~95% with seroconversion).

c. 0.5% with post-injection discomfort.

d. Three injection series (birth, 1-2 months, 6-18 months).

e. Cost limits use in developing countries.

8. Haemophilus influenzae type b

a. Very safe, even in HIV + individuals.

b. Very effective in preventing invasive disease (meningitis, pneumonia).

c. Essentially no significant adverse reactions.

d. Given with DTP during first year, then a single dose after age 12 months.

e. A single dose between 12 and 60 months of age is protective.

f. Used in some developing countries.

9. Varicella (Chicken Pox)

a. Live virus vaccine. Use in HIV + individuals only if no signs of AIDS.

b. Generally safe and effective, but about 5% with mild post-vaccine varicella.

c. Does not prevent zoster (shingles).

d. One injection between 12 months and 12 years of age.

e. Two injections one month apart if initiated after 12 years of age.

10. Pneumococcus

a. Recommended for patients at risk of disease, such as:

(1) Young children (at risk for meningitis, bacteremia, pneumonia, otitis).

(2) Patients with sickle cell disease, nephrotic syndrome or other chronic conditions.

(3) Older adults.

b. Two vaccines available:

(1) 23-valent vaccine

(a) Not effective in young children.

(b) Used for at-risk older children.

(2) Newer 7-valent conjugate vaccine

(a) Effective, even in infancy.

(b) Protects against 93% of all invasive pneumococcal disease.

(c) Prevents about 7% of otitis media.

(d) Now incorporated into routine US infant vaccine schedule.

(e) Expensive but useful, if available.

11. Influenza vaccine

  a. For use annually, when available, for children with chronic health problems such as asthma, sickle cell disease, and diabetes.

  b. Two injections one month apart the first year vaccine is used if age < 9 years, otherwise a single annual injection.

  c. Safe with no chance of causing influenza.

12. Meningococcus

  a. Vaccine effective against strains A, C, Y, and W135 (not B).

  b. Vaccine only partially effective before age 4 years.

  c. Consider use for high risk individuals:

    (1) During local outbreaks.

    (2) Residence in college dorm, military camp.

  d. Single injection, repeat dose each 3-5 years.

13. Yellow Fever

  a. Live virus vaccine, some risk in HIV + individuals.

  b. Need for vaccine limited to some areas of South America and Africa.

  c. Vaccine dangerous in early months of life (may cause encephalitis).

  d. Given at or after 9 months of age, repeat dose every 10 years.

  e. Used for travelers and in some endemic countries.

14. Japanese Encephalitis

  a. Biggest risk of disease in rural areas of some Asian countries.

  b. Three dose vaccine schedule.

  c. Allergic-type reaction in up to 10% of recipients.

  d. Part of routine childhood schedule in some countries.

15. Rabies (see also Chapter 1, section IX, H)

  a. Effective pre-and post-exposure (specific immune globulin, too, if post-exposure without pre-exposure prophylactic vaccination).

  b. Consider for high risk individuals (children in areas of rabid, stray animals).

  c. Consider booster (or serological testing) every three years.

  d. Not a routine immunization except for some travelers.

II. MALNUTRITION

A. General

  1. According to WHO, malnutrition is one of the most common causes of morbidity and mortality among children throughout the world.

  2. Approximately 9% of children <5 years of age suffer from wasting, an inadequate body mass for length. These children are at risk of death or severe impairment of growth and psychological development.

  3. Screening for malnutrition can be done using mid upper arm circumference in children 12-60 months. <12.5cm indicates severe malnutrition, 12.5-14.5cm suggests moderate malnutrition with significant health risk and >14.5cm is considered "normal". Weight for length is more precise and may be performed on those with arm circumference <14.5cm.

4. Etiology of poor weight gain
   a. By far the most important is inadequate nutritional intake, due to poverty with nutrients being unavailable and family choices limiting child's intake. Inability to eat normally (swallowing problem, such as with cleft palate or developmental delay) is important, but rare.
   b. Loss of nutrients can occur with gastroesophageal reflux, vomiting, malabsorption or renal wasting (sugar loss with diabetes).
   c. Increased energy needs occur with chronic infections, such as tuberculosis or osteomyelitis, or chronic diseases such as asthma or renal failure.
   d. Inefficient energy use may occur with heart failure or anemia.

5. Malnutrition results from chronic nutritional and, often, emotional deprivation of the child. Successful management requires that both medical and social problems be recognized and corrected.

B. Initial phase of management of severe malnutrition (hospital)

1. Children whose weight-for-height is below -3 standard deviation (SD) or <70% of the median National Center for Health Statistics/WHO reference values are termed "severely wasted". (see Appendix II) Those who have symmetrical edema involving at least the feet are termed "edematous malnutrition". Both groups are considered to be severely malnourished and should be admitted to the hospital initially for treatment.

2. History should include information about usual diet, recent food and fluids, breastfeeding history, presence and duration of vomiting or diarrhea, recent weight loss, birth weight, immunizations, developmental milestones, exposure to measles or tuberculosis.

3. Examination should evaluate weight and height, edema, jaundice or hepatomegaly, abdominal distension, pallor, hypothermia or fever, signs of shock, corneal lesions, skin rashes, mouth infections and respiratory status.

4. Suggested laboratory studies (to diagnose specific associated problems):
   a. Glucose - hypoglycemia
   b. Hemoglobin/hematocrit - anemia
   c. Malaria smear
   d. Urinalysis - infection
   e. Stool exam - blood, parasites
   f. Chest x-ray - pneumonia, heart failure
   g. Skin test for tuberculosis

5. Hypoglycemia
   a. All severely malnourished children are at risk of developing hypoglycemia (glucose <54mg/dl or <3mmol/l). This is an important cause of death in the first 2 days of treatment.
   b. To prevent hypoglycemia, the child should be fed every 2-3 hours day and night.

c. If hypoglycemia is suspected or confirmed, give 50cc of 10% glucose or sugar water (1 rounded teaspoon of sugar in 3 ½ tablespoons water) to drink. If the child is not arousable, this may be given NG or 5cc/kg 10%dextrose may be given IV. Recheck blood glucose again after 30 minutes and after two hours. If it is low again, repeat the 50cc glucose solution or sugar water.

d. When the child regains consciousness, immediately begin giving food or glucose in water (60gm/l).

e. Consider treating with broad-spectrum antibiotics all malnourished children with hypoglycemia.

6. Hypothermia

a. Infants <12 months, those with marasmus, large areas of damaged skin or infections are susceptible to hypothermia.

b. If the rectal temperature is <35.5° C. (95.9° F.) the child should be warmed externally. Put the child on the mother's bare chest or abdomen (skin-to-skin contact) and cover them. If the mother is absent, clothe the child, including the head, and cover with a warmed blanket. Keep the room warm. Do not use hot water bottles.

c. Check for hypoglycemia whenever hypothermia is found.

7. Dehydration and septic shock.

a. These two entities are difficult to differentiate.

b. Many signs used to assess dehydration are unreliable in the child with severe malnutrition. Many signs of dehydration are also seen in septic shock.

c. The following may be helpful:
(1) History of diarrhea - dehydration
(2) History of thirst - dehydration
(3) Hypothermia - septic shock
(4) Sunken eyes - dehydration
(5) Weak or absent radial pulse - both
(6) Cold hands and feet - both
(7) Decreased urine flow - both

d. When possible, a dehydrated child with severe malnutrition should be hydrated orally. IV rehydration may cause over-hydration and should be used only when there are definite signs of shock.

e. Because severely malnourished children are deficient in potassium and have high levels of sodium, the oral rehydration salts (ORS) solution should be modified. This modified solution is called ReSoMal. ReSoMal can be obtained commercially or made by diluting one packet of standard ORS in 2 liters of water and adding 50gm sucrose and 40cc of mineral mix solution. (see Appendix III)

f. 70-100cc/kg of ReSoMal given over 12 hours should restore normal hydration to the dehydrated child. It may be given as 5cc/kg q30 minutes for the first 2 hours po or NG, then 5-10cc/kg/hour for the next 4-10 hours. Stop when the child is no longer thirsty, urine is passed and signs of dehydration resolve, or if there are signs of volume overload (increased heart rate, rapid breathing or increased edema). Maintenance fluids should be based on the child's willingness to drink.

g. Monitor the progress of rehydration every 30 minutes for the first two hours, then every hour for the next 6-12 hours. Check pulse, respiratory rate, and how often urine, stool and vomit are passed.

h. If diarrhea is present, children < 2 years of age should be given 50-100cc of ReSoMal after each loose stool. Older children should receive 100-200cc. Continue until diarrhea stops.

i. Children who are weak or exhausted, and those who vomit, have tachypnea or painful stomatitis should be given ReSoMal by NG tube.

j. The only indication for IV fluids in the severely malnourished child is circulatory collapse. One of the following solutions should be used:
  (1) ½ strength Darrow's solution with 5% glucose.
  (2) Ringer's lactate with 5% glucose.
  (3) ½ normal saline with 5% glucose.
  (4) Give 15cc/kg IV over 1 hour. Repeat, then switch to ReSoMal orally or NG (10cc/kg/hour). If the child fails to improve, treat for septic shock. (see 9, b)

k. Breast feeding should not be interrupted during rehydration. Begin feeding orally or by NG tube within 2-3 hours after starting rehydration. The diet and ReSoMal may be given in alternate hours. If the child vomits, give the diet by NG tube.

8. Feeding

a. All severely malnourished children have electrolyte imbalance and are unable to tolerate the usual amounts of dietary protein, fat and sodium. They must be fed a diet low in these nutrients and high in carbohydrate. Two formula diets, F-75 and F-100 are used for severely malnourished children, F-75 in the initial phase of treatment and F-100 in the rehabilitation phase. These formulas can be prepared using dried skimmed milk, sugar, cereal flour, oil, mineral mix and vitamin mix.

b. Food should be given frequently, every 2-3 hours and in small amounts. Children who are unwilling to eat should be fed by NG. If vomiting occurs, decrease the amount given at each feed and the interval between feeds. Each child should be given 130cc/kg/day of the F-75 diet or its equivalent. (see Appendix IV)

c. Children may be fed from cup and spoon, or dropper or syringe, if they are very weak. Bottles should be avoided.

d. Significant milk intolerance is unusual and should be diagnosed only if copious diarrhea occurs promptly after milk-based feeds and improves when milk intake is reduced. In these cases a lactose-free formula may be given, if available.

9. Infections
   a. Most severely malnourished children have bacterial infections when first admitted to the hospital. Signs of infection may be difficult to detect.
   b. All children should routinely receive broad-spectrum antibiotics on admission. Those without apparent signs of infection may be given TMP/SMX orally twice a day for 5 days. Children with sepsis or specific infections should be given ampicillin 50mg/kg IM q6hours x 2 days, then amoxicillin 15mg/kg q 8 hours for 5 days, and gentamicin 7.5mg/kg IM q day for 7 days.
   c. If the child fails to improve in 48 hours, add chloramphenicol 25mg/kg po or IV q6 hours x 5 days. Chloramphenicol is unreliably absorbed following intramuscular injection. Oral doses, if not vomited, are comparable to IV.
   d. Other specific infections such as dysentery, malaria, and helminthiasis should be treated as well.
   e. All malnourished children should receive measles vaccine, if available, on admission to the hospital.
10. Vitamin and mineral deficiencies
    a. Vitamin A
       (1) Severely malnourished children are at risk of developing blindness due to vitamin A deficiency.
       (2) A large dose of vitamin A should be given routinely to all malnourished children on the day of admission. Give 50,000 IU for age <6months, 100,000 IU 6-12months, 200,000 IU >12months.
       (3) If there are clinical signs of vitamin A deficiency, a large dose should be given on the first 2 days, followed by a 3rd dose 2 weeks later.
       (4) Vitamin A-rich foods include eggs, liver, oils, fruits.
    b. Folic acid deficiency causes macrocytic anemia. Folate 5mg should be given on day 1 followed by 1mg daily thereafter. Folate rich foods include green, leafy vegetables.
    c. Vitamin C deficiency can cause leg pain, petechiae and hemorrhages. 100-200mg may be given daily. Vitamin C-rich foods include citrus fruits.
    d. Vitamin D deficiency can cause tetany, perhaps with seizures and rickets with weak, deformed bones. It may be treated with vitamin D 600,000 units IM once or vitamin D3 100mcg po daily. Sunlight exposure (face and head for 40 minutes/week at equator) may also help. Adequate dietary calcium should be assured, as well.
    e. Calcium deficiency can lead to rickets also, as well as pathologic fractures. If diet is inadequate, supplemental calcium 400-800mg/day may be given.

f. Zinc deficiency may cause facial and perianal rash and poor healing from infections. Treatment is with zinc 1mg/kg/day orally.

g. Deficiencies in these vitamins can be corrected by adding the vitamin mix to the malnourished child's diet. (see Appendix III)

11. Severe anemia

a. Children with very severe anemia (Hgb <4 g) need blood transfusion. Give 10cc/kg packed cells or whole blood over 3 hours.

b. If heart failure is present, furosemide 1mg/kg may be given IV.

c. Do not give iron until the child has a good appetite and starts gaining weight (usually during the second week of treatment). Then give 3mg/kg/day elemental iron.

C. Rehabilitative phase of management (hospital)

1. The malnourished child is said to have entered the rehabilitative phase when his or her appetite has returned.

2. Nutritional rehabilitation - the most important determinant of the rate of recovery is the amount of energy consumed by the child. Children in the rehabilitative phase of recovery should receive the F-100 diet which contains more kcal than the F-75 diet.

a. Children <24 months

(1) F-100 diet should be given every 4 hours day and night. The quantity should be progressively increased with each feed by 10cc until the child is taking 150-220 kcal/kg per day (4-6gm protein/kg/day).

(2) F-100 diet should be continued until the child achieves -1SD of the median NCHS/WHO reference values for weight-for-height.

b. Children >24 months

(1) Can also be treated with increasing quantities of F-100 diet. For older children, solid food may be introduced.

(2) Local foods should be fortified to increase their energy content, minerals and vitamins. Oil should be added to increase the energy content and the mineral and vitamin mixes used in the F-100 diet should be added to the food after cooking.

(3) Local food diets should be alternated with F-100 diet to make 6 feeds per day. Once growth occurs, one of the night-time feeds can be omitted.

c. Iron should be given during the rehabilitation phase (should never be given during the initial phase). It should be given as elemental iron 3mg/kg/day in 2 divided doses for 3 months. Meat and green leafy vegetables are rich in iron. Folic acid 1mg per day should also be given.

d. Assess progress by plotting weight daily on a graph. Usual weight gain is 10-15gm/kg/day. Target weight is the -1SD median reference value for weight-for-height.

3. Emotional and physical stimulation
   a. Emotional and physical stimulation can reduce the risk of mental retardation and emotional impairment in the future.
   b. Sensory deprivation should be avoided. The child must be able to see and hear what is happening around him or her.
   c. The caregiver (usually mother) should stay with the child in the hospital and be encouraged to feed, hold, comfort and play with her child.
   d. Toys should be available and play activities encouraged. Mothers can be taught to make some simple toys to use at home also.
4. Teaching parents to prevent malnutrition
   a. Parents should be taught the causes of malnutrition and how to prevent its recurrence. They must also know how to treat diarrhea and other infections. They should understand the importance of every 6 month treatment for intestinal parasites.
   b. After discharge, the child should be fed at least 3 times a day. Supplementary feeds of F-100 diet should be gradually reduced prior to discharge.
   c. Immunizations should be given prior to discharge. A follow-up appointment should be made for 1 week.

III. FEVER

A. Importance of fever
1. A sign of illness.
2. Reminder that supportive care is needed.
3. A cause of other complications, such as increased fluid losses, decreased appetite and febrile seizures.
4. Rectal temperature >38° C. (100.4° F.) is considered a significant fever.

B. Approach to the febrile child
1. Evaluation and treatment of the febrile infant or child is determined by the following factors:
   a. Evidence of "toxicity", based on overall appearance and activity of the child. It is generally recommended that toxic-appearing children be admitted to the hospital for work-up and treatment.
   b. Age of the child. The potential for serious bacterial infection (especially sepsis and meningitis) is greatest in the newborn and young infant, and can be difficult to diagnose, especially where cultures are unavailable. As the infant gets older, not only is the risk of serious bacterial infection decreased, but clinical signs and symptoms are easier to evaluate.
   c. The differential diagnosis of the febrile child in developing countries must include acute illnesses such as malaria, typhoid fever, dengue, and chronic infections, such as tuberculosis and brucellosis. Therefore, suggested guidelines for work-up must be tailored to rule

out the diseases which are endemic or most common in the region in which the practitioner is working.

2. Diagnostic considerations

a. CBC is often helpful in evaluating a febrile child. WBC > 15,000, especially with a left shift, or <5000 may be seen in sepsis. Anemia may suggest malaria (malaria smear may be diagnostic).

b. Spinal tap if meningitis is a consideration. Check CSF for glucose, protein, WBC count, Gram stain.

c. Urinalysis may show indicators of infection, such as WBC's, nitrates, leukocyte esterase, bacteria.

d. Chest x-ray should be considered in patients with respiratory symptoms, such as cough, wheezing or respiratory distress. It is also helpful to exclude serious bacterial infection in newborns and young infants.

e. Blood, urine and CSF cultures are helpful, if available. If not, a full course of antibiotics is usually given in situations where bacterial infection or sepsis is likely.

3. General treatment measures

a. Remove excess clothing and blankets.

b. Tepid water sponging may be done. Do not bathe with alcohol.

c. Hydrate with cool oral liquids.

d. Antipyretics

   (1) Paracetamol (acetaminophen) 10-15mg/kg/dose every 4-6 hours.

   (2) Ibuprofen 10mg/kg/dose every 6 hours (for age >6 months).

   (3) Aspirin is less frequently used as an antipyretic in children because of the association with Reye's syndrome.

e. Febrile seizures

   (1) Seizure without other pathology, stimulated by rising temperature. Febrile seizures usually occur between 3 months and 6 years of age (especially 6 months to 3 years).

   (2) Immediate care

     (a) Position to avoid trauma.

     (b) Keep patient on side to facilitate respiration and avoid aspiration.

     (c) No need to manipulate tongue.

   (3) Longer-term care

     (a) No need for anticonvulsants unless seizures occur frequently or are more than 10 minutes in duration.

     (b) Only small risk of ongoing epilepsy.

C. Evaluation of fever according to age

1. Newborn (0-4 weeks of age)

a. Febrile infants in this age group are at high risk of serious bacterial infection (sepsis or meningitis). Pneumonia and congenital malaria are also considerations.

b. Symptoms of infection may be very nonspecific and include lethargy, poor feeding or irritability.

c. All febrile infants in this age group should have a sepsis workup (CBC, urinalysis, chest x-ray, spinal tap and cultures, if available). They should be hospitalized for parenteral antibiotics for presumed sepsis (ampicillin and gentamicin). If cultures are available, the antibiotics can be stopped if cultures come back negative in 1-2 days and the infant is doing well. If cultures are not available, these infants should be treated with a full course of antibiotics for sepsis or meningitis. Duration of treatment for sepsis is 7 days, for meningitis 10 -14 days.

2. **Infants 4-12 weeks of age**

a. The risk of occult bacteremia and serious bacterial infection increases with increasing degree of fever in this age group (10% of children with a temperature >40.5° C. have bacteremia).

b. The response to an antipyretic is not useful in identifying those with serious bacterial infection or in differentiating viral from bacterial infection.

c. Another bacterial focus of infection (i.e. otitis media) does not exclude serious illness in children < 3 months of age.

d. In the US, it is generally recommended that febrile infants from 4-8 weeks of age should have a sepsis workup, including CBC, urinalysis, spinal tap, chest x-ray and cultures. Infants in the 8-12 week age group fall into a gray area, where sepsis workup is not necessary, if the practitioner feels comfortable in assessing the infant clinically. For non-pediatricians, this can be a problem, however, and work-up may be indicated in order to avoid missing signs of a serious bacterial infection. In developing countries, diseases such as malaria must be considered in the differential diagnosis, and work-up must be tailored to rule out the most likely infectious diseases for that region.

e. Infants who appear toxic, have focal bacterial infection, such as meningitis, pneumonia, osteomyelitis, or laboratory studies suggestive of sepsis, should be hospitalized and treated with parenteral antibiotics (chloramphenicol or ceftriaxone). Toxic appearance includes altered mental status, lethargy/unresponsiveness, poor skin perfusion, hypo- or hyperventilation, cyanosis, abnormal vital signs.

f. Infants who do not appear toxic, have normal laboratory studies and no bacterial focus of infection may be considered for outpatient therapy with amoxicillin or penicillin and close follow-up.

3. **Infants 3 - 24 months of age**

a. Differential diagnosis includes viral illness, pharyngitis, otitis, pneumonia, osteomyelitis, meningitis, urinary tract infection, malaria and typhoid fever.

b. Patients in this age group are easier to evaluate clinically than younger infants.

c. Laboratory testing

(1) If the temperature is <39° C. (102.2° F.) without a source of infection on physical examination, no laboratory tests or workup needs to be done. Paracetamol (acetaminophen) may be given for fever and the child re-evaluated if the fever persists >48 hours or the child's clinical condition worsens.

(2) If the temperature is > 39° C, laboratory studies may be helpful in determining the etiology of the fever. CBC with differential may be helpful in evaluating for possible sepsis. WBC> 15,000, especially with an increase in immature neutrophils, or <5000 may be an indication of significant bacterial infection or sepsis. Blood and urine cultures should be done, if available. Consider malaria smear if consistent fever pattern/exposure. Chest x-ray may be done if there are respiratory symptoms or signs. Urinalysis should be considered in males < 12 months and females < 2 years. Stool examination for WBCs may be helpful if diarrhea is present.

(3) Lumbar puncture should be considered in those patients with a toxic appearance or abnormal neurologic examination.

(4) Malaria smear should be considered in endemic areas.

d. Treatment

(1) All toxic patients should be hospitalized.

(2) If a non life-threatening source of fever is identified and the patient is not toxic, treat according to the source as an outpatient.

(3) If no source of fever is identified and the temperature is > 39° C. and WBC > 15,000, treat with oral amoxicillin 50-100mg/kg/day (occult bacteremia in this age group is usually due to *S. pneumoniae*). An alternative is not to treat, and to follow closely as an outpatient. Always consider antimalarial treatment in areas where malaria is prevalent.

(4) All patients need close follow up.

D. Evaluation of fever according to source of infection

1. Acute febrile illnesses with localized source include otitis media, streptococcal pharyngitis, pneumonia, bacterial meningitis, urinary tract infection, osteomyelitis/septic arthritis, etc. These are bacterial infections which usually need to be treated with antibiotics.

2. Acute febrile illnesses without localized source include malaria, typhoid fever, viral infections such as rubeola, rubella, varicella, roseola, dengue, etc. These infections produce systemic, non-localized symptoms.

3. Chronic febrile illnesses include tuberculosis, brucellosis and collagen vascular diseases. They should be considered in patients with symptoms of long duration.

IV. RESPIRATORY PROBLEMS
A. Stridor
1. Definition
  a. Stridor is a harsh inspiratory noise caused by inflammation of the larynx, trachea or epiglottis.

  b. Croup is the clinical syndrome most often characterized by stridor. It is most common in children 3 months - 3 years of age.

2. Pathogenesis
  a. In developed countries, stridor is usually due to viral croup. Occasionally, congenital malformations or foreign body can cause stridor.

  b. In developing countries, stridor is usually due to bacterial croup involving the epiglottis (acute epiglottitis) or the trachea (bacterial tracheitis). Less common causes of stridor are viral croup, measles or diphtheria.

3. Management
  a. Severe croup

  (1) Characterized by stridor, retractions, hoarseness. In bacterial croup, there may be purulent sputum, fever, drooling, or airway obstruction. Examination of the throat should be avoided to prevent gagging and complete airway obstruction. Severe croup and epiglottitis may be difficult to distinguish clinically.

  (2) Patients with severe croup should be admitted to the hospital. If there are signs of impending airway obstruction, measures must be taken to protect the airway before any diagnostic or therapeutic interventions are started.

  (3) If available and appropriate, soft tissue neck x-rays may be obtained. In croup, subglottic narrowing (steeple or hour-glass sign) will be present. In epiglottitis, the x-ray will show a swollen epiglottis (thumb sign) on the lateral film.

  (4) Antibiotic therapy with chloramphenicol 25mg/kg q 6 hours IV or po should be given in developing countries. Antibiotics are not necessary when viral croup is suspected (developed countries).

  (5) Humidified air or oxygen may improve respiratory distress. If available, racemic epinephrine 0.25-0.5cc diluted in 2cc of normal saline may be given by nebulizer.

  (6) Dexamethasone 0.6mg/kg IM or po may reduce the severity and duration of viral croup.

  b. Acute epiglottitis

  (1) Usually caused by *H. influenzae* type B. May occur in adults.

  (2) Symptoms include acute onset of sore throat, fever, stridor and respiratory distress. Typically, the child with epiglottitis sits with head forward, mouth open, drooling and anxious. The child looks toxic.

(3) The most important aspect in management of the child with suspected epiglottitis is to protect the airway. If there are signs of airway obstruction (severe retractions, cyanosis, poor air exchange, agitation and anxiety), intubation or tracheostomy should be done immediately. Once the airway is secured, CBC, blood cultures, if available, and lateral neck x-rays can be done. The epiglottis may be visualized while the airway is being secured, obviating the need for further diagnostic studies, such as x-rays.

(4) Antibiotic therapy with chloramphenicol 25mg/kg q 6 hours IV or po should be given. Patients usually improve in 36-48 hours and the artificial airway can be removed. Antibiotics should be given orally to complete a 7-10 day course.

(5) Household contacts <4 years of age may be given rifampin 20mg/kg/d x 4 days (maximum 600mg/day) as prophylactic therapy. Infants < 1 month of age should receive 10mg/kg/day x 4 days. Hospitalized patients may receive rifampin prior to discharge in order to eliminate the carriage of pathogens that could be shared with household contacts.

c. Acute diphtheria

(1) Laryngeal diphtheria may present with inspiratory stridor, harsh cough, hoarse voice. It can be distinguished from other causes of croup by the presence of a grayish, adherent pharyngeal membrane in the throat.

(2) Patients with suspected diphtheria should be admitted to the hospital.

(3) Procaine penicillin 50,000 units/kg IM should be given daily for 7 days. Diphtheria antitoxin 40,000 units IM should also be given.

(4) Airway obstruction should be treated with intubation or tracheostomy.

B. Pneumonia

1. General

a. Acute respiratory infections are a common cause of death in children in developing countries.

b. According to WHO, most cases of severe pneumonia in children in developing countries are caused by bacteria, usually *Strep pneumoniae* or *H. influenzae*. This is in contrast to the developed world, where the majority are due to viruses.

c. Early treatment with antibiotics can reduce mortality from pneumonia.

d. Most cases of pneumonia can be detected using clinical signs and symptoms, in areas where x-rays are limited. CBC is not helpful in the management of respiratory illnesses.

2. Clinical

a. Pneumonia in neonates and young infants may present with nonspecific symptoms, such as poor feeding or irritability. Fever may be present, as well as lethargy, grunting and retractions. Tachypnea (respiratory rate > 60/minute) is one of the most sensitive clinical signs of lower respiratory tract illness. Rales or decreased breath sounds may be heard on exam, and cyanosis may be present.

b. Older infants and children who present with cough or difficulty breathing should be suspected of having pneumonia. Tachypnea (respiratory rate > 50/minute 2 months - 12 months, > 40/minute 1-5 years) and subcostal retractions (chest indrawing) are common. Fever, dehydration and cyanosis may be present in severe pneumonia.

c. Examination should be done to look for other illnesses which may be associated with pneumonia, such as measles, or other diseases. Evaluate for measles rash. Look for apneic spells and listen for the "whoop" of pertussis. If stridor is present, consider croup.

d. Danger signs, indicating the need for more extensive evaluation and hospitalization, include stridor when calm, severe malnutrition, lethargy and convulsions. These symptoms may indicate very severe pneumonia, sepsis or meningitis.

3. **Management in neonates and infants < 2 months**

a. The normal respiratory rate in the young infant is higher (up to 60/minute) and more variable than in the older infant, so more than one respiratory rate measurement is recommended in evaluating these patients. In the neonate and young infant with pneumonia, cough may be absent. Either fever or hypothermia may be present. Respiratory distress is usually manifested by grunting. Feeding problems, abdominal distension, apnea or cyanosis may be present.

b. It is difficult to distinguish between pneumonia, sepsis and meningitis in the young infant < 2 months. Those with fever should be managed according to the fever guidelines in section III. Infants < 2 months of age with suspected pneumonia (poor feeding, rapid breathing, grunting, cyanosis or apnea, or infiltrate on chest x-ray) should be admitted and given antibiotics (ampicillin and gentamicin IM or IV).

c. Supportive care includes maintaining a neutral thermal environment (room temperature 25° C.). The infant should be kept dry, well wrapped, with a hat or bonnet on the head. Breast feeding should be continued, unless the child is in respiratory distress. If unable to drink, expressed breast milk or formula may be given by NG tube 20cc/kg q 4 hours (120cc/kg/day).

4. **Management in children 2 months to 5 years** (WHO classification)

a. Very severe pneumonia

(1) Cough and difficult breathing associated with central cyanosis, inability to eat and drink. Retractions are usually present also.

(2) Admit to the hospital.

(3) Give oxygen, if available.

(4) Antibiotics - chloramphenicol 25mg/kg q 6 hours IV initially, then oral for 10 days. Benzylpenicillin 50,000 units/kg q 6 hours IM and gentamicin 2.5mg/kg q 8 hours IM or IV are an alternative. Suspect staph pneumonia if there is clinical deterioration or if chest x-ray shows pneumatocele or empyema. Treat with cloxacillin 25-50mg/kg q 6 hours IM or IV and gentamicin for 3 weeks.

(5) Treat associated symptoms such as fever or wheezing.

(6) Give supportive care.

b. Severe pneumonia

(1) Cough or difficult breathing associated with retractions but no central cyanosis and able to drink.

(2) Admit to the hospital unless very close follow up can be arranged.

(3) Give oxygen if the respiratory rate is > 70/minute or there are severe retractions.

(4) Antibiotics - benzylpenicillin 50,000 units/kg or ampicillin 25-50mg/kg q 6 hours IV or IM for 3 days, then oral amoxicillin or daily procaine penicillin IM to finish 5-10 days. Continue antibiotics for 3 days after the child is well. If the child is severely malnourished, treat as for very severe pneumonia with chloramphenicol.

(5) Treat fever and wheezing.

(6) Supportive care.

(7) If no improvement after 48 hours, change to chloramphenicol and examine for complications.

c. Pneumonia

(1) Cough or difficult breathing associated with tachypnea but no retractions or cyanosis.

(2) May be treated as an outpatient.

(3) Antibiotics - TMP/SMX 4mg of trimethoprim/kg q 12 hours, amoxicillin 15mg/kg q 8 hours or procaine penicillin 50,000 units/kg IM once daily may be given for 5-10 days.

(4) Advise the mother to give home care as follows:

   (a) Feed during the illness, increase feeding after.

   (b) Clear nose if it interferes with feeding.

   (c) Increase fluids.

   (d) Soothe the throat and relieve the cough with safe home remedies such as tea with sugar. Avoid antihistamines.

   (e) Bring the child back if breathing becomes difficult or fast, child is unable to drink or looks sicker.

5. Management in children > 5 years

a. *Strep. pneumoniae* is the most common bacterial pathogen. *Mycoplasma pneumoniae* is common in school-age children up to young adulthood.

> **b.** Treat with erythromycin 250mg po qid. Tetracycline 250mg po qid or doxycycline 100mg po bid may be given to children > 8 years of age.

6. Special considerations/associated conditions

> **a.** Persistent pneumonia - symptoms persisting despite 10-14 days of antibiotic treatment should prompt search for the following:
>> (1) Tuberculosis - skin test, chest x-ray.
>> (2) Foreign body - inspiratory and expiratory chest x-ray.
>> (3) *Chlamydia* pneumonia - especially in infants < 6 months of age. Treat with oral erythromycin.
>> (4) Pneumocystis pneumonia - in malnourished infants and children with AIDS.
>> (5) Heart failure.

> **b.** Wheezing
>> (1) Causes include bronchiolitis (consider with first episode of wheezing in an infant < 6 months of age), pneumonia and asthma (recurrent wheezing). History and chest x-ray may help differentiate these.
>> (2) Treat as for asthma. (see Chapter 4, section I)

> **c.** Measles-associated pneumonia
>> (1) Most measles-associated respiratory deaths are from pneumonia, which may be caused by the measles virus itself or bacterial superinfection. Laryngotracheitis (croup) can cause fatal airway obstruction also.
>> (2) Children with measles and pneumonia, especially if accompanied by dehydration or malnutrition, should be admitted to the hospital.
>> (3) Treat the pneumonia as above. Give supportive care according to the management of measles (see Chapter 1, section IX, E, 4).

7. Supportive care in the treatment of pneumonia

> **a.** Feeding
>> (1) Anorexia is common, especially if fever is present. Breast-feeding should be encouraged. If the child is too ill to breast-feed, expressed milk can be given by spoon or NG tube.
>> (2) Older children should be given small meals frequently. They should not be forced to eat.

> **b.** Fluids
>> (1) Increased fluid loss occurs during acute respiratory infections, especially when fever and tachypnea are present. Some patients with sepsis may develop shock, which needs to be treated aggressively.
>> (2) Children with severe pneumonia may secrete a large amount of anti-diuretic hormone and are at risk of fluid overload and pulmonary edema. Oral or NG fluids should be given unless the child is in shock or has respiratory distress (risk of aspiration with

feeding). Dehydration should be corrected more slowly than in a patient with diarrhea.

(3) Fluid management in severe respiratory illness without diarrhea:

Shock and/or severe dehydration	
Shock	RL 30cc/kg IV over 1 hour Repeat if signs of shock persist
No shock	ORS 15-20cc/kg/hr for 2 hours (may give NG) Encourage breastfeeding
Followed by	ORS 10cc/kg/hr for 4 hours (may give NG) Encourage breast feeding
If signs of dehydration persist after 4 hours, repeat ORS 10cc/kg/hr for another 4 hours	
If no signs of dehydration, give frequent breast feeding or milk or formula	5cc/kg/hr for age < 12 months 3-4cc/kg/hr for age 12 months-5years

(4) Secretions - nasal secretions may prevent an infant from feeding adequately. A plastic syringe or bulb syringe may be used to aspirate secretions from the nose. Saline nose drops may be used to soften dry mucus.

(5) Thermal environment - it is important not to overheat or chill a child with pneumonia. This is especially important for the neonate. The child should be lightly clothed in a warm room (25° C).

C. Bronchiolitis
1. General
a. Clinical syndrome in infancy characterized by rapid respirations, chest retractions and wheezing.

b. Occurs most frequently in infants < 2 years of age (usually 2-6 months).

c. Mortality is highest in infants < 2 months.

d. Usually caused by respiratory syncytial virus (RSV).

2. Clinical
a. Symptoms begin with upper respiratory infection, low-grade fever, and decreased appetite. Lower respiratory symptoms such as dyspnea, retractions, and wheezing occur over a few days, more rapidly in severe cases.

b. Examination can show tachypnea, respiratory distress, nasal flaring and subcostal retractions. Cyanosis may be present. Respirations are shallow and rales and wheezes are common. Dehydration may be present.

c. Chest x-ray shows hyperinflation of the lungs. Small areas of atelectasis may be present. CBC is usually normal and not helpful.

3. Management
a. Patients with significant respiratory distress should be hospitalized. Those with very mild disease and who are alert, playful, feeding well and well-hydrated may be managed as outpatients.

      b. Hypoxia is common and oxygen is helpful, if available. Indications for its use include tachypnea with flaring or retractions. Mist may be helpful.

      c. ß 2-agonists (albuterol, salbutamol) are helpful in the 10% of patients who have concurrent reactive airway disease. The nebulized form is most helpful in severe cases. Subcutaneous epinephrine or terbutaline may be used in cases of respiratory failure. Outpatients can be given oral salbutamol 0.1mg/kg/dose tid.

      d. Steroids are not helpful. Antibiotics are not necessary, unless there is secondary bacterial infection.

      e. Consider inpatient isolation for all patients hospitalized with bronchiolitis (as well as those with cough, measles and the first day of meningitis treatment).

D. Pertussis

  1. General

      a. Pertussis (whooping cough) is a highly communicable bacterial respiratory illness that is most common and severe in infants and young children.

      b. Etiologic agent is *Bordetella pertussis*, a Gram-negative pleomorphic bacillus.

  2. Clinical

      a. Incubation period is 7-14 days.

      b. Three phases

         (1) Catarrhal phase - characterized by rhinorrhea, malaise, conjunctivitis, low-grade fever. Infectivity is greatest at this stage. Lymphocytosis is often seen at the end of this stage. May last 1-2 weeks.

         (2) Paroxysmal stage - cough becomes paroxysmal. A typical paroxysm consists of a series of short coughs of increasing intensity and then a deep inspiration (the "whoop") or apnea in infants. Vomiting frequently follows. During the attack, the infant may be cyanotic. Between paroxysms, the child will appear well. This phase may last 4-6 weeks.

         (3) Convalescent phase - paroxysms gradually decline in frequency and intensity. Recovery may take 4-12 weeks.

      c. Treatment

         (1) Supportive care - oxygen, gentle suction, maintenance of nutrition and hydration.

         (2) Look for associated pneumonia or otitis media if high fever is present.

         (3) Antibiotics may help shorten the clinical illness if given during the catarrhal phase. They also help limit contagiousness, even if given later in the disease. Macrolides are helpful in decreasing spread of disease to other people. Erythromycin 15mg/kg/dose

qid x 14 days may be given. Clarithromycin and azithromycin are effective, if available. If pneumonia is present or suspected give chloramphenicol.

(4) Consider admission for infants < 6 months of age, presence of pneumonia, dehydration, malnutrition, prolonged apnea or cyanosis after coughing. Maintain droplet precautions for 5 days after starting erythromycin or 3 weeks post onset of paroxysms.

E. Tuberculosis (see Chapter 1, section VIII)

F. Respiratory distress

1. Differential diagnoses

   a. Pneumonia, especially if fever present.

   b. Asthma if patient is wheezing.

   c. Heart failure

   d. Intoxication - tachypnea is seen with aspirin overdose.

   e. Pneumothorax - spontaneous in young teens or asthmatics. May be post-traumatic.

2. Treatment according to underlying cause.

V. CARDIOLOGY

A. Pediatric heart murmurs

1. General

   a. Approximately 1/3 of all children have a heart murmur at some time during childhood.

   b. <5% of heart murmurs are caused by cardiac pathology.

   c. The majority of children with heart murmurs are asymptomatic.

   d. One third of newborns who have serious heart malformations do not have a detectable murmur during the first two weeks of life.

2. Clinical evaluation of heart murmurs

   a. Cyanosis, exercise intolerance, feeding difficulty, dyspnea or syncope suggest cardiac dysfunction. Failure to thrive, diaphoresis, lethargy and chest pain may also be present.

   b. ¼ of children with congenital cardiac disease will have extracardiac anomalies.

   c. Auscultatory findings suggestive of cardiac disease include loud, pansystolic, late systolic, diastolic or continuous murmurs, abnormally loud or single second heart sound, fourth heart sound or S4 gallop.

   d. In the newborn, persistent tachycardia after birth is frequent with cardiac disease. A persistently hyperdynamic precordium is also suggestive of organic heart disease.

3. Organic murmurs (most common - see also Chapter 13)

   a. Ventricular septal defect (VSD)

      (1) Most common form of congenital heart disease. Presents from first month of life.

(2) Patients with small defects have normal growth and development. Those with moderate to large defects have decreased exercise tolerance, repeated pulmonary infections, delayed growth and development and may develop heart failure early in infancy (sometimes by 2-3 months of age).

(3) Loud, holosystolic murmur at the left sternal border.

(4) ECG in moderate disease shows left ventricular hypertrophy.

(5) Chest x-ray shows cardiomegaly of varying degrees and pulmonary vascular congestion.

(6) Spontaneous closure occurs in 30-40% of patients, usually in the first year of life. Large defects tend to become smaller with age. Surgical repair is recommended electively at age 2-4 years or if heart failure is not responding to medical therapy.

b. Atrial septal defect (ASD)

(1) Often presents in the 3rd or 4th year of life. Infants and children are usually asymptomatic.

(2) Systolic ejection-type murmur along the upper left sternal border, and a widely split second heart sound.

(3) ECG shows right axis deviation and right ventricular hypertrophy.

(4) Chest x-ray shows cardiomegaly with enlargement of right atrium and right ventricle.

(5) Adults may develop atrial arrhythmias, heart failure and pulmonary hypertension.

(6) Treatment is surgical repair.

c. Patent ductus arteriosus.

(1) More common in premature infants.

(2) Asymptomatic when small. May cause heart failure when defect is large.

(3) Continuous murmur at the upper left sternal border. Hyperactive precordium and bounding peripheral pulses are present.

(4) ECG and chest x-ray findings similar to VSD.

(5) Treatment is surgical repair, done electively age 2-5 or at any time in infants with complications.

d. Coarctation of the aorta

(1) Systolic ejection murmur at the upper left sternal border and left back. Can be diagnosed any time in childhood.

(2) There is a pulse disparity with missing or decreased pulses below the waist. There may be hypertension in the arms.

(3) Symptoms depend on where the coarctation occurs in the aorta. Those with preductal coarctation (proximal to the ductus arteriosus) become symptomatic early in infancy, with heart failure developing by 3 months of age. They usually have early death from heart failure. Those with postductal coarctation may be asymptomatic in infancy. They should have elective surgical repair in childhood.

e. Tetralogy of Fallot
  (1) The most common cyanotic cardiac defect beyond infancy. A right-to-left shunt is present.
  (2) Most patients are symptomatic with cyanosis, dyspnea on exertion, squatting or hypoxic spells ("tet" spells).
  (3) Varying degrees of cyanosis and clubbing are seen on examination.
  (4) Systolic ejection murmur at the mid and lower left sternal border. S2 is usually single.
  (5) ECG may show right axis deviation and right ventricular hypertrophy.
  (6) Chest x-ray shows smaller than normal heart with decreased pulmonary vascular markings.
  (7) Treatment is surgical repair.

4. Innocent murmurs
  a. Vibratory - low-pitched midsystolic ejection murmur at the lower left sternal border and apex.
  b. Venous hum - medium pitched, continuous diamond-shaped murmur in the subclavicular area. Disappears in the supine position.
  c. Pulmonary flow murmur - medium-pitched, systolic flow murmur in the upper left sternal border. S2 is split normally.
  d. Physiologic branch pulmonary artery stenosis - medium-pitched, systolic ejection murmur across the entire chest. Disappears by 4-6 months of age.

5. Acquired murmurs (see Chapter 3)

B. Heart failure
  1. Causes
    a. Cardiac malformation (VSD, ASD).
    b. Acquired valvular heart disease (mitral regurgitation, mitral stenosis, aortic valve disease).
    c. Arrhythmias, especially supraventricular tachycardia.
    d. High-output states (anemia, vascular malformation).
    e. Hypertension (coarctation of the aorta, post-streptococcal glomerulonephritis, essential hypertension).
  2. Diagnosis
    a. Clinical - tachycardia, tachypnea, weakness, fatigue, poor activity tolerance (feeding in infants) and perspiration while feeding (infants).
    b. Chest x-ray shows cardiomegaly (normal infant heart may measure up to 55% of thoracic span). Severe heart failure may present with bilateral perihilar infiltrates consistent with pulmonary edema.
  3. Treatment
    a. Specific to cause, if possible.
    b. Salt and fluid restriction.
    c. Furosemide 1mg/kg/dose daily to qid. Follow serum potassium or consider supplementation, especially if furosemide >2mg/kg/day.

d. Digoxin 5-10mcg/kg/day, divided bid if < 10 years old.

C. Hypertension

1. General

a. In children, blood pressure should be measured using a cuff with a bladder that covers approximately 2/3 the distance from the elbow to the shoulder and that goes around ¾ of the arm.

b. "Normal" blood pressure varies by age. On average, systolic blood pressures should be less than (110 + age in years) in 95% of prepubertal children.

c. Repeated blood pressure measurements over time are important to determine if significant hypertension (rather than a temporary response to anxiety) is present.

2. Causes

a. Renal (see also VII, C)

(1) Post-infectious glomerulonephritis

    (a) Hypertension is often an important presenting symptom, associated with nephritis, and often uremia.

    (b) Treat with fluid and salt restriction and antihypertensive medication. Parenteral therapy is often necessary initially, followed by oral medication until the hypertension resolves.

(2) Henoch-Schönlein purpura

    (a) Purpuric rash, abdominal pain, arthritis and nephritis, often with hypertension.

    (b) Sustained, significant hypertension should be treated until the illness resolves (usually several months).

(3) Hemolytic-uremic syndrome

    (a) Microangiopathic hemolytic anemia, thrombocytopenia and uremia.

    (b) Treatment includes fluid and salt restriction and control of hypertension and edema.

(4) Chronic pyelonephritis

    (a) Antibiotic treatment for infection.

    (b) Surgically manage obstructive lesions and severe vesicoureteral reflux.

(5) Reflux nephropathy

    (a) Voiding cystoureterogram to diagnose reflux, then follow annually with possible spontaneous resolution.

    (b) Antibiotic prophylaxis to prevent UTI, if mild reflux.

    (c) Antibiotic prophylaxis and surgical reimplantation of ureter(s) if severe reflux.

    (d) Antihypertensive medication if persistent hypertension.

b. Vascular

(1) Coarctation of the aorta (see also V, A, 3, d)

    (a) Diagnosed by absent (or weak, delayed) pulses below the waist.

   (b) Antihypertensives if significant, sustained upper extremity
      hypertension.
   (2) Renal artery anomaly/obstruction
      (a) Plasma renin level is often elevated, if available.
      (b) Diagnosis is made by doppler ultrasound and/or arteriography.
      (c) Medical management if mild hypertension. Consider surgical
         management if sustained, severe hypertension.
   c. Endocrinopathy
      (1) Hypertension is possible with hyperthyroidism, adrenal
         dysfunction, pheochromocytoma.
      (2) Primary treatment of cause, if possible.
      (3) Antihypertensive medication if significant sustained hypertension.
   d. Essential
      (1) Unusual prior to adolescence.
      (2) Antihypertensive medication if significant sustained hypertension.
3. Treatment
   a. General
      (1) Fluid and salt restriction is useful when there is an associated
         renal problem.
      (2) Weight loss (if obese) and regular physical activity can be helpful
         adjuncts to treatment.
   b. Urgent
      (1) Nifedipine sublingual 0.2-0.5mg/kg/dose (max 10mg).
      (2) Hydralazine 0.1-0.5mg/kg IV.
      (3) Diazoxide 1-5mg/kg/dose IV, max 150mg.
      (4) Furosemide 1mg/kg IV.
   c. Non-urgent (chronic)
      (1) Propranolol 0.5-1.0mg/kg/dose tid to qid.
      (2) Captopril 0.1-0.5mg/kg/dose with increases as needed to max
         4mg/kg/day divided bid to tid. Especially helpful in patients with
         renal disease associated with high renin levels.
      (3) Furosemide 1mg/kg/dose up to qid or hydrochlorothiazide
         1mg/kg/dose bid to qid are useful if fluid retention is present.
      (4) Nifedipine 0.2-0.5mg/kg/dose (max 10mg) qid.
      (5) Alpha methyldopa 10mg/kg/day (increased if needed to
         50mg/kg/day) divided bid to qid.

D. Rheumatic fever
   1. General
      a. Acute rheumatic fever (ARF) is a delayed, nonsuppurative sequela of
         a pharyngeal infection with *group A streptococcus*. Pharyngitis
         usually occurs 2-4 weeks prior to onset of ARF symptoms.
      b. Most common between ages 5 and 15 years.
      c. Due to abnormal immune response following streptococcal infection.
      d. Prevented with appropriate antibiotic treatment for streptococcal
         pharyngitis.

2. Clinical
a. Major criteria
- (1) Arthritis - usually the earliest symptomatic manifestation of ARF. Affects several joints in quick succession, each for a short time (migratory arthritis). Joint involvement is more common and more severe in teenagers and young adults than in children.
- (2) Carditis - pancarditis, with a variety of signs and symptoms. New or changing murmurs may be present, especially mitral regurgitation. Isolated aortic regurgitation and stenotic lesions of the aortic or mitral valves are unusual at presentation. Mitral stenosis, especially, is a manifestation of late scarring rather than acute injury. Myocarditis can lead to congestive heart failure.
- (3) Sydenham chorea (St. Vitus dance) - abrupt, purposeless, non-rhythmic involuntary movements, often more marked on one side. Muscular weakness and emotional disturbance may be present also.
- (4) Subcutaneous nodules - firm, painless, most common over a bony surface or near tendons. Size varies from a few millimeters to 1-2 cm. Nodules are present for 1-2 weeks and are usually symmetric. Usually occur only in patients with carditis.
- (5) Erythema marginatum - evanescent, non-pruritic rash affecting the trunk and proximal limbs, but not the face. The lesions are pink or light red, with central clearing. Usually occur early in the disease, and only in patients with carditis.

b. Minor criteria
- (1) Arthralgia
- (2) Fever
- (3) Previous rheumatic fever or rheumatic heart disease.

c. Diagnosis is confirmed by the presence of two major or one major plus two minor criteria.

3. Treatment
a. Treat untreated streptococcal infection.

b. Aspirin 15mg/kg/dose q4-6 hours for acute rheumatic fever with carditis, chorea or arthritis.

c. Prednisone 1mg/kg/dose bid for two weeks, then tapered, is given if heart failure is present. Heart failure is treated with diuretics and digoxin as needed. (see V, B)

d. Rheumatic heart disease is the most severe sequela of ARF. It occurs 10-20 years after the original attack and is the major cause of acquired valvular heart disease in the world. Valvular damage occurs in almost half of all patients with evidence of carditis at the time of initial diagnosis. The mitral valve is more commonly involved than the aortic valve. Mitral stenosis is the classic finding in rheumatic heart disease and often requires surgical correction. The new technique of percutaneous mitral balloon valvotomy has potential for treatment of patients with mitral stenosis in countries where cardiac surgery is unavailable.

VI. GASTROINTESTINAL PROBLEMS
A. Diarrhea
1. General
  a. Diarrheal diseases cause much morbidity (3-6 illnesses per year per child) and over a million pediatric deaths per year in developing countries.

  b. Prevention is critically important and involves good water and food hygiene as well as ensuring adequate nutritional status.

  c. Diarrhea is defined as 3 or more loose or watery stools in a day. Diarrhea is classified as acute (lasts <2 weeks) or persistent (2 weeks or longer). It may further be classified as watery (noninflammatory) vs. bloody (inflammatory, dysentery).

  d. The major dangers of diarrhea are death from dehydration and malnutrition. Dehydration can be prevented at home if the child is given extra fluids as soon as the diarrhea starts (ORS solution, soup, rice water and yogurt drinks or water).

  e. Feeding during episodes of diarrhea will help prevent malnutrition. After the diarrhea has stopped, an extra meal should be given each day for 2 weeks to help the child regain weight lost during the illness.

  f. Antidiarrheal drugs and antiemetics should not be given to infants and children.

  g. Antibiotics are not effective against most organisms which cause diarrhea. They should be given only in cases where there is high suspicion for bacterial etiology (such as shigella dysentery). For further discussion of enteric infections, see Chapter 1.

2. Fluid management of a child with diarrhea
  a. Assess hydration status (see chart below)

Degree of Dehydration			
	Mild	**Moderate**	**Severe**
Weight loss	3-5%	6-9%	10% or more
Pulse	Normal	Rapid	Rapid, weak
Fontanel	Normal	Sunken some	Sunken much
Eyes	Decreased tears	Dry, sunken	Dry, very sunken
Mouth	Moist to slightly dry	Dry	Very dry
Urine output	Slightly reduced	Reduced	Nearly none

  b. Fluid requirements (cc/kg/day)
    (1) Maintenance fluids per day, based on patient's weight:
      (a) 100cc/kg for each of first 10 kg.
      (b) 50cc/kg for each of second 10 kg.

(c) 20cc/kg for each kg after 20kg.

(2) Maintenance calories are roughly equivalent to maintenance fluids (i.e. 1 kcal of energy for each 1cc of maintenance fluid). This does not take into account increased metabolic needs.

(3) Excessive losses - approximate quantity of fluid loss via emesis and diarrhea.

(4) Oral rehydration solution (ORS) is adequate and desirable in all but the most severe cases of dehydration. Families should be taught to prepare and give the solution. It should be given to infants and young children using a clean spoon or cup. Children under 2 years of age should be offered a teaspoonful every 1-2 minutes. Older children may take sips directly from the cup.

c. Fluid therapy for the child who is not dehydrated

(1) Maintenance rate plus replacement of excessive losses.

(2) Give slow, frequent drinks, sips, spoonfuls, or syringefuls.

(3) Concurrent vomiting is a reason to continue oral fluids aggressively, not a reason to seek another route of hydration.

(4) Maintain usual, age-appropriate diet.

d. Fluid therapy for the child who is mildly or moderately dehydrated

(1) Give oral fluids 50-100cc/kg over 4-6 hours initially to correct dehydration.

(2) Give ongoing maintenance rate plus replacement of excessive losses daily. Up to 2 years of age, give 50-100cc after each loose stool. Over 2 years, give 100-200cc after each loose stool.

(3) Give slow, frequent drinks, sips, spoonfuls or syringefuls. If the child vomits, wait 5-10 minutes and start giving fluids again, but more slowly (a spoonful every 2-3 minutes).

(4) WHO-type rehydration solution for initial replacement, otherwise any fluid the child likes. Children should continue their usual diet even when they have diarrhea.

(5) Maintain usual, age-appropriate diet after initial rehydration is complete.

e. Fluid therapy for the child who is severely dehydrated

(1) IV fluids if possible (normal saline or lactated Ringers) - bolus with 20cc/kg rapidly, repeat if still lethargic or hypotensive. If IV access cannot be accomplished, intraosseous route should be considered. ORS can be given by NG tube in the meantime (20cc/kg/hour for 6 hours).

(2) Transition to oral fluids and feedings as soon as possible.

3. Causes of diarrhea

a. Infectious - by far the most important cause of diarrhea in children. (see Chapter 1)

b. Intussusception - see C, 2, c below.

c. Food intolerance

(1) Transient post-viral lactose intolerance - give trial without dairy products for 3-5 days, then resume usual diet, if better.

(2) Chronic lactose intolerance - rare in first 5 years of life. Chronic avoidance of lactose is effective.

(3) Fat malabsorption with cystic fibrosis - uncommon except in lightly-pigmented ethnic groups.

(4) Gluten-sensitive enteropathy - diagnosis by duodenal biopsy. Serologic tests useful, if available. Treat by avoiding gluten-containing foods.

d. Chronic illnesses, such as tuberculosis and HIV disease.

B. Constipation

1. Acute treatment of impaction

a. Glycerin or bisacodyl suppository.

b. Fleet's enema (pediatric).

c. Mineral oil 15cc po.

d. Soapsuds enema or manual disimpaction in resistant cases.

2. Chronic treatment

a. Increase fluids and fiber in diet.

b. Barley malt extract 1-2 teaspoons can be added to a feeding 2-3 times a day to treat infants with unusually firm stools. A bulking agent such as Metamucil, may be given to older children.

c. Routine suppositories or stimulant laxatives should be avoided.

3. Hirschsprung disease

a. Suspect in infants with delayed first stool, irregular stooling since.

b. Most develop symptoms within the first month of life.

c. Plain x-rays and barium enema may be helpful in establishing the diagnosis.

d. Rectal biopsy is definitive.

C. Abdominal pain

1. General

a. History should ascertain if the pain is acute in onset vs. chronic or recurrent. Other important factors are the location of the pain, whether it radiates and where, the quality of pain, constant vs. intermittent, duration, associated symptoms, such as nausea, vomiting, diarrhea, fever, cough, rash. Determine if any medications or home remedies have been tried. Does the child have any underlying medical illnesses? Is there a history of trauma? Is anyone else at home ill?

b. Physical examination should include evaluation of the heart and lungs, and evaluation for the presence of rash, fever, joint swelling. Abdominal exam should evaluate for bowel sounds, areas of tenderness, presence of organomegaly or masses, guarding or other signs of peritoneal irritation. A rectal exam may be helpful and a pelvic examination in female adolescents, if culturally appropriate.

c. Laboratory tests are determined by the findings on history and physical exam. If a surgical problem is suspected, CBC with differential, electrolytes, BUN, creatinine and glucose, urinalysis and abdominal x-rays may be helpful. Ultrasound should be done, if available, for suspected gallstones, kidney stones, ectopic pregnancy and, possibly, trauma.

2. Surgical causes (see Chapter 20, section I)

  a. Acute appendicitis

    (1) Often "atypical" presentation in children.

    (2) Consider in patients with acute onset of abdominal pain which progressively worsens, settling in the right lower quadrant of the abdomen. Anorexia and vomiting are often present.

    (3) Focal right lower quadrant tenderness on abdominal and rectal exams is suggestive.

    (4) White blood cell count is usually mildly elevated, higher if the appendix is perforated.

    (5) X-ray may show appendicolith and ultrasound an edematous appendix, if the diagnosis is in question.

    (6) Surgical intervention is necessary.

  b. Volvulus

    (1) Often associated with malrotation in children.

    (2) High level of concern if bilious emesis in the early months of life.

    (3) Diagnosis by contrast upper intestinal x-rays.

    (4) Surgical correction necessary.

  c. Intussusception

    (1) Common from 6 months to 2 years of age. May occur later if "lead point" is a node or tumor.

    (2) Characterized by intermittent, spasmodic, severe spasms of abdominal pain. Patient is often calm between spasms. Younger infants may have lethargy, dehydration or obtundation.

    (3) Fever is common. "Currant jelly" stools may be present.

    (4) The abdomen may be non-tender between episodes of pain, but eventually becomes distended. A sausage-shaped mass in the right upper quadrant may be palpable.

    (5) Diagnosis and treatment can be accomplished by careful barium enema. If unsuccessful, surgery may be necessary.

  d. Mesenteric adenitis

    (1) Pain with spasmodic cramping.

    (2) Perforation may occur with findings of an acute abdomen.

3. Medical causes

  a. Gastritis, with or without ulcer

    (1) Burning upper abdominal pain which often varies with food intake.

    (2) Sometimes associated blood loss. Reflux may also be present.

(3) *H. pylori* infection is possible in children.

(4) Treatment similar to adults, with dosages adjusted for size.

b. Hepatitis

(1) Abdominal pain usually not a prominent symptom. There may be mild right upper quadrant pain or tenderness.

(2) Jaundice and elevated liver function tests establish the diagnosis.

c. Parasitic infestation

(1) Intestinal worms, such as ascaris, may cause chronic abdominal discomfort and abdominal distension and bloating. Hookworm may cause GI bleeding and severe anemia.

(2) Diagnosis can be made on examination of a fresh stool specimen.

(3) Treatment is often presumptive.

d. Malabsorption

(1) May cause bloating, discomfort after eating and loose stools.

(2) Giardiasis, lactose intolerance are possible causes.

4. Gynecological causes - see Chapter 20 Surgery

5. Trauma

a. Consider with direct blow to the abdomen or back, or with fall. May have splenic, liver or pancreatic injury.

b. Ultrasound or CT scan helpful, if available.

c. Renal injury may cause hematuria.

6. Infectious

a. Pneumonia

(1) Basilar pneumonia can present with abdominal pain. Fever, cough and respiratory difficulty can suggest the diagnosis.

(2) Chest x-ray is diagnostic, if available. Clinical symptoms should prompt treatment.

b. Acute pyelonephritis

(1) Causes pain in the flank, usually with fever. Costovertebral angle tenderness is usually present on exam.

(2) Urinalysis with WBCs and bacteria is suggestive, especially if WBC casts are present, as well.

c. Urinary tract infection

(1) May cause vague abdominal discomfort, especially in the suprapubic region. Dysuria is usually present in older children.

(2) Diagnose by urinalysis (WBCs, bacteria).

d. Pelvic inflammatory disease

(1) Causes lower abdominal pain, usually with vaginal discharge.

(2) Cervical motion tenderness and adnexal tenderness on pelvic or rectal exam is suggestive and should prompt treatment for gonorrhea and chlamydia infection, even if cultures are unavailable.

7. Emotional causes

a. Often vague, mid-abdominal discomfort.

b. Deal with underlying concerns.

8. Tumor
a. Unusual cause of abdominal pain, but Wilms tumor and neuroblastoma possible.
b. Diagnosis by palpation, perhaps ultrasound.

D. Jaundice
1. General
a. Important historical information includes duration of jaundice, associated GI or systemic symptoms, stool color change, darkening of urine, pruritus, weight loss, exposure to persons with known hepatitis or jaundice, drug exposure, sexual activity.
b. Physical examination should look for color of skin and sclera, liver size, abdominal tenderness or masses and distension.
c. Laboratory tests should include CBC, reticulocyte count, bilirubin, liver function tests, Coombs test, hepatitis serology and coagulation tests (if available). Ultrasound will be helpful if surgical cause is suspected.

2. Elevated indirect bilirubin
a. Hemolysis
(1) Anemia and high reticulocyte count are usually present.
(2) Causes include sickle cell disease, malaria, drug reactions, and autoimmune factors (positive Coombs test).
b. Physiologic jaundice in the newborn and hypothyroidism in the newborn.
c. Hereditary hepatic dysfunction.

3. Elevated indirect and direct bilirubin
a. Infections
(1) Hepatitis A, B, C - treatment is supportive. Hepatitis A is self-limited. B and C can persist long-term and lead to chronic liver disease. Fulminant, severe cases are possible.
(2) Epstein-Barr virus (infectious mononucleosis) can cause hepatitis which is self-limited and treated supportively.
(3) Other infectious causes include congenital rubella, leptospirosis, syphilis and sepsis.
b. Cirrhosis - usually the sequela of hepatitis (or alcohol abuse in developed countries).
c. Cholelithiasis (gallstones) - diagnosed by ultrasound, if available. Treatment is surgical.
d. Chemicals (heavy metals, drugs, cleaning fluids).
e. Congenital - biliary atresia, cystic fibrosis, Dubin-Johnson syndrome.
f. Neoplasms - benign or malignant.

VII. GENITOURINARY AND RENAL PROBLEMS
A. Urinary tract infection
1. Clinical

a. Typical symptoms include dysuria, frequency, urgency, enuresis. Many UTIs are asymptomatic.

b. Nonspecific symptoms, especially in infants, may include vomiting, diarrhea, fever, lethargy, irritability and abdominal pain.

c. Physical exam is usually normal. Suprapubic tenderness may be present. CVA tenderness associated with fever and leukocytosis suggests pyelonephritis. Blood pressure should be checked (recurrent UTIs can cause chronic renal failure and hypertension). Genitalia should be examined for vaginitis, local irritation or phimosis in males.

2. Diagnosis

a. Clean-catch or catheterized U/A may show pyuria and bacteriuria.

b. Culture is most definitive, if available, to identify specific organism and susceptibility.

3. Treatment

a. Neonatal - UTI is often associated with sepsis. Patients should have full septic work-up and be hospitalized for parenteral antibiotics.

b. Children > 3 months

(1) Parenteral antibiotics if toxic or high fever or in cases of suspected upper tract disease (IV ampicillin and gentamicin, followed by full course of oral antibiotics).

(2) Oral regimens include TMP/SMX, amoxicillin/clavulanate, nitrofurantoin or cephalosporin. A full 10 day course is recommended. Short courses may be used only in older children.

4. Special considerations

a. Vesicoureteral reflux

(1) Found in 30-50% of children with UTI. These children have a higher incidence of renal scarring than those without reflux.

(2) Diagnosed with voiding cystourethrogram (VCUG) and IVP or renal ultrasound. This should be done on all males, all infants and females < 5 years of age or those with recurrent infection.

(3) Mild reflux (grades 1-3) usually disappears with increasing age. These patients may be followed with radiologic testing every few years. Antibiotic prophylaxis (such as nitrofurantoin 1.5mg/kg q hs) may be helpful.

(4) Severe reflux usually persists and requires urologic evaluation and surgical correction.

b. Followup

(1) All children with UTI should have a repeat U/A 1-3 weeks after completion of therapy.

(2) Patients with 3 infections in a year should be on prophylactic therapy for 6 months to 2 years

B. Abnormal urinary symptoms

1. Pain with urination

a. Trauma - protect child if concern about non-accidental trauma, abuse.

    b. Urinary stones - urinalysis usually shows blood. Acute treatment with increased fluids, pain control. Intravenous pyelogram or ultrasound helpful with diagnosis, if available.

    c. Urinary tract infection - see VII, A above.

2. Decreased urination

    a. Dehydration - treat with fluid challenge (should lead to increased urine output).

    b. Bladder outlet obstruction - large bladder, relieved by catheterization. Surgery if posterior urethral valves (usually newborn boys). Dilatation if stricture (usually post-trauma or infection).

    c. Glomerulonephritis - hematuria, oliguria, hypertension possible. Usually self-limited. Treat hypertension, order fluid restriction to avoid overload.

3. Increased urination

    a. Excessive drinking - rule out inability to concentrate urine (fast overnight and check concentration of the urine in the morning).

    b. Diabetes mellitus - check urine sugar and/or blood sugar. Treat with fluids, insulin, dietary management.

    c. Diabetes insipidus - high serum sodium or failure to raise urine specific gravity >1.010 after restricting fluid intake. Treat with desmopressin (DDAVP) to maintain normal serum sodium. Ensure adequate fluid availability.

4. Colored urine

    a. Bloody - evaluate for urinary tract infection (hemorrhagic cystitis) or glomerulonephritis.

    b. Dark without blood - consider dehydration with concentrated urine or hepatitis (positive urine urobilinogen).

C. Hematuria

1. Acute post-streptococcal glomerulonephritis

    a. Clinical

        (1) Child may present with tea-colored or grossly bloody urine 1-3 weeks after a streptococcal sore throat or skin infection. Nephritis may develop despite antibiotic treatment of the infection.

        (2) Oliguria, edema (especially periorbital), hypertension and heart failure may be present.

        (3) Physical findings vary with the severity of the disease.

    b. Laboratory

        (1) Urine usually shows hematuria with RBC casts and proteinuria. WBCs may be present.

        (2) Anemia and electrolyte abnormalities may be present.

        (3) Chest x-ray may show heart failure.

    c. Treatment

        (1) Admit patients with oliguria, edema or hypertension.

(2) Oral intake of fluid, salt and potassium should be restricted.
(3) Treat edema and heart failure with furosemide (1-5mg/kg/day orally).
(4) Hypertension can be treated acutely with hydralazine 0.5mg/kg IV. Oral hydralazine, captopril or nifedipine can be used to treat hypertension until it is resolved. (see V, C, 3)

d. Outcome
(1) 90% of patients completely recover within a short time (6-18 months).
(2) Hematuria and proteinuria may persist in some patients. Rapidly progressive glomerulopathy develops rarely.

2. Henoch-Schönlein purpura
a. Nonthrombocytopenic purpuric rash, abdominal pain, arthritis and nephritis are the hallmarks of the disease. Rash is usually on the lower extremities and buttocks. Persistence of the rash for 2-3 months is associated with nephropathy.
b. Renal disease may be transient hematuria, nephritic syndrome, or nephritic-nephrotic syndrome (nephrosis more predictive of chronic renal disease).
c. Etiology uncertain. It is thought to be a vasculitis. Usually occurs in children 2-11 years. May follow seemingly minor infectious illnesses.
d. No specific treatment is indicated. Prednisone may help abdominal pain and joint symptoms. Significant, sustained hypertension should be treated with antihypertensive medication.
e. Often resolves over 6-18 months.

3. Hemolytic-uremic syndrome
a. Characterized by microangiopathic hemolytic anemia (fragmented red cells on smear), thrombocytopenia and uremia, often with oliguria and even anuria for weeks.
b. It is associated with infectious agents, such as cytotoxic *Escherichia coli, Shigella dysenteriae*, and *Streptococcus pneumoniae*.
c. The illness usually begins with diarrhea (watery or bloody), with or without vomiting or abdominal pain several days before the hemolytic-uremic symptoms begin. These include irritability, restlessness, oliguria, edema and signs of fluid overload.
d. Laboratory studies should include CBC, platelet count, peripheral smear examination, BUN, creatinine and electrolytes, if available. Liver function tests may be elevated.
e. Treatment includes fluid and salt restriction, IV furosemide, correction of electrolyte abnormalities, control of hypertension (hydralazine, captopril or nifedipine) and transfusion, if necessary. Antibiotics are not indicated if *E.coli* is the cause. Dialysis may be necessary for uncontrollable hypertension, fluid overload or electrolyte imbalance.
f. There is full resolution in the majority of patients if oliguria/anuria is not fatal.

4. **Urologic causes** - trauma, tumors, urinary stones, hematospermia (in adolescent males).

5. **Infectious** - renal tuberculosis, malaria, hemorrhagic cystitis, schistosomiasis.

VIII. ORTHOPEDIC PROBLEMS
A. Pediatric limp
1. **Transient tenosynovitis**
   a. Occurs in ages 2-12 years.
   b. Frequently follows an upper respiratory or other viral infection.
   c. No systemic signs of toxicity, such as fever, elevated white count.
   d. Mild discomfort and limitation of hip motion.
   e. Resolves within a week.
   f. Treat with anti-inflammatory agent and activity as tolerated.
2. **Septic hip joint/osteomyelitis**
   a. Patient looks sick and keeps the hip in flexion and external rotation. Severe pain on adduction, internal rotation. Child refuses to bear weight.
   b. Fever is usually, but not always present.
   c. WBC usually >10,000, but may be normal. Sed rate is usually increased (>25mm/hr). X-ray is not usually helpful.
   d. Joint/bone aspiration is helpful to identify the etiologic agent. Surgical drainage should be done if septic arthritis is confirmed (purulent fluid on aspiration). Cultures should be done, if available. AFB smear can be done to look for tuberculosis, but yield is low (usually presents with less acute onset).
   e. Antibiotics to cover staphylococcus (nafcillin, dicloxacillin, chloramphenicol, amoxicillin/clavulanate, cephalosporins) should be given initially IV and continued for 3 weeks for septic arthritis. If osteomyelitis is suspected, antibiotics should be continued for at least 6 weeks. Surgical debridement should be done if chronic osteomyelitis with sequestrum is present.
   f. If the patient is not responding to IV antibiotics, surgical drainage of the joint is indicated.
3. **Legg-Calve-Perthes disease** (aseptic necrosis of the femoral head)
   a. Occurs in ages 5-10 years.
   b. More frequent in patients with sickle cell disease.
   c. Patients develop slow onset of hip pain and limp. The hip pain is progressive. Pain may be felt in the knee or thigh.
   d. Physical exam shows limited motion of the hip. There may be flexion contracture (especially rotation and abduction).
   e. X-ray in the early stage shows widening of the joint space and subcortical fractures. Late changes are flattening of the femoral head and sclerosis of the epiphysis.

f. Treatment is with immobilization and, sometimes, surgical correction.

4. Slipped capital femoral epiphysis

   a. Most common in ages 8-15 years. More common in obese patients and those with thyroid disease.

   b. Slip of the head of the femur at the proximal physis. The onset may be acute or chronic.

   c. Passive range of motion causes pain, and hip motion is limited.

   d. Diagnosis is made by x-ray. There is irregularity and widening of the growth plate of the proximal femur or displacement of the femoral head.

   e. Treatment is with immobilization and immediate surgical stabilization.

5. Osgood-Schlatter disease

   a. Occurs in ages 10-15 years.

   b. Caused by repeated quadriceps stress. Patients complain of pain below the knee, which is increased with activity and kneeling.

   c. Physical exam shows pain on palpation of the tibial tubercle (usually unilateral).

   d. X-rays are not helpful.

   e. Treatment consists of rest and anti-inflammatory medication. The condition resolves when the proximal tibial epiphysis closes (age 14-16 years).

6. Juvenile rheumatoid arthritis (JRA)

   a. Pauciarticular arthritis involving one large joint is the most common form of the disease in children.

   b. Need to rule out a septic joint.

   c. Treat with aspirin 80-125mg/kg/day or anti-inflammatory agents. Steroids may be used for patients who do not respond adequately to initial treatments.

B. Pediatric fractures

   1. Young children are more likely to break a bone than to sprain ligaments. Immobilization is as for adults, but young children often heal well with just 3-4 weeks of immobilization.

   2. Unusual fractures (multiple fractures, varied ages of fractures, spiral fractures of long bones, "bucket handle" break of knees, rib fracture, injury out of proportion to the fracture, and unusual bruising in a child with a fracture) should raise the question of child abuse and the need for changing the child's environment.

   3. Frequent fractures, especially in a child with bluish sclerae, raises the possibility of osteogenesis imperfecta.

C. Congenital hip dislocation (developmental dysplasia of the hip)

   1. Clunking dislocation and/or relocation noted on hip exam in newborns.

   2. Often associated with asymmetric skin folds on the thighs.

   3. Sometimes not evident until several months of age or when child has delayed initiation of walking. Repeated screening exams can help, especially if special risk (girls, breech delivery, positive family history).

4. Diagnosis confirmed by x-ray.
5. Treatment with harness to hold hips in abduction ("frog leg" position) for several months. Surgery is required when the diagnosis is delayed or in cases which present later.

D. Rickets
1. **Causes**
   a. Nutritional
      (1) Vitamin D deficiency - especially in darker pigmented breastfed babies kept out of the sun.
      (2) Calcium deficiency - usually after first year of life, with dietary insufficiency of calcium. More common in some countries (Nigeria, Bangladesh).
   b. Renal - associated with renal failure.
   c. Hereditary - various forms, some with phosphate wasting.
   d. Hepatic - rare, but possible with severe hepatic insufficiency.
   e. Iatrogenic - unusual complication of phenytoin therapy.
2. **Diagnosis**
   a. Clinical features include widened wrists, beaded ribs, curved legs (bow leg, knock knees, windswept deformity), sometimes other chest and head deformities, short stature.
   b. Hypocalcemic tetany is possible.
   c. Laboratory - high alkaline phosphatase, calcium normal to low. 25 hydroxy-vitamin D is low if vitamin D deficiency is present. Phosphorous is very low if hypophastemic rickets is present; normal to low if other cause.
   d. X-rays - knees and wrists with widened, frayed epiphyses, sometimes cupping.
3. **Treatment**
   a. Specific, if etiology determined.
   b. Phosphorous supplements if hypophastemic rickets.
   c. Manage renal disease and supplement 1,25 dihydroxy- vitamin D if renal failure.
   d. Vitamin D orally each day (100mug vitamin D or 1 mug per 25 OHD) or 600,000 IU vitamin D IM as single one-time dose.
   e. Ensure adequate sun exposure.
   f. Calcium - to assure at least 1000 mg elemental calcium intake per day.
   g. Surgery only if needed for severe deformities after resolution of medically active rickets.
4. **Prognosis** - good with resolution of nutritional deficiencies, life-long treatment if hereditary or renal rickets.

IX. DERMATOLOGY (see also Chapter 12)
A. Exanthems
1. **Scarlet fever**

   a. Acute febrile illness caused by group A, *beta-hemolytic streptococci.*
   b. Symptoms begin with fever, sore throat, headache and abdominal pain, followed by an exanthem in 1-2 days. Tonsils and pharynx are red and covered with exudate. The tongue has a white coating, which disappears in 4-5 days, leaving a bright red "strawberry tongue".
   c. The rash starts on the neck, axillae, and groin first and then spreads to the trunk and extremities. It is red, with tiny papules, giving a sandpaper feel.
   d. Treat as for streptococcal pharyngitis
2. Staphylococcal scalded-skin syndrome (SSSS)
   a. Febrile illness of neonates and young children.
   b. Symptoms begin with fever, malaise, irritability, skin tenderness. Then, a diffuse macular erythematous rash develops on the face, neck, axillae, and groin. Within 1-3 days, large, flaccid bullae appear and rupture spontaneously, leaving large denuded areas, which dry and desquamate.
   c. Treatment consists of parenteral antistaphylococcal antibiotics (cloxacillin, nafcillin), fluids, and wound care. Steroids should not be used.
3. Viral exanthems
   a. Enterovirus infections commonly cause illness with rash in children.
   b. Hand, foot, and mouth disease is caused by an enterovirus. Symptoms include fever, anorexia, malaise, and sore mouth. Oral lesions (vesicles that ulcerate) appear in 1-2 days, followed by cutaneous lesions (red papules, which change to gray vesicles on the hands, feet, and occasionally buttocks). The lesions heal in 7-10 days.
   c. Herpangina is associated with coxsackie and echovirus infection. Symptoms of fever (to 40° C.), headache, sore throat, anorexia develop acutely. The pharynx may have yellowish-white vesicles, which ulcerate and persist for 5-10 days.
4. Erythema infectiosum (fifth disease)
   a. Caused by a parvovirus.
   b. Symptoms begin with a fiery red rash on the cheeks, which fades after 4-5 days (slapped cheek appearance).
   c. 1-2 days after the facial rash, a nonpruritic erythematous, maculopapular rash occurs on the trunk and limbs. This may last a week.
   d. Associated symptoms may include fever, malaise, headache, sore throat, cough, coryza, nausea, vomiting or diarrhea.
   e. Treatment is symptomatic.
5. Roseola infantum (exanthem subitum)
   a. Common acute febrile illness of childhood (6 months - 3 years).
   b. Caused by a herpes virus.

c. Characterized by a febrile period of 3-5 days (temperature up to 40° C.), defervescence and the appearance of a rash for 1-2 days. The rash is an erythematous maculopapular rash on the neck, trunk, buttocks. May be present on the face and extremities. The patient may have cough, coryza, anorexia, and abdominal discomfort.

d. There is no specific treatment.

6. Pityriasis rosea

a. Age range of 10-35 years.

b. May be a few prodromal symptoms (malaise, headache, sore throat, arthralgias).

c. The rash begins with a herald patch (solitary, erythematous patch with raised border) occurring on the chest or back. About 1-2 weeks later, there is a widespread, symmetrical eruption of pink maculopapular lesions. The patches are oval and dry. The long axes of the patches run parallel to lines of skin tension. Successive crops of lesions may occur, and the rash may last 3-8 weeks.

d. Treat with oral antihistamines and emollients for the itching.

B. Diaper dermatitis

1. General guidelines

a. Avoid continuous moisture and excessive heat with frequent diaper changes.

b. Cleanse diaper area with water at each diaper change.

c. Apply protective ointment with petrolatum or zinc oxide base as needed.

d. Secondary bacterial infection is uncommon but can be treated with local care and oral antibiotics for strep and staph. Topical antibiotics are very sensitizing and should not be used.

2. Primary irritant dermatitis

a. Most common form of diaper dermatitis.

b. Varies from mild erythema to papules and macerated lesions.

c. Treat according to general guidelines (above). In severe cases, a low-potency corticosteroid cream (hydrocortisone 1%) can be applied with each diaper change for 5-7 days. A rash lasting more than 4 days is usually colonized with Candida.

3. Candida diaper dermatitis

a. Characterized by bright, red plaques with satellite papules and pustules, usually involving inguinal creases.

b. Topical nystatin, miconazole, clotrimazole or ketoconazole can be applied 3-4 times a day.

X. OTHER PEDIATRIC SYMPTOMS

A. Chest pain

1. Costochondritis

a. Exacerbated by movement and associated with pain on sternal compression.

    b. Treat with rest, gradually increasing activity as tolerated. Anti-inflammatory medication, such as ibuprofen 10mg/kg 3-4x/d may help the pain.

  2. Trauma, with rib fracture
    a. Pain with movement. Concern for non-accidental trauma with rib fracture in infant (possible child abuse).
    b. Treat with analgesic and activity as tolerated.

  3. Gastritis, esophagitis, gastroesophageal reflux
    a. Burning pain, often associated with eating.
    b. *Helicobacter pylori* possible. Can confirm with serology, if available. Treat as in adults with weight-modified dosing.
    c. Reflux can be treated with antacids, ranitidine 1-2mg/kg bid or tid or metoclopramide 0.1mg/kg/dose qid before meals.

  4. Pleural effusion or pneumonia
    a. Pleuritic chest pain.
    b. Chest x-ray useful in diagnosis.
    c. Thoracentesis may be useful if effusion is present to evaluate for infection vs. neoplasia. Placement of a drainage tube may be helpful if respiratory distress is present or purulent effusion.

B. Colic
  1. By definition, infants with colic cry inconsolably more than 3 hours a day, at least three days a week for at least 3 weeks.
  2. Usually occurs from 2 weeks to 3 months of age in normal, healthy babies.
  3. Etiology is uncertain. Hunger, swallowed air, milk intolerance or associated acute illness should be excluded.
  4. Typical pattern is that a previously calm infant suddenly screams, draws knees up to the abdomen, and cries for 30 minutes to 2 hours. Flatus or feces may be passed during these episodes.
  5. Management
    a. Avoid underfeeding and overfeeding.
    b. Hold and rock the infant.
    c. Allow the infant to cry.
    d. Minimize parental anxiety.
    e. Sedatives and anticholinergic drugs are not recommended.

C. Fatigue
  1. Any infection can cause fatigue. Common infectious causes of fatigue that might not be clinically obvious include sinusitis, urinary tract infection, anicteric hepatitis, tuberculosis.
  2. Poor nutritional status.
  3. Poor sleep from sleep apnea.
  4. Psychosocial stress and/or imbalance, depression.

D. Mouth sores
  1. Acute, vesiculo-ulcerative lesions

    a. Often viral (herpes or other).
    b. No specific treatment.
    c. Provide good oral hygiene. Nutritional support as needed.
    d. Symptomatic care - "painting" or rinsing with mixture of diphenhydramine and liquid antacid sometimes helpful.
  2. Acute, white exudate
    a. Most likely monilial (yeast).
    b. Treat with gentian violet (daily topical application for 1-5 days) or nystatin (rinse tid until lesions resolved).
    c. Concern for possible immune suppression if present after age 18 months.
E. Swelling
  1. Neck
    a. Bacterial adenitis
      (1) Tender, swollen mass.
      (2) Usually staphylococcal or streptococcal in origin.
      (3) Treatment with penicillin if local staphylococci susceptible (15mg/kg/dose tid x 10 days). Otherwise, cephalexin or amoxicillin/clavulanate each dosed as 15mg/kg/dose tid x 10 days.
    b. Mycobacterial disease
      (1) Chronic, slightly tender mass unresponsive to adenitis treatment. Mass may suppurate.
      (2) Diagnose with excisional biopsy.
      (3) Treat as for pulmonary tuberculosis.
    c. Infected branchial cleft cyst
      (1) Recurrent inflammatory, pustular, cystic lesions.
      (2) Treat with antibiotics as for adenitis.
      (3) Surgical excision after medical therapy for recurring lesions.
    d. Benign adenopathy
      (1) 0.5 - 3cm non-tender, soft, mobile nodes.
      (2) Viral origin common.
      (3) Can persist for years.
      (4) No specific evaluation or therapy needed.
    e. Malignant adenopathy
      (1) Non-tender, large, fixed lesion.
      (2) Diagnosis and treatment depends on biopsy results.
  2. Extremity edema
    a. Trauma.
    b. Cellulitis, osteomyelitis, septic arthritis.
    c. Sickle cell crisis.
  3. Generalized edema
    a. Nephrotic syndrome.
    b. Protein-calorie malnutrition (kwashiorkor).

CHAPTER 15

OBSTETRICS

I. PRE-NATAL CARE
A. Objectives
1. Vaccination
2. Dating
3. Detect high risk conditions
   a. Multiple births
   b. Malpresentation
   c. Hypertension/pre-eclampsia
   d. Large for gestational age (LGA)/ Small for gestational age (SGA)
   e. Medical problems (diabetes, anemia, UTI, malaria)
4. Screen for STDs
5. Patient education
B. History
1. Gravity/Parity
   a. Gravity = total number of pregnancies, including current one.
   b. Parity = pregnancy outcome
      (1) Term (>37 weeks)
      (2) Preterm (28-37 weeks)
      (3) Abortions (<28 weeks)
      (4) Living children
2. Dating (gestational age)
   a. Last menstrual period (Nägele's rule) - take 1st day of LMP date, add 7 days, subtract 3 months to get the estimated date of confinement (EDC).
   b. First fetal movement
      (1) Primigravida - 18-20 weeks
      (2) Multipara - 16-18 weeks
   c. Fetal heart tones
      (1) Fetoscope - 17-20 weeks
      (2) Doppler - 12 weeks
   d. Fundal height measurement
      (1) 12 weeks - symphysis
      (2) 16 weeks - halfway between the symphysis and umbilicus.
      (3) 20 weeks - umbilicus
      (4) 20-36 weeks - height from symphysis pubis to top of fundus in cm = gestational age in weeks.
   e. Ultrasound
      (1) 6-10 weeks - gestational sac measurement (2cm at 6 weeks, 5cm at 10 weeks).
      (2) 7-13 weeks - crown-rump length + 6.5 = gestational age.
      (3) >13 weeks - biparietal diameter (BPD) chart. From 13-20 weeks, BPD chart is accurate +/- 7-10days, from 20-28 weeks, chart is accurate +/- 2 weeks, >28 weeks, chart is accurate +/- 3 weeks.

3. Factors suggesting high risk pregnancy
   a. History of preterm delivery (<36 weeks or weight <5.5 pounds or 2500gm).
   b. Prior stillbirth, intrauterine fetal demise or miscarriage.
   c. Multiple gestation.
   d. Third trimester bleeding.
   e. Rh negative blood type.
   f. Previous ectopic pregnancy, myomectomy, C-section.
   g. Medical illness.
C. **Physical exam**
   1. **Weight**
      a. Average overall weight gain - 10-18 kg (25-40 pounds), 1# or 0.5 kg per week.
      b. Weight gain >1 kg (2#) per week in third trimester may be a sign of pre-eclampsia, especially if it is a sudden increase.
   2. **Blood pressure**
      a. Abnormal if diastolic > 85mmHg, systolic >140mmHg, or if there is a rise in diastolic of 15mmHg or a rise in systolic of 20mmHg.
      b. Repeat in both arms, and if still abnormal, check urine protein.
      c. High BP early in pregnancy suggests chronic hypertension.
   3. **Fundal height measurement**
   4. **Presentation** - Leopold's maneuvers.
      a. First maneuver - palpate the fundus with the tips of the fingers of both hands, to define which fetal pole is present in the fundus.
      b. Second maneuver - place the palms of the hands on both sides of the abdomen and palpate deeply to determine which side the fetal back and small parts are on.
      c. Third maneuver - using the thumb and fingers of one hand, grasp the lower portion of the maternal abdomen, just above the symphysis pubis to differentiate between head and breech presentation.
      d. Fourth maneuver - facing the mother's feet, pressure is applied with the fingers of each hand, in the direction of the pelvic inlet, to determine the direction of the face.
   5. **Fetal heart tones** (should be heard with fetoscope after 20 weeks).
   6. **Pelvic exam** - check for vaginal lesions, estimation of pelvic adequacy.
D. **Laboratory**
   1. **Hematocrit** - initially and again in the third trimester, if normal. All patients should be on iron and multivitamins. Add folate if anemic.
   2. **Blood type** - discuss potential need for Rhogam if patient is Rh negative.
   3. **U/A** - protein, glucose, WBCs. Give antibiotics for pyuria even if asymptomatic (ampicillin or nitrofurantoin). If Trichomonas is found, treat with metronidazole after the first trimester.
   4. **Fasting blood sugar** - check at 26-30 weeks, especially in patients with

a history of large babies. Abnormal is >90mg%. If there is a history of diabetes in the family, or the patient has had hyperglycemia in the past, screen for diabetes on the first visit.

5. RPR or syphilis test - initial visit.

E. Preventive measures

1. **Tetanus toxoid immunization** - assure primary series (give 3 doses during pregnancy if unsure). Booster if > 5 years since last immunization.

2. **Malaria prophylaxis** - weekly chloroquine should be considered in pregnant patients from malaria-endemic areas. See Chapter 1, section V, F.

II. VAGINAL BLEEDING

A. General evaluation

1. Pregnancy test to confirm pregnancy (bleeding may be normal menses).
2. Determine gestational age (categorize into first, second, third trimester).
3. Vital signs, orthostatic pulse and blood pressure will help determine volume status, severity of blood loss.
4. Speculum examination (except in third trimester) to evaluate for vaginal laceration, cervical lesion, presence of tissue, severity of bleeding. Abdominal and bimanual exam to assess uterine size, adnexal masses.
5. CBC to assess for blood loss, possible infection.
6. Ultrasound helpful in determining intrauterine pregnancy vs. ectopic, gestational age, fetal viability, presence of placenta previa, etc.

B. First trimester bleeding

1. **Threatened abortion**

   a. Diagnosis
   (1) Vaginal bleeding which may or may not be accompanied by mild cramping pain.
   (2) Cervix closed, vital signs stable, mild bleeding, no tissue passed.
   (3) R/O ectopic pregnancy clinically or with ultrasound (identify intrauterine gestational sac).

   b. Management
   (1) Mild symptoms and patient lives close - bedrest at home, return if increased bleeding.
   (2) If significant bleeding has occurred, admit for observation, bedrest, oral iron therapy.
   (3) Start IV and order blood for transfusion if bleeding warrants.

2. **Inevitable or incomplete abortion**

   a. Diagnosis
   (1) Dilated cervix, ruptured membranes, tissue passed.
   (2) Usually with uterine contractions.

   b. Management
   (1) Assess cardiovascular stability (pulse, BP, mucous membranes, rate of bleeding).

(2) If evidence of volume depletion, start IV with RL or NS, order stat Hgb/Hct and type and crossmatch.

(3) Methergine 0.2mg IM or oxytocin 20-40 units/1000ml RL IV if bleeding is heavy.

(4) If tissue is present in the cervical os, remove it with ring forceps. If bleeding persists or is heavy and does not seem to be stopping, do D&C.

3. Complete abortion

a. Diagnosis

(1) Uterus small for dates, cervix closed with mild bleeding.

(2) History of heavy bleeding or tissue passed, or products of conception examined.

b. Management

(1) Observation for increased bleeding, CBC, iron therapy.

(2) If cervix is dilated, tissue present or bleeding persists, assume incomplete abortion and consider D&C.

4. Ectopic pregnancy

a. Diagnosis

(1) Consider in any pregnant patient with abdominal pain and/or vaginal bleeding or spotting. Symptoms may be very subtle.

(2) Uterine size may be smaller than expected for dates.

(3) Cervix is usually not dilated and tissue will not be present in the os or vaginal vault.

(4) Adnexal fullness or tenderness may be present. If ruptured, the patient will have signs of an acute abdomen (guarding, rigidity, hemodynamic instability).

(5) Ultrasound is helpful, if available. The presence of an intrauterine pregnancy makes ectopic unlikely (heterotopic pregnancy with intrauterine pregnancy and ectopic together is very rare). Adnexal mass may be visualized. Occasionally, the ectopic fetus will have cardiac activity on ultrasound (abdominal pregnancy).

b. Management

(1) Start IV, give IV fluids (saline or RL) to support blood pressure.

(2) CBC, type and crossmatch, if available.

(3) Surgical exploration (vs. laparoscopy, if available).

5. Septic abortion

a. Diagnosis

(1) Likely if delayed evacuation >48 hours, or if induced abortion.

(2) Signs - slight bleeding, pus from the cervix, fever, leukocytosis and/or left shift, tender uterus.

b. Management

(1) Admit - CBC, U/A, cervical Gram stain and culture (if available).

(2) If induced abortion, consider plain and upright x-ray of the

abdomen for look for free air secondary to perforation. Air in the uterus may indicate anaerobic gas-forming bacteria.
(3) IV fluids to assure a urine output of 30-60cc/h. May need Foley catheter to monitor.
(4) Monitor vital signs closely.
(5) Broad spectrum antibiotics - ampicillin 2gm IV q6h plus gentamicin 1.5mg/kg IV q8h plus either metronidazole 500mg IV q8h or clindamycin 600mg IV q8h. High dose penicillin plus chloramphenicol IV may be used as an alternative.
(6) D&C may be necessary to remove retained products of conception. Start antibiotics well in advance of the procedure, and do carefully, since the infected uterus is soft and easy to perforate.

C. Second trimester bleeding
1. Threatened abortion
a. R/O other causes of irritable uterus, such as UTI.
b. Treat as in first trimester. May try tocolytic after 24 weeks, to stop contractions.
2. Inevitable or incomplete abortion
a. Give oxytocin 10-20 units/1000ml RL and remove the placenta with ring forceps, if needed.
b. Make sure completely delivered. If not, needs D&C.
3. Complete abortion
a. Some abortions are complete in the second trimester. Try to examine what is passed or get a good history to insure completeness. Consider D&C if uncertain or if bleeding heavy, without signs of slowing down.
b. If there is a history of painless dilatation, consider incompetent cervix. May need cerclage with the next pregnancy.
4. Ectopic pregnancy
a. Unlikely if fetal heart tones are heard (should be audible with Doppler at 10-12 weeks).
b. Evaluate with ultrasound, if available, and FHTs not audible.
5. Placenta previa/abruptio - rule out with ultrasound.

D. Third trimester bleeding
1. General
a. Admit and put at bedrest.
b. Monitor the degree of bleeding.
c. No vaginal or rectal exams.
d. Ultrasound - estimate gestational age, presentation, amount of amniotic fluid present, placental location, retroplacental clot.
e. Document fundal height, fetal presentation on exam.
f. VS q hour on mother and fetus if bleeding significantly.
g. Serial Hgb/Hct, type and crossmatch 2-3 units.
h. IV with large bore needle (RL or NS).

     i. Sterile speculum exam, GENTLY (no manual or speculum exam if confirmed previa). Check dilatation (may be a heavy bloody show). R/O cervical lesion, carcinoma.

2. Placenta previa

  a. Diagnosis

    (1) Sudden painless bleeding in the third trimester (first bleed is usually mild, self-limited; second bleed more ominous and unexpected).

    (2) Risk factors - multiparity, previous C/S, advancing age.

    (3) Confirmed by ultrasound.

  b. Management

    (1) If a previa is present and bleeding stops, there is no labor and mother and fetus are stable, but pre-term - watch and give oral iron.

    (2) If severe bleeding, mother in labor or fetal distress - immediate C/S. General anesthesia is preferred over spinal, to avoid hypotension.

3. Abruptio placenta

  a. Predisposing factors

    (1) Multiparity, pre-eclampsia/eclampsia, overdistended uterus.

    (2) HTN, renal disease, advanced age, malnutrition, diabetes, abdominal trauma.

  b. Diagnosis

    (1) May have external (painless) hemorrhage.

    (2) Internal (concealed) hemorrhage - more hazardous.

      (a) Pain can be severe if rapidly separating; mild if not.

      (b) Uterus tender and firm and fails to relax. Backache or pelvic pain if posterior abruption.

      (c) Fetal distress/death.

      (d) Anemia/DIC.

  c. Management

    (1) Transfuse earlier than normal.

    (2) If near term, rupture membranes and closely monitor the fetus.

    (3) If no fetal distress and delivery anticipated in <6h, deliver vaginally even if oxytocin has to be used. Especially try to deliver vaginally if coagulation abnormalities are present.

    (4) If fetus is dead, deliver vaginally if it can be done in <6h.

    (5) If fetal distress is present, do a C/S if mother's coagulation status permits.

4. No placenta previa or abruption

  a. Admit for observation, bedrest.

  b. Check Hgb/Hct, platelets.

  c. Speculum exam to check cervical dilatation and evaluate for a cervical lesion or infection.

d. If the patient remains stable for several days with no bleeding, she may be discharged with instructions to remain at bedrest, with no intercourse, if the following conditions are met:
(1) <37 week gestation.
(2) Estimated fetal weight <5# (2200 gm).
(3) Bleeding moderate and decreasing.
(4) Not in labor.
(5) No fetal distress.
(6) No placenta previa on ultrasound.

III. NORMAL LABOR AND DELIVERY (see Appendix V)
A. Diagnosis
1. Uterine contractions with progressive increase in frequency, duration and quantity.
2. Progressive cervical dilatation and effacement.
3. Descent of the presenting part.
B. Stages
1. **First stage** - cervical effacement and dilatation up to complete dilatation.
   a. Latent phase - begins with cervical change in the presence of regular contractions.
   b. Active phase - begins with increasing rate of cervical dilatation. Usually considered active at 4 cm dilatation in nullipara, 3cm in multipara.
2. **Second stage** - complete dilatation up to birth of the infant. Stage of pushing with subsequent expulsion of the fetus.
3. **Third stage** - begins with delivery of the infant and ends with delivery of the placenta.
C. Normal parameters of labor

NORMAL PARAMETERS OF LABOR		
Stage	Nullipara	Multipara
First stage		
Latent phase	< 20 hours	< 14 hours
Active phase		
Onset	3-4 cm	3 cm
Dilatation (slope on Friedman curve)	1.2 cm/hr	1.4 cm/hr
Duration	< 12 hours	< 5 hours
Second stage	< 3 hours	< 1 hour

D. Principles of normal labor management
1. Non-narcotic analgesia until the active phase.
2. Use sterile gloves for vaginal exams. Minimize vaginal exams after membranes are ruptured, since repeat exams significantly increase the risk of chorioamnionitis.
3. Chart all findings at least every 4 hours.

E. Delivery

1. Take to the delivery room or prepare for delivery when the primigravida is crowning and the multigravida is 8cm to complete.
2. Dorsal lithotomy position (depending on cultural norms), wash the perineum and catheterize the bladder, if distended.
3. Determine fetal position and establish position of both fontanels.
4. If episiotomy is necessary, inject 1-2% lidocaine for anesthesia when perineum is distended, then cut in midline or mediolateral position. This may be avoided in many patients, especially multiparas.
5. Modified Ritgen maneuver for delivery of the head (moderate upward pressure is applied to the fetal chin by the posterior hand, while the other hand exerts pressure superiorly against the occiput).
6. Allow external rotation of the head before delivering the shoulders. Check for nuchal cord.
7. Suction the pharynx first and then nares.
8. Deliver the anterior shoulder until it clears the symphysis by deflecting the head downward.
9. Deliver the posterior shoulder while observing the perineum by elevating the head.
10. Deliver the body with a double hold behind the head and at the ankles. Lay baby on sterile towels on the table or the mother's abdomen.
11. Deliver the placenta using one of the following methods:
    a. Modified Crede (massage uterus while taking up slack on the cord).
    b. Brandt-Andrews (push the uterus away with gentle traction on the cord).
12. Do not use excessive traction, as uterine inversion may occur.
13. Avoid manual removal except with retained placenta (as evidenced by >30 minute delay in delivery, or excessive vaginal bleeding).
14. Remove all membranes with Kelly clamp or ring forceps.
15. Massage the uterus until firm. Give oxytocin 10-20u/1000ml RL IV. Can give 10u oxytocin IM if no IV.
16. For extremely heavy bleeding, give methergine 0.2mg IM or ergometrine 0.5mg q 2-4 hours up to a maximum of 5 doses. Can be given IV in emergency situations, but blood pressure should be monitored closely. Do not use methergine or ergometrine in patients with pre-eclampsia, eclampsia, or hypertension.
17. Examine cord for 2 arteries and 1 vein (if not present, the fetus may have other abnormalities).
18. Visualize the cervix and vagina and repair with 2-0 or 3-0 chromic, if lacerated.
19. Examine the extent of the episiotomy and look for tears, especially around the urethra and rectum.
20. Repair lacerations with 2-0 or 3-0 chromic suture.
21. Do a digital rectal exam to insure that no sutures entered the rectum.

IV. NORMAL POSTPARTUM CARE
A. General
1. Complete recovery from the changes of pregnancy usually occurs within 6 weeks of delivery.
2. Extracellular volume decreases back to normal over several days.
3. The patient may note increased urinary frequency initially.
4. The uterus begins to involute. It is palpated midway between the umbilicus and symphysis at one week. Not usually palpable by 4 weeks.
5. Vaginal discharge (lochia) is initially bloody but changes to brown, then white over 2-6 weeks.

B. Routine care - first 24 hours
1. Monitor the patient's vital signs frequently during the immediate postpartum period.
2. Monitor to ensure the uterus remains firmly contracted. Massage the uterus to maintain contraction. Use oxytocin IM or IV drip, if necessary.
3. Analgesics - painful uterine contractions may occur requiring analgesics (paracetamol or acetaminophen). They usually subside within 48-72 hours.
4. Minor temperature elevation may occur (less than 38°C., 100.4°F.).
5. Leukocytosis may be present, occasionally up to WBC of 20,000/mm3.
6. The patient should be encouraged to eat as desired.
7. Ambulate the patient early.
8. Encourage early breast feeding.
9. Perineal care
   a. Ice packs may reduce swelling.
   b. Cleanse the perineum frequently.
   c. Sitz baths prn (3-4 times daily).

C. Subsequent care
1. Laxatives are not routinely necessary.
2. Watch for anemia.
3. Watch for signs of infection.
4. Breast care - see Chapter 16.
5. Contraception - see Chapter 16, section IX.

V. LABOR ABNORMALITIES
A. Prolonged latent phase (>24 hours without progress at term)
1. **Cervix unfavorable**
   a. Sedate - this will stop contractions if in false labor. Meperidine 50-100mg IM or morphine 5-10mg IM are recommended, and may have less toxicity than nalbuphine.
   b. Give fluid load or hydrate.
   c. If contractions continue without progress, or ROM 12-24 hours, do amniotomy and begin oxytocin augmentation. Then, if still no progress, do C/S.

2. **Cervix favorable**
   a. Amniotomy
   b. Oxytocin augmentation.
   c. If still no progress, do C/S.
B. **Arrest of active phase**
   1. **Hypotonic uterine contractions**
      a. Hydrate (500cc RL bolus)
      b. Amniotomy
      c. Oxytocin augmentation
   2. **Fetopelvic disproportion**
      a. Suspect if adequate uterine contractions and no progress in 2-3h.
      b. CPD is unusual before 4cm dilatation. Be sure the patient is not in the latent phase of labor and that the head is engaged.
      c. Complications of obstructed labor include:
         (1) Fetal death
         (2) Uterine rupture
         (3) Infection
         (4) Vesicovaginal fistula formation
      d. If CPD is felt to be present, do C/S.
C. **Protracted active phase** (no arrest of progress but low slope of active phase)
   1. Oversedation - expectant management.
   2. Hypotonic uterine contractions - hydrate, amniotomy, oxytocin augmentation.
   3. Fetopelvic disproportion or malposition - C/S.
D. **Prolonged or arrest of descent phase** (1 hour after good pushing begins)
   1. Exhaustion - apply vacuum or forceps.
   2. Malposition or frank disproportion - vacuum (if +2 station), forceps, symphysiotomy or C/S.
E. **Meconium**
   1. May indicate fetal distress.
   2. Thick or early heavy meconium is especially associated with asphyxia and acidosis.
   3. Monitor fetal heart tones closely. Consider C/S.
   4. Suction nose and mouth prior to delivery of shoulders.

VI. PRETERM LABOR
A. **Definition**
   1. Onset of regular contractions prior to 37 weeks and after 20 weeks, accompanied by cervical dilatation and effacement.
B. **Management**
   1. Bedrest.
   2. IV hydration.

3. Sedation.
4. Ultrasound to assess gestational age.
5. If >32-34 weeks, consider amniocentesis for shake test to assess fetal lung maturity (see Section XVI, C), Gram stain and culture.
6. Tocolytics (if <35 weeks)
   a. Terbutaline 0.25mg SQ q1h x 3 doses, maintaining maternal heart rate < 120. Oral terbutaline may quiet the uterus, but is ineffective in prolonging labor.
   b. Albuterol 0.5mg IM or 4mg po q6h may also be effective.
   c. MgSO4 4gm IV over 20 minutes, then 1-3 gm/h infusion or 4gm IV plus 4gm IM stat, then 4gm IM q4h. Maintain at least 24h, then D/C.

C. Other considerations
1. If cervix ≥ 5cm with contractions, unlikely to stop labor.
2. If rupture of membranes occurs, stop tocolytics.
3. Steroids may be used to improve fetal maturity at 26-34 weeks gestation, if no infection is present. One of the following may be used:
   a. Betamethasone 12mg IM q24h x 2 doses.
   b. Dexamethasone 6mg IM q12h x 4 doses.

VII. PREMATURE RUPTURE OF MEMBRANES

A. General
1. **Definition** - rupture of membranes prior to the onset of labor.
2. **Diagnosis**
   a. History
   b. Sterile speculum exam shows pooling fluid in the vaginal vault. Fluid has a pH >8 with Nitrazine paper. There is also ferning seen on examination of a dried thin smear.
   c. Ultrasound - minimal fluid present.
   d. **DO NOT PERFORM VAGINAL EXAM UNTIL LABOR IS ESTABLISHED.**

B. Management
1. **<24 weeks** - consider termination of pregnancy vs. expectant management.
2. **24-34 weeks**
   a. Bedrest.
   b. CBC periodically (if WBC normal initially, check 2-3x/week).
   c. Daily exam for uterine tenderness, fetal or maternal tachycardia, examination of fluid (foul-smelling or purulent).
   d. Temperature q6h.
   e. Delivery for any suspicion of chorioamnionitis.
   f. No tocolysis.
   g. Consider prophylactic antibiotics - ampicillin IV for 24-48 hours, followed by po amoxicillin for 5 days. Erythromycin can be used in penicillin-allergic patients.

h. Consider corticosteroids if no evidence of chorioamnionitis.

3. 34-37 weeks - try to induce after 24 hours even if the cervix is unfavorable (hyaline membrane disease is low after this amount of time has elapsed with ROM).

4. Term

a. Induce labor.

b. Try to deliver in <24h.

c. Start antibiotics (IV ampicillin) if membranes ruptured >18 hours.

5. For ROM >24h, the infant needs CBC and prophylactic antibiotics (ampicillin 50mg/kg IM q12h plus gentamicin 2.5mg/kg IM q12h x 7-10d) after delivery to prevent sepsis.

6. If chorioamnionitis is present, treat with IV ampicillin and gentamicin prior to delivery.

VIII. BREECH PRESENTATION

A. Causes of breech presentation

1. Placenta previa.

2. Fetal anomalies (hydrocephalus, anencephalus).

3. Multiple fetuses.

4. Uterine anomalies.

B. Possible complications associated with breech presentation

1. Perinatal morbidity and mortality from a difficult delivery. The major concern with breech presentation is head entrapment if the head is large or the cervix is not adequately dilated.

2. Low birth weight from prematurity, growth retardation or both.

3. Prolapsed cord.

C. Classification

1. Frank - lower extremities are flexed at the hips and extended at the knees. Feet are close to the head (buttocks only as presenting part).

2. Complete - flexed thighs, flexed knees (buttocks and feet as presenting part).

3. Footling - one or both legs extend below the buttocks (one or both feet as presenting part).

D. General considerations

1. Be prepared for potential problems.

2. Possible indications for C-section (not universally agreed upon by all OBs)

a. Breech with large fetus.

b. Footling breech.

c. Breech with hyperextended head.

d. Breech and uterine dysfunction.

e. Breech and unfavorable pelvis.

f. Breech with premature fetus in active labor.

g. Breech not in labor with maternal indications for delivery (ROM >12h, hypertension, etc.).

h. Primipara breech.

3. Look for a reason to do a C/S. If none, give a trial of labor. Expect to assist delivery.

E. Vaginal delivery

1. Place in dorsal lithotomy position and empty the bladder.

2. Large episiotomy is usually necessary, if full term.

3. Breech of the fetus should be allowed to deliver spontaneously to the umbilicus.

4. Downward traction on sacrum and hips until ribs and scapulas are visible.

5. Slight rotation should bring the bisacromial diameter of the fetus into the AP diameter of the pelvic outlet.

6. Downward traction to deliver the anterior shoulder and arm. If unsuccessful, lift the infant upward to release the posterior shoulder and arm.

7. Extraction of the head with forceps or the Mauriceau maneuver, as follows:

   a. The operator's index and middle finger of one hand are applied over the fetal maxilla, while the body rests upon the palm of the hand and forearm.

   b. Two fingers of the operator's other hand are hooked over the fetal neck and downward traction is applied by grasping the shoulders.

   c. When the suboccipital region appears under the symphysis, the body of the fetus is then elevated toward the mother's abdomen and the mouth, nose, brow and occiput emerge over the perineum.

   d. Suprapubic pressure applied by an assistant helps keep the head flexed, and aids in delivery.

IX. TWINS

A. Determination of zygosity

1. Monozygotic - juxtaposed amnions not separated by chorion.

2. Dizygotic - adjacent amnions separated by chorion (occasionally monozygotic).

B. Delivery

1. Potential complications

   a. Premature labor.

   b. Uterine dysfunction.

   c. Abnormal presentations.

   d. Prolapse of the umbilical cord.

   e. Premature separation of the placenta.

   f. Postpartum hemorrhage.

2. Ascertain presentation and position of both fetuses (by x-ray or ultrasound).

3. Dilute oxytocin can be used to augment labor, if necessary.

4. First twin
   a. Usually larger.
   b. Rare problems with delivery if cephalic.
   c. If breech - problem if the fetus is very large or very small. Watch for cord prolapse. Have a low threshold for C/S.
   d. "Locked twins" - first is breech, second is cephalic. Rarely causes a problem.
5. Second twin
   a. Determine the presenting part and size.
   b. If the presenting part is fixed in the birth canal, the membranes can be ruptured. Check for prolapse of the cord immediately after rupture.
   c. If no contractions in 10 minutes, start dilute oxytocin.
   d. If the occiput or breech cannot be positioned over the pelvic inlet, or if there is excess uterine bleeding, internal podalic version may be done or immediate C/S.
6. Possible indications for C-section
   a. Twin A - breech, fetal distress, prolapsed cord, delivery before 33 weeks gestation or fetal weight <1500 gm.
   b. Twin B - fetal distress, prolapsed cord, constricted uterine ring, persistent abnormal presentation (breech or transverse), larger with failure to descend.

X. CORD PROLAPSE
A. Viable fetus
   1. Elevate the presenting part with hand to prevent occlusion of the cord during contractions.
   2. Large bore IV.
   3. Foley catheter.
   4. Avoid touching the cord (may cause spasm).
   5. To OR for immediate C/S. If there is delay in getting to the OR, fill the bladder with 300cc of fluid.
   6. Pre-op ampicillin 1gm IV.
B. Non-viable fetus
   1. Attempt vaginal delivery if presentation is favorable.
   2. If unsuccessful, do C/S.

XI. POST-TERM PREGNANCY
A. Definition
   1. Pregnancy that persists for 42 weeks or longer without labor.
   2. Establishment of accurate dates is important.
B. Management
   1. There is greater risk of fetal morbidity and mortality if the fetus remains in the uterus more than 42 weeks. Ultrasound may be done to check for decreased amniotic fluid.

2. If post-term and favorable for induction, induce with oxytocin. If unsuccessful, wait 1 week and try again.

3. If post-term but unfavorable for induction, no intervention if there are no maternal complications, fetus is active and adequate amniotic fluid is present. If not, attempt induction with oxytocin.

4. If > 44 weeks, deliver promptly. Induce, if possible. If unsuccessful, do C/S.

5. Possible post-term, without confirmation of dates and with adequate amniotic fluid present - follow weekly.

C. Special considerations

1. Close monitoring of fetal heart tones is necessary to detect fetal distress early.

2. Avoid meconium aspiration with thorough suctioning. If thick meconium appears early in labor, consider C/S.

3. Macrosomia is sometimes present with post-term infants, leading to shoulder dystocia.

XII. PREVIOUS C-SECTION

A. Possible VBAC candidate

1. Obtain old record to document transverse uterine incision.

2. Consider VBAC for prior C/S with non-recurrent indication (fetal distress, placenta previa, placenta abruptio, breech, abnormal presentation).

3. If previous CPD, carefully evaluate current size of the fetus, gestational age, pelvimetry and progress of labor before considering VBAC.

B. Not a VBAC candidate

1. Prior vertical uterine incision or extension of transverse uterine incision into the upper uterine segment (T-incision).

2. History of hysterotomy, deep myomectomy, cornual resection, repaired uterine rupture.

C. Labor management for VBAC

1. CBC, type and cross 2 units.

2. Large bore IV.

3. NPO.

4. Foley catheter ready for placement, if necessary.

5. Monitor fetal heart rate q 30 minutes in first stage, at least q 15 minutes in second stage of labor (auscultation immediately after contractions).

6. VS q1h.

7. Be alert for excessive pain, bleeding, fetal distress or inadequate cervical dilatation or descent of the presenting part.

8. Pitocin may be used to augment labor, with close monitoring of uterine contractions.

D. Delivery considerations

1. After delivery of the placenta, do an intra-uterine exam to document intact scar.

2. If retained placenta with anterior low segment implantation, consider possible placenta accreta.

XIII. PRE-ECLAMPSIA
A. Diagnosis
1. Hypertension (diastolic BP>90, systolic BP>140) with proteinuria (2+ or greater) and edema or both.
B. Other symptoms and signs
1. Hyperreflexia.
2. RUQ pain (tense liver capsule) - may be indicative of imminent convulsions.
3. Hand and face edema (mild pretibial edema is normal finding and not significant), excess fluid retention.
4. Headache, visual symptoms (scotoma or blurring).
5. Lab - hemoconcentration, decreased platelets, elevated AST, BUN, creatinine.
C. Management
1. **Mild** (BP <160/100, trace or no proteinuria, mild edema)
   a. Strict bedrest - encourage lying on the left side.
   b. BP q4h if hospitalized.
   c. Daily weights and fetal heart tones.
   d. Urine protein measurement q2d.
   e. Induce labor if no improvement and the fetus is term.
2. **Severe** (BP>160/100, proteinuria, edema, symptoms)
   a. Admit.
   b. No added salt diet.
   c. Seizure precautions.
   d. Examine eyegrounds.
   e. Daily weights, BP q1-4h, FHT at least daily.
   f. Place Foley, monitor I&O.
   g. Lab - CBC, U/A, BUN, creatinine, electrolytes, AST, platelets.
   h. Magnesium sulfate (may give IM or IV):
      (1) IV: 4-6 gm IV stat over 20 minutes, then constant infusion of 1-3gm/hr (in 100cc D5W). Check levels if available.
      (2) IM: load with 4-6 gm IV over 20 minutes plus 4-5 gm IM, then continue with 4gm IM q4h if the following conditions are met: reflexes are present, urine output >25cc/hr or 100cc/4h, respiratory rate >16/min.
      (3) Continue MgSO4 24 hours after delivery or 24 hours after last seizure.
      (4) Mg toxicity (decreased respirations) - treat with calcium gluconate 10ml IV slowly (should be kept at the bedside).
   i. Hydralazine 5-10mg IV or IM q2-4h for BP control. Diuretics are not recommended, unless pulmonary edema is present.

j. IV fluids at 60-150cc/hr unless there are excessive losses of fluid or blood.

k. TREATMENT OF PRE-ECLAMPSIA AND ECLAMPSIA IS DELIVERY

(1) If fetus viable, cervix ripe, head down, pelvis adequate - induce

(2) If fetus viable, cervix not ripe, pelvis inadequate - C/S

(3) If fetus not viable, mother stable or improving - monitor

(4) If fetus not viable, mother deteriorating - deliver anyway

XIV. ECLAMPSIA

A. Diagnosis

1. Some or all symptoms of pre-eclampsia.
2. PLUS the mother has had a seizure or is comatose.

B. Management

1. MgSO4 stat if not already started.
2. Hydralazine for BP control.
3. Diazepam IV slowly until the seizure stops.
4. Deliver as soon as the mother is stabilized (C/S usually necessary).
5. General anesthesia is preferred.

C. Complications

1. Acute renal failure - give IV fluids at a moderate rate (100-150cc/hr) unless excessive losses.
2. Malignant hypertension - treat with hydralazine as needed.
3. DIC - follow platelets, clotting time.
4. CVA may result from high BP and DIC.
5. Pulmonary edema - result of too-aggressive hydration. May need digitalization. Be cautious with diuretics. Poor prognostic sign.

XV. POSTPARTUM COMPLICATIONS

A. Postpartum fever

1. **Definition** - puerperal infection is defined as a temperature greater than 38°C. (100.4°F.) on two successive days after the first 24 hours without other apparent causes.
2. **Differential diagnosis**
   a. Dehydration
   b. UTI, pyelonephritis.
   c. Malaria
   d. Lower respiratory infection.
   e. Genital tract infection (endometritis).
3. **Evaluation**
   a. Look for non-GYN source of infection (get CBC, U/A, malaria smear).
   b. In endometritis, the uterus is usually enlarged, boggy, tender.
   c. Lochia may increase in amount, become malodorous.

4. Treatment
    a. Rule out non-genital tract sources.
    b. Treat empirically for malaria.
    c. If fever persists, begin broad spectrum antibiotics to cover gm (+), gm(-) rods, *Enterococcus*, and anerobes (ampicillin + gentamicin, add metronidazole or chloramphenicol for serious infections).
    d. Watch closely for progression of infection to pelvic cellulitis or peritonitis.

B. Postpartum hemorrhage
  1. Definition - blood loss in excess of 500cc in the first 24 hours following delivery. Late postpartum hemorrhage (occurring after 24 hours) occasionally occurs.
  2. Etiology
    a. Most common
      (1) Genital tract trauma - episiotomy, lacerations of vagina or cervix, uterine rupture.
      (2) Uterine atony - more common with overdistended uterus (polyhydramnios or twins), prolonged labor, rapidly progressive labor, high parity.
    b. Less common
      (1) Incomplete removal of placenta.
      (2) Placenta accreta.
      (3) Coagulation defects.
  3. Evaluation
    a. Palpate the fundus of the uterus. If soft or boggy, bleeding is likely due to uterine atony.
    b. If the fundus is firm, bleeding is likely due to genital trauma.
      (1) Bright red blood suggests lacerations. Inspect vulva and vagina for lacerations.
      (2) Inspect the cervix carefully using ring forceps (use adequate retraction and light). Provide adequate analgesia during the exam.
  4. Treatment
    a. Obtain help.
    b. Start large bore IV.
    c. Use bimanual uterine massage.
    d. Begin oxytocin drip. Methergine with continued uterine atony.
    e. Repair episiotomy, vaginal or cervical tears, if present.
    f. Replace blood.
    g. If uncontrolled bleeding, do hypogastric artery ligation, then hysterectomy, if needed.

XVI. PROCEDURES
  A. Oxytocin drip
    1. Indications

a. Ruptured membranes at term or premature ruptured membranes with high amnionitis risk.

b. Hypotonic uterine contractions with adequate pelvis.

c. Medical induction for post-dates, diabetes, pre-eclampsia, etc.

2. **Contraindications**
   a. Abnormal presentation
   b. CPD
   c. Cord prolapse (viable fetus)
   d. Prior transfundal uterine surgery
   e. Placenta previa

3. **Method**
   a. Oxytocin 5u/500cc RL or 10u/1000cc RL.
   b. Start at 5 drops/minute and increase by 5 drops/minute every 30 minutes to a maximum of 20 drops/minute. Titrate according to the contraction pattern.
   c. Stop oxytocin if no relaxation between contractions or if fetal distress occurs.

B. **Bishop Score** (for assessing the favorability of the cervix before induction of labor)

Score	0	1	2	3
Dilatation (cm)	Closed	1 - 2	3 - 4	5 - 6
Effacement (%)	0 - 30%	40 - 50%	60 - 70%	80 - 100%
Station	-3	-2	-1, 0	+1, +2
Consistency	Firm	Medium	Soft	-
Position	Posterior	Mid	Anterior	-

A Bishop score of 9 or greater indicates that induction should be successful. A score <4 is unfavorable.

C. **Shake test** (Foam Stability Test)

1. **Test of fetal lung maturity.**

2. **Amniocentesis:**
   a. Local anesthesia.
   b. 20 or 22g needle, 3-6 inches long (spinal needle is good).
   c. Insert suprapubically, pushing the head up out of the way or identify pocket of fluid on ultrasound which is free of cord or body parts.

3. **Shake test:**
   a. Tube #1 - 1ml amniotic fluid + 1 ml 95% ethanol.
   b. Tube #2 - 0.5 ml fluid + 0.5 ml 0.9% saline + 1 ml 95% ethanol.
   c. Shake each tube vigorously for 15 seconds and place upright in a rack for 15 minutes.
   d. The persistence of an intact ring of bubbles at the air-liquid interface after 15 minutes is considered a positive test (risk of fetal respiratory distress is low).

CHAPTER 16

GYNECOLOGY

I. BREAST DISEASE
A. Benign diseases of the breast
1. Fibrocystic changes
  a. Represent exaggerated physiologic responses to changing hormonal environment. Estrogen-progesterone imbalance is usually present.
  b. Include painful, lumpy breasts (mastodynia, mastalgia), masses and nipple discharge.
  c. Most common at 30 - 50 years of age.
  d. Pre-menstrual breast tenderness may be present.
  e. Physical exam reveals irregular thickening of the breasts, especially in the upper outer quadrants. There may be multiple lumps which are diverse in size and show marked variation in tenderness and size throughout the menstrual cycle.
  f. There is an increased risk of breast cancer. New masses should be aspirated or biopsied.
  g. Treatment includes pre-menstrual analgesics or diuretics, low estrogen, high progesterone oral contraceptives or medroxy-progesterone (Provera) 5-10mg/d x 10d before menses.
2. Mastodynia (mastalgia)
  a. Common complaint. Cause is usually unclear.
  b. May be due to cyclic mastalgia occurring prior to menses, fibrocystic changes or referred pain (such as costochondritis).
3. Nipple discharge
  a. Galactorrhea - spontaneous secretion of a milky discharge not associated with pregnancy. Usually persistent and may be a large quantity. May be associated with elevated prolactin levels. The following drugs can increase prolactin and should be discontinued: digoxin, marijuana, heroin, phenothiazines, haloperidol, metoclopramide, isoniazid, tricyclic antidepressants, reserpine, methyldopa, cimetidine, benzodiazepines.
  b. Serous or bloody breast discharge must be investigated. Usually caused by benign intraductal papilloma, but may be carcinoma. Needs biopsy.
  c. Postmenopausal nipple discharge - suggestive of carcinoma. Must be investigated.
  d. Duct ectasia (comedomastitis) - occurs in older, multiparous women. Characterized by thick, white or discolored, cheesy material draining from the nipple, with induration under the areola. No treatment is necessary unless it is bothersome. May cause repeated infections, in which case local excision may be done.
4. Mass
  a. May be cystic, solid, benign or malignant. Fibroadenoma is most common.

    b. Aspirate with 23 g needle. If fluid is obtained and is clear or cloudy, with resolution of the mass, the patient should be re-examined in 1 month. If the fluid is bloody or if there is residual mass present after aspiration, a biopsy is necessary.

   5. Infection - acute mastitis usually occurs in lactating women. If no history of lactation or trauma, be suspicious of inflammatory breast cancer.

B. Breast cancer

  1. Findings suggestive of malignancy

    a. Solitary mass with induration.

    b. Lack of tenderness.

    c. Axillary lymph node enlargement.

    d. Overlying skin changes.

    e. Mammogram, if available, showing mass with irregular borders and clustered microcalcifications especially within the mass.

  2. Evaluation of a breast mass

    a. History and physical.

    b. If the mass is not suspicious, watch through 1 menstrual cycle.

    c. If it persists, do a fine needle aspiration. If fluid is obtained and the mass disappears and does not recur in 3 months, assume a benign cyst.

    d. If the mass is solid or recurs, do a biopsy.

C. Common breast-feeding problems

  1. Sore nipples

    a. Symptoms of cracking, bruising, bleeding and soreness.

    b. Prevented by using nipple rolling beginning at 35 weeks to prepare them.

    c. Proper positioning of the infant's mouth.

  2. Engorgement

    a. Occurs on the third or fourth postpartum day.

    b. The breast becomes large and hard.

    c. Treat with hand expression or pumping before nursing to soften the breast.

  3. Blocked ducts

    a. Cause a smooth, tender lump in the breast that does not decrease after nursing.

    b. Apply local heat, massage the lump toward the nipple, frequent nursing.

  4. Candida infection

    a. Causes intense, burning nipple pain, papules.

    b. Treat with topical nystatin.

  5. Mastitis

    a. Symptoms of breast pain, erythema, fever, body aches, chills, malaise.

    b. Continue nursing and/or expression of milk, local heat, hydration, bedrest, paracetamol (acetaminophen).

    c. Antibiotics (cloxacillin or dicloxacillin 500mg po qid; erythromycin if PCN-allergic) should be given for 7-10 days. Initiate as soon as possible to reduce abscess formation.

II. DISEASES OF THE VULVA
A. Bartholin's gland cyst
1. Asymptomatic and small - need no treatment.
2. Symptomatic and/or recurrent with abscess formation - need surgical therapy (consider cancer if patient >40 years old).
   a. Marsupialization - portion of the cyst wall is excised and the edges of the cyst lining are everted and fixed to the skin and mucous membrane. Heal within 6 weeks.
   b. Word catheter - bulb tip is put in thru a stab wound and inflated with 2-4cc of water. The plugged end is placed in the vagina. Catheter is kept in at least 4-6 weeks, then removed.
B. Bartholin's gland abscess
1. Develops over 2-3 days.
2. Usually has spontaneous rupture in 72 hours.
3. Management
   a. Bedrest, analgesics, hot wet dressings or Sitz baths qid.
   b. Tetracycline 500mg po qid x 7-10d.
   c. I & D (pack with iodoform gauze or put in Word catheter).
   d. If recurrent abscesses, do a definitive procedure.

III. VAGINITIS
A. General
1. Vulvovaginitis is a common outpatient gynecologic complaint.
2. Symptoms include discharge, pruritus, odor.
3. Physical examination and wet prep (with saline and KOH) usually give the diagnosis.
4. Characteristics of vaginal discharges

	Candidiasis	Trichomonas	Gardnerella
Character	Thick, cheesy, white	Copious, thin, foamy, green/yellow	Watery
Symptoms	Pruritus	Pruritus	Fishy odor
pH	4.5	5-7	5-6
Wet prep	Hyphae	Trichomonads	Clue cells
KOH prep	Positive	Negative	Negative

B. Candidiasis
1. Causes a thick, cheesy discharge with much itching.
2. Commonly seen in association with pregnancy, antibiotic usage, diabetes and HIV infection.
3. On exam, there is usually erythema, with white patches on the vaginal wall.

4. Diagnosis is confirmed with KOH prep.

5. Treatment

    a. Antifungal vaginal suppositories or cream (nystatin, clotrimazole, miconazole, butoconazole or terconazole).

    b. Fluconazole 200mg po as a single dose may be used, if available.

C. Trichomoniasis

  1. Causes a copious, foamy discharge with soreness and itching. Frequently there is an odor. May have urinary symptoms.

  2. 10% of patients are asymptomatic.

  3. The exam shows yellow, frothy discharge and inflammation.

  4. Diagnosis is confirmed by the wet prep showing the organism.

  5. Treatment

    a. Metronidazole 2 gm po x 1 dose or 500mg po bid x7d (15mg/kg/d tid x7d).

    b. Tinidazole 2gm po x 1 (50mg/kg once) is available in other countries.

    c. Avoid in the first trimester of pregnancy. May use 20% saline douche or clotrimazole 100mg intravaginally q hs x7d.

    d. D/C breast feeding for 24 hours after giving metronidazole.

    e. Treat the sexual partner.

D. Bacterial vaginosis (*Gardnerella vaginalis*)

  1. Causes a scanty, malodorous discharge with a fishy smell.

  2. The exam is nonspecific.

  3. Diagnosis is suspected on wet prep with the finding of "clue cells".

  4. Treatment

    a. Metronidazole 500mg po bid x7d or metronidazole vaginal cream 5 gm bid x 5d.

    b. Clindamycin 300mg po bid x 7d or clindamycin vaginal cream 5gm qd x7d may be used in pregnancy.

E. Atrophic vaginitis

  1. Thin watery discharge or dryness +/- spotting.

  2. Seen in postmenopausal women.

  3. Exam shows dryness and thinning of the vaginal mucosa.

  4. Treatment is with topical estrogen creams (Premarin 0.1% cream) 1-2x/d or oral estrogens.

IV. UTERINE ENLARGEMENT

A. Normal uterine measurements

  1. Nulliparous - 8 cm long, 5cm wide, 2.5 cm AP diameter.

  2. Multiparous - 9 cm long, 6 cm wide, 3.5 cm AP diameter.

  3. On ultrasound, the normal uterus appears 8x4x4 cm.

B. Causes of uterine enlargement

  1. Pregnancy

    a. Normal

    b. Missed abortion - uterus is smaller than expected.

    c. Molar pregnancy - uterus may be larger than expected, heart tones are absent.

2. Adenomyosis

    a. Benign condition characterized by endometrial glands and stroma within the myometrium.

    b. 30% are asymptomatic. Can cause menorrhagia or dysmenorrhea.

    c. Management - hysterectomy.

3. Leiomyomas (fibroids)

    a. Benign condition. Contain smooth muscle with some fibrous connective tissue elements.

    b. Abnormal bleeding is the most common symptom. Pain is not characteristic, but may be present in up to 1/3 of patients. Rarely causes infertility.

    c. Management - surgery if >12 week size (hysterectomy vs. myomectomy depending on desire for future pregnancy). If asymptomatic, and < 12 week size, follow q 6 months.

    d. After menopause, leiomyomas usually shrink.

    e. Rapid growth, or any growth after menopause is cause for hysterectomy to rule out sarcoma.

    f. Estrogens may cause leiomyomas to grow.

4. Uterine cancer

    a. Endometrial carcinoma is a common pelvic genital cancer in older women.

    b. Risk factors include obesity, nulliparity, late menopause. Diabetes and hypertension may be associated.

    c. Painless vaginal bleeding is the hallmark of endometrial cancer. Postmenopausal or abnormal perimenopausal bleeding should always be assumed to be an underlying malignancy. Pain is a late symptom.

    d. Evaluation

        (1) Endometrial biopsy or fractional D&C for diagnosis. U/S may be helpful.

        (2) IVP, chest x-ray to evaluate for metastatic disease and tumor extension.

    e. Management

        (1) Hysterectomy (TAH-BSO).

        (2) Pelvic and lymph node dissection in selected cases.

        (3) Radiation, progestins or chemotherapy.

V. ADNEXAL MASSES

A. History

    1. Determine if premenopausal or postmenopausal.

    2. Ask about associated vaginal bleeding.

    3. Look for factors which suggest non-gynecologic cause of mass (GU, GI).

B. Physical exam
1. Determine if uterine vs. adnexal enlargement.
2. Do wet mount, cultures for *N. gonorrhea*, *Chlamydia*, if available.
3. Benign tumors are usually unilateral, cystic and mobile.
4. Malignancies are usually solid, fixed and nodular and may cause ascites.

C. Diagnostic tests
1. Urine pregnancy test.
2. Pelvic ultrasound - do emergently in the patient with tender adnexal mass and purulent cervical discharge (R/O tubo-ovarian abscess), and those with a positive pregnancy test or vaginal bleeding and adnexal mass (R/O ectopic pregnancy).

D. Management
1. Masses which are >10cm, septated or solid have a high likelihood of being malignant. They should be removed surgically.
2. Any enlarging mass should be removed surgically.
3. Premenstrual and postmenopausal females are at high risk for malignancy. Any mass in these age groups should be evaluated immediately and probably removed.
4. Masses presenting with acute pain and/or fever need immediate evaluation for infection (PID, tubo-ovarian abscess), ectopic pregnancy, torsion of an adnexal mass or ruptured ovarian cyst (clear fluid on culdocentesis).
5. Functional ovarian cysts are the most common cause of adnexal masses in the reproductive years. If <6cm they can be watched over 1-2 cycles. If they persist unchanged, ovarian suppression with oral contraceptives may be tried for 1-2 cycles.
   a. Follicular cysts
      (1) Torsion and rupture produce acute pain.
      (2) Cysts smaller than 6-8cm usually resolve after 1-2 cycles. Cysts > 6-8cm have a higher suspicion of neoplasm and should be evaluated by U/S, laparoscopy or laparotomy.
      (3) Clear or serosanguineous fluid on culdocentesis is consistent with a ruptured cyst.
   b. Corpus luteum cysts
      (1) Occur after ovulation. May disappear over 1-2 cycles or with oral contraceptives.
      (2) Can occur with early pregnancy, and usually disappear by the end of the first trimester.
   c. Luteoma of pregnancy
      (1) Benign, solid tumor 5-10cm in size.
      (2) Occasionally produces testosterone.
      (3) Regresses after pregnancy.
   d. Theca lutein cysts
      (1) More common with trophoblastic disease or multiple gestation.

(2) Multiple cysts 1-15 cm. Ovaries enlarge rapidly. No treatment unless torsion occurs.

  e. Endometriomas (chocolate cysts)

    (1) Formed by cyclic menstrual bleeding into endometrial tissue that has implanted on the ovaries or the pelvis.

    (2) Usually immobile, due to scarring.

    (3) May be asymptomatic, or give history of severe cyclic pain and severe dysmenorrhea.

    (4) Require removal if larger than 2 cm.

  f. Polycystic ovaries (Stein-Leventhal syndrome)

    (1) Abnormality in the hypothalamic-pituitary-ovarian axis. Luteinizing hormone is increased several times above normal.

    (2) Clinical findings include obesity, hirsutism, irregular menses and infertility secondary to anovulation.

    (3) Treat with ovarian suppression (birth control pills or depot progesterone).

    (4) Usually require clomiphene to conceive.

    (5) Risk of endometrial carcinoma if amenorrhea prolonged (>12 months).

  g. Ovarian cancer

    (1) Often presents with fixed pelvic mass and ascites.

    (2) Surgery should include TAH-BSO, omentectomy, and excision of all tumor, if possible.

    (3) Staging includes biopsies of pelvis, gutters, diaphragms, and washings.

VI. ABNORMAL UTERINE BLEEDING

Causes of Uterine Bleeding		
Age Group	**Etiology**	**Treatment**
Peri-menarcheal	Anovulatory DUB	OCs x several cycles
	R/O pregnancy	Provera 10mg/d x 10d/month
Reproductive	Ovulatory DUB:	-
	Mid cycle bleeding	Premarin 1.23-2.5 mg/d from 3d before to 2d after ovulation
	Short cycles	Clomiphene or OCs
	Anovulatory DUB:	-
	>30 years old	Endometrial biopsy
	Pregnancy desired	Clomiphene
	Pregnancy not desired	Provera 10mg/d x 10d/month or low dose estrogen OCs
	Menorrhagia or intermenstrual bleeding	R/O anatomic abnormalities Premarin and Provera, OCs
Peri-menopausal	Anovulatory DUB	Provera 10mg/d x 10d/month
Postmenopausal period	Atrophic changes	Estrogen cream, Premarin and Provera
	Endometrial hyperplasia or malignancy	Surgery

A. Patterns of abnormal bleeding
  1. **Amenorrhea** - no menstrual flow for more than 90 days.
  2. **Menorrhagia** - excessive bleeding at the time of menses, either number of days, amount of blood, or both.
  3. **Metrorrhagia** - bleeding occurring irregularly between menstrual cycles.
  4. **Menometrorrhagia** - prolongation of the menstrual flow associated with irregular intermenstrual bleeding.
  5. **Oligomenorrhea** - menstrual bleeding occurring at intervals > 35 days.
  6. **Polymenorrhea** - menstrual bleeding occurring at intervals < 22 days.
B. Normal menstruation
  1. Normal volume of blood loss - 20-80 ml (average 30 ml).
  2. Normal interval between cycles - 28-30 days (may be 21-35 days).
  3. Duration of flow - 3-5 days (1-8days).
C. General etiologies for abnormal bleeding
  1. **Pregnancy** - including ectopic pregnancy, threatened abortion, placenta abruptio and placenta previa.
  2. **Organic pelvic lesions** (neoplasm or infections).
  3. **Coagulopathies** (especially Von Willebrand's disease).
  4. **Dysfunctional uterine bleeding** (no evidence of organic lesions)
    a. Dysfunctional uterine bleeding (DUB) is usually associated with anovulatory cycles, but can be seen with ovulatory cycles.
    b. In an anovulatory cycle, the prolonged effect of estrogen on the endometrium results in abnormal proliferation and hyperplasia. Irregular endometrial shedding occurs when the endometrial height is greater than the stromal support. This can cause prolonged bleeding.
    c. Ovulatory DUB can cause mid-cycle bleeding or abnormal cycles. It occurs when estrogen levels are reduced at ovulation.
D. Evaluation
  1. Careful history and physical examination, including pelvic examination.
  2. CBC, platelet count. Bleeding time and clotting time should be done if coagulopathy is suspected.
  3. U/A, urine pregnancy test.
  4. GC and *Chlamydia* cultures, if available.
  5. Pelvic ultrasound, if a mass is present.
  6. Endometrial biopsy or D&C in peri-menopausal or postmenopausal patients.
E. Management of abnormal bleeding
  1. **Peri-menarcheal period**
    a. Anovulatory DUB is the most common cause of abnormal bleeding in this age group. Usually, there are irregular menses with menorrhagia. Rule out pregnancy.
    b. If excessive bleeding occurs, resulting in anemia, coagulation defects should be ruled out (especially Von Willebrand's disease).

c. Oral contraceptives (OC) are the treatment of choice. One 5μg estrogen pill is given qid for 5-7d, then low estrogen (35μg) pill for 21d. After 7 days of withdrawal, heavy menses should follow. Continue OCs through several cycles (normal doses). Periods should get lighter with each cycle. Stop after several cycles to see if regular menses will start.

d. Progestational agents - medroxyprogesterone (Provera) 10mg/d or norethindrone 5mg qid may be given for 10 days, after which withdrawal bleeding should occur (may be heavy). Oral contraceptives can then be used cyclically, or medroxyprogesterone 10mg may be given daily for 10 days at the beginning of each month to cause regular withdrawal bleeding.

e. Profuse, persistent bleeding.
  (1) Consider transfusion if anemic or hemodynamically unstable.
  (2) Premarin 25 mg IV q4h up to 3 doses can be given to stop the acute bleeding. If unsuccessful or unavailable, do a D&C.
  (3) Once the acute bleeding stops, OCs or progestational agents should be started.

2. Reproductive period
  a. <20% of abnormal bleeding in this group is due to anovulatory DUB. Pregnancy, PID, IUDs, OCs, neoplasm, thyroid disease, endometriosis and adenomyosis are common etiologies.
  b. Ovulatory DUB
    (1) Mid cycle bleeding - occurs at the time of ovulation when the level of estrogen drops. If spotting only, it doesn't need treatment. If treatment is required, use Premarin 1.25-2.5mg qd from 3 days before to 2 d after ovulation.
    (2) Abnormal corpus luteum function - suspected with menstrual cycles that are abnormally short (<24d). May cause infertility. Results in inadequate progesterone levels or shortened progesterone secretion. Diagnosed with an endometrial biopsy. It does not necessarily need treatment, unless bothersome to the patient. Can use clomiphene citrate (Clomid) if pregnancy is desired or OCs if not.
  c. Anovulatory DUB
    (1) General
      (a) Anovulatory DUB is often due to polycystic ovarian syndrome or obesity. Infertility is a common problem in these patients, as is hirsutism.
      (b) Anovulatory cycles associated with amenorrhea or oligomenorrhea lead to an excess of estrogen exposure of the endometrium. This causes an increased risk of developing hyperplasia or cancer.
      (c) Endometrial biopsy is indicated in patients >30 years old with anovulatory DUB.

(2) Treatment of anovulatory DUB
   (a) Pregnancy desired - ovulation induction. Clomiphene citrate (Clomid) 50mg qd is given on days 5-9 of the cycle. Ovulation should occur 3-10 days after the last dose. Increase by 50mg increments each cycle to a maximum of 200mg. The patient should have intercourse q2d beginning 3 days after the last Clomid tablet. Most pregnancies will occur within 6 ovulatory cycles of therapy. Other ovulation-inducing drugs include human menopausal gonadotropin (Pergonal) and bromocriptine mesylate (Parlodel). These should be given by a specialist.
   (b) Pregnancy not desired - medroxyprogesterone 10mg qd x 10d each month followed by withdrawal bleeding. Alternative - low estrogen dose OCs cyclically. This is especially helpful with hirsutism.

d. Functional ovarian cysts (follicular cysts or persistent corpus luteum cysts). See section V.

e. Functional ovarian tumors
   (1) May cause abnormal menses.
   (2) Not suppressible with OCs.
   (3) Need surgical evaluation.

3. Peri-menopausal period
   a. Anovulatory DUB is a common cause of abnormal bleeding in this age group. Other causes listed in the reproductive age group need to be considered.
   b. Treatment
     (1) Medroxyprogesterone 10mg/d 10-14 days per month until menopause.
     (2) Hysterectomy if biopsy shows atypical hyperplasia or cancer.

4. Postmenopausal period
   a. Any bleeding that occurs after a 12 month cessation of regular menstrual flow, or after the onset of vasomotor changes, needs investigation.
   b. Etiologies
     (1) Benign - atrophic vaginitis, atrophic endometrium, endometrial or endocervical polyps, endometrial hyperplasia.
     (2) Malignant - endometrial adenocarcinoma, cervical cancer.
   c. Management
     (1) Atrophic changes
       (a) Estrogen cream short term for vaginitis.
       (b) Conjugated estrogens (Premarin) 0.625 mg/d plus medroxyprogesterone 10mg/d 10-14 days per month. (Medroxyprogesterone is given to reverse the estrogen effect on the uterus and reduce the risk of developing endometrial cancer.)

    (c) Continuous estrogen and progesterone (Premarin 0.625mg plus medroxyprogesterone 2.5-5.0mg/d every day). There may be irregular spotting in the first 3-6 months. A baseline endometrial biopsy is not necessary before starting therapy.

  (2) Adenomatous hyperplasia

    (a) Surgery - TAH-BSO.

    (b) High dose progesterone in patients who are not good surgical candidates.

  (3) Malignancies - surgery, radiation or chemotherapy.

VII. MENOPAUSE

A. General

1. **Definition** - menopause is that time when spontaneous menstruation ceases for 6 months to 1 year.
2. **Etiology** - caused by the progressive loss of ovarian follicular units. The ovary eventually ceases estrogen production. There is a subsequent rise in levels of serum gonadotropins (FSH).

B. Symptoms

1. Menstrual irregularities, leading to complete cessation of menses.
2. Vasomotor instability (may precede menopause by months to years) - hot flashes, night sweats.
3. GU atrophy - vaginal dryness, pruritus, irritation, dyspareunia, urinary frequency and dysuria.
4. Emotional symptoms - depression, lability, irritability, insomnia.
5. Cardiovascular disease (increased LDL, decreased HDL).
6. Osteoporosis - 50% bone loss in the first 7 years.

C. Diagnosis

1. History and physical exam, including pelvic exam.
2. Negative pregnancy test.
3. Increased FSH levels (>40), decreased estradiol, if available.

D. Estrogen replacement therapy

1. Best management of menopause for those without contraindications. Definitely indicated for patients with premature menopause. Reduces the post-menopausal loss of bone mass.
2. Contraindicated in patients with estrogen-dependent neoplasms or undiagnosed vaginal bleeding. May be contraindicated in patients with acute and chronic liver disease, thromboembolic disease, and endometrial hyperplasia.
3. Risk of endometrial cancer with use of unopposed estrogen is 3-8x. This risk is reduced when progestins are given with the estrogens. Breast cancer risk is elevated. Baseline mammography should be obtained, if available.
4. Routine pretreatment endometrial biopsy is unnecessary. Biopsy is indicated in patients on cyclic estrogen replacement therapy with unscheduled bleeding, and in patients on unopposed estrogens.

5. Dosage regimens (treat for 5-10 years)
   a. Intact uterus (choose one regimen):
      (1) Conjugated estrogen 0.625mg qd day 1-25 plus medroxyprogesterone 10mg qd day 13-25, with a 3-6 day break at the end of each cycle.
      (2) Continuous conjugated estrogen 0.625mg qd plus medroxyprogesterone 2.5mg qd. Most women become amenorrheic in 1 year.
      (3) Lower dose estrogen 0.3mg cyclically with progesterone may reduce bleeding. Give with calcium to offer osteoporosis protection.
   b. Absent uterus
      (1) Estrogens should be given in doses to prevent osteoporosis (conjugated estrogen 0.625mg/d).
      (2) Progestins are not needed except to treat estrogen side-effects (such as breast tenderness), but progestins will adversely affect serum lipids.
6. Special considerations
   a. Vasomotor symptoms will be reduced after 3-6 months of estrogen therapy.
   b. GU atrophy - vaginal estrogen creams (Premarin cream applied 1-2x/d are effective, but do not prevent the systemic effects of estrogen, because levels of estrogen in the circulation are as high or higher than with oral therapy).
   c. Osteoporosis prevention - the minimum effective dose of conjugated estrogens in preventing osteoporosis is 0.625 mg/d. Lower doses (0.3mg) combined with calcium 1000 - 1500mg/d may be equally effective. The risk of osteoporosis should be evaluated for each patient. Estrogens should be started at menopause, but are still effective if started years later. Treatment should be continued long term.

VIII. INFERTILITY
A. Definition
   1. One year of unprotected intercourse without conception.
   2. Common causes include male factors, ovulation disorders and tubal disease.
B. Objectives of evaluation
   1. Document ovulation.
   2. Establish patency of the female reproductive tract.
   3. Evaluate sperm production, interaction and survival within the female reproductive tract.
C. Female evaluation
   1. History - fertility, overall health status, menstrual history, sexual history, gynecologic history, drugs and medications.

2. Physical exam and pelvic.

3. Ovulation detection

  a. History of regular menstruation is highly suggestive of ovulation. Cycles <21 days or >35 days suggest ovulatory dysfunction.

  b. Ovulation symptoms - mittelschmerz, premenstrual syndrome.

  c. Basal body temperature (BBT) - should see a 0.5 - 1°F. rise in temperature with ovulation. There should be 11 or more days between the temperature rise and onset of menses with a normal luteal phase.

  d. Cervical mucus

    (1) Evaluate for infection (*Chlamydia, Ureaplasma*). Treat with tetracycline or erythromycin 250-500mg qid x 7-14d.

    (2) Increased mucus quality, clarity and stretchability is present in the peri-ovulatory period (vs. thick, cloudy, scant mucus with anovulation).

    (3) Fern pattern can be seen when peri-ovulatory cervical mucus is dried on a slide and observed under the microscope (absent when estrogen levels are low).

4. Patency of the female reproductive tract

  a. Hysterosalpingography demonstrates abnormalities within the uterus and tubes.

  b. Laparoscopy or laparotomy is done when tubal or intraperitoneal pathology is suspected.

D. Male evaluation - (semen analysis)

  1. Obtain semen following 2-4 days of abstinence.

  2. Analysis should be performed within 1 hour of obtaining the specimen.

  3. Normal values:

    a. Semen volume: 2.0-5.0 ml

    b. Sperm concentration: 20-250 million/ml

    c. Percentage motility: >40-60%

    d. Progression: >50% progressing

    e. Sperm morphology: >50% oval

  4. If semen analysis is abnormal, repeat in 2-3 months and refer to a urologist if still abnormal.

E. Management

  1. Anovulation - clomiphene citrate (Clomid) 50mg po qd days 5-9 of the cycle. Ovulation should occur 3-10 days after the last tablet is taken. Increase the dose by 50mg increments each cycle to a maximum of 200mg. Intercourse on alternate days beginning 3 days after the last tablet, until ovulation has occurred (BBT rise, mid-luteal progesterone levels). Most pregnancies will occur within six ovulatory cycles.

  2. Luteal phase defects - vaginal progesterone suppositories 25mg bid starting 3d after ovulation and continued until menses or until week 10 of pregnancy.

  3. Damaged Fallopian tubes - surgical repair, if available.

4. **Male infertility** (low sperm counts, abnormal postcoital tests) - artificial insemination, if available.

IX. CONTRACEPTION

Contraception			
Method	**Failure rate**	**Contraindications**	**Side-effects**
Natural methods	20%	None	Difficult in women with irregular menses
Oral contraceptives	0 - 3%	Thromboembolic dis., CVA, coronary artery dis., breast ca., pregnancy, liver disease, HTN, smoker, immobility, headaches, abn. vag. bleeding	Thromboembolic dis., HTN, hepatic adenoma, GB dis., depression, headache, weight gain, nausea, fluid retention, breast tenderness, menstrual irregularities
Depo-Provera	0 - 1%	Same as above	Heavy or irregular bleeding, amenorrhea
Norplant	0 - 0.5%	Same as above	Irregular bleeding
IUD	3%	PID, pregnancy, previous ectopic pregnancy	PID, perforation, spotting and bleeding
Diaphragm	18%	Allergy to latex or spermicide, recurrent UTI, TSS, pelvic pain	Irritation, vaginal discharge, allergic reaction, pelvic discomfort, TSS
Spermicides and contraceptive sponge	18 - 28%	None	Irritation, allergic reaction
Condom	5 - 10%	None	None

A. Natural methods
1. **Failure rate** - 20%.
2. **Calendar method**
   a. Count cycle length for 8 cycles prior to using the method.
   b. Calculate first fertile day by subtracting 18 from the length of the shortest cycle (during the preceding 8 months). Last fertile day is calculated by subtracting 11 from the length of the longest cycle.
3. **Basal body temperature method**
   a. Retrospective method.
   b. Avoid intercourse on day 4 until 4 days after ovulation (as determined on the basis of the preceding 3-4 BBT charts, or 3 days of successive temperature elevation).
4. **Cervical mucus charting** (Billings method)
   a. Avoid intercourse at the onset of any vaginal moisture or cervical mucus.
   b. Continue until the evening of the 4th day after the "peak day" of maximum mucus secretion associated with ovulation.

B. Hormonal (oral contraceptives)
1. **Failure rate** - 0 - 3%
2. **Types**
   a. Combined pills - daily dosage of estrogen (ethinyl estradiol) and progestin (norethindrone or norgestrel) for 21 days in each 28 day cycle.
   b. Minipills - progestin only, taken continuously with no cyclic interruptions. High incidence of irregular and unpredictable vaginal bleeding.
3. **Contraindications to oral contraceptives**

Absolute contraindications	Relative contraindications
Thrombophlebitis or thromboembolic disorder	Severe headaches
Cerebrovascular accident	Hypertension
Coronary artery or ischemic heart disease	Long-leg cast or forced immobility
Known or suspected breast carcinoma	> 40 years old plus risk factor for CV disease
Pregnancy	> 35 years old and smoker
Liver tumor or impaired liver function	Abnormal vaginal bleeding

4. **Dosage**
   a. Choose the lowest dosage that provides effective protection from pregnancy.
   b. Usually start with 30-35µg pills.
   c. Progestin-only (minipill) may be the best choice for postpartum or nursing mothers, women >30-35 years old, women who have vascular headache, and those who do not tolerate combined pills.
5. **Follow-up**
   a. Check BP and tolerance at 3 months.
   b. Annual exam and Pap smear, if available.
   c. Breast exam q 2 years in patients >35 years old.
6. **Major side effects** - venous and arterial thromboembolic disease, hypertension, hepatic adenoma, gallbladder disease, depression. Minor side effects include nausea, weight gain, fluid retention, breast tenderness, menstrual irregularities.
7. **Patient instructions**
   a. Five pill danger signs (**ACHES**)
      Abdominal pain
      Chest pain or shortness of breath
      Headaches
      Eye problems
      Severe leg pain
   b. Start the first pill pack on the first day of normal menstrual period or anytime in the following 6 days. Backup contraception should be used in the first 2 weeks. Triphasic pills do not need a backup method if started on the first day of menses.

    c. Forgotten pills
      (1) One pill missed - double up the next day.
      (2) Two pills missed - double up for 2 days and use backup method until the next menstrual period.
      (3) Three or more pills missed - start a new pack of pills and use backup method.
    d. Skipped period
      (1) Obtain a pregnancy test.
      (2) If the patient is amenorrheic, increase the estrogen or progestin potency for 6 months or more, evaluate for other causes of amenorrhea.
    e. Spotting
      (1) Watch and wait.
      (2) Take pills at the same time daily.
      (3) May require switching to a triphasic pill or higher dosage (up to 50μg estrogen).
    f. Hypertension or headaches
      (1) Change to minipills.
      (2) Stop OCs altogether.
  8. Other hormonal methods
    a. Medroxyprogesterone acetate (Depo-Provera) 150mg IM q3 months. May have heavy or irregular bleeding. Best given within 5-7 days of the last menstrual period. Most women stop menstruating after 1 year.
    b. Progestin implants (Norplant) placed subcutaneously in 6 plastic cylinders provides contraception for 5 years. May be removed at any time. Nearly 100% effective.
C. IUD's
  1. Failure rate - 3%
  2. Types
    a. Copper T-380A - replace every 7 years.
    b. Progestasert - contains progestin. Requires removal and reinsertion each year.
    c. Copper-7 - should be removed and replaced with another type or alternate contraceptive method.
    d. Lippes Loop - does not require reinsertion.
    e. Saf-T-Coil - does not require reinsertion.
  3. Contraindications
    a. Active PID
    b. Pregnancy
    c. Previous ectopic pregnancy
  4. Side effects - PID, uterine or cervical perforation, IUD expulsion, spotting and bleeding which may lead to anemia, and pregnancy (including ectopic).
  5. Patient instructions

a. IUD's may be inserted and removed at any time in the menstrual cycle, but most physicians prefer to insert them at the end of a menstrual period.

b. IUD danger signs for patients (**PAINS**)
Period late or missing
Abdominal pain
Increased temperature
Noticeable discharge
Spotting

D. Diaphragm

1. Failure rate - 18%

2. Effect - serves as an inefficient barrier preventing sperm from reaching the cervix. Spermicide used with it kills any sperm that get past the diaphragm rim.

3. Needs to be fitted by the practitioner. The largest that will fit comfortably should be prescribed.

4. Contraindications
  a. Allergy to latex or spermicide.
  b. Recurrent UTI.
  c. History of toxic shock syndrome.
  d. Introital or pelvic pain.
  e. Anatomic abnormalities.

5. Side effects - irritation, vaginal discharge, allergic reactions, pelvic discomfort and (rarely) toxic shock syndrome.

6. Patient instructions
  a. Apply 1 tablespoon of contraceptive cream or gel to the inner dome.
  b. Insert by pushing the rim downward and toward the back wall of the vagina. Check to be sure the diaphragm is covering the cervix.
  c. Leave in place at least 6 hours after intercourse. Wash with soap and water and let it dry. Avoid leaving in place > 24 hours.
  d. Do not use talcum or perfumed powder or any petroleum products on the diaphragm.
  e. Signs of toxic shock syndrome include fever of 100°F. or more, diarrhea and vomiting, muscle aches and rash.

E. Spermicides and contraceptive sponge

1. Failure rate - 18-28%

2. Types
  a. Foam
  b. Cream and gel - often used with a diaphragm.
  c. Suppositories and tablets - dissolve over a period of 10-30 minutes after placement in the vagina. Effective for 1 hour.
  d. Contraceptive sponge - acts as a barrier, traps sperm and kills them.

3. Side effects - irritation and allergic reaction.

4. Patient instructions
   a. Follow package instructions carefully.
   b. Insert before intercourse.
   c. No douching for at least 6 hours after intercourse.
   d. Sponges should not be worn > 24 hours.
   e. Review the danger signs of toxic shock syndrome.

F. Condoms
  1. Failure rate - 5 - 10%
  2. Types
    a. Most are latex.
    b. Lubricated or non-lubricated.
    c. Straight or tapered.
    d. With or without a reservoir tip.
  3. No major side effects. Provide the best protection against STDs.
  4. Patient instructions
    a. New condom must be used for every act of intercourse and placed on the penis before vaginal entry.
    b. After intercourse, the penis should be withdrawn soon and carefully, so as not to spill any semen.
    c. Store condoms in a cool, dry place.
    d. Don't use with petroleum jelly.

CHAPTER **17**

OPHTHALMOLOGY

I. THE EYE HISTORY AND EXAMINATION
A. History - check for:
1. Vision changes - blurred or decreased vision, duration, rate of onset, one or both eyes, severity.
2. Eye pain - foreign body (FB) sensation, irritation or burning, severity.
3. Discharge - quantity, appearance, duration.
4. Swelling - eyelids, face, facial trauma.
5. Use of contact lenses or glasses.
6. Previous eye disease, injury, or surgery.
7. Family history of eye disease.
8. Medical history, especially diabetes, hypertension, stroke, TB, HIV disease.
B. Eye exam
1. **Visual acuity (VA)**
2. **Pupil size and reaction**
3. **External appearance** - redness, discharge, swelling of eyelids, swelling of conjunctiva (chemosis), proptosis, ptosis.
4. **Fundi** - disc, macula, vessels, background.
5. **Other items** - as necessary:
   a. Alignment and motility.
   b. Confrontation visual fields.
   c. Upper eyelid eversion to look for FB.
   d. Slit lamp exam, or exam with magnifying lens
      (1) Fluorescein stain to check cornea for abrasions.
      (2) Look for corneal FB.
   e. Tonometry for intra-ocular pressure (IOP).

II. DIFFERENTIAL DIAGNOSIS OF THE RED EYE

	Acute Conjunctivitis	Acute Iritis	Acute Glaucoma (Angle Closure)	Corneal Trauma and/or Infection
Incidence	Extremely common	Uncommon	Uncommon	Common
Pain	None or slight	Moderate	Severe	Moderate to severe
Vision	Normal	Slightly blurred	Markedly blurred	Usually blurred
Pupil size	Normal	Small	Mid-dilated and fixed	Normal or small; irregular if corneal perforation
Pupil reaction	Normal	Decreased	Poor or none	Usually normal
External - conjunctival redness	Diffuse, redness mostly away from cornea, in fornices	Circum-corneal (Limbal flush)	Circum-corneal (Limbal flush)	Circum-corneal (Limbal flush)

	Acute Conjunctivitis	Acute Iritis	Acute Glaucoma (Angle Closure)	Corneal Trauma and/or Infection
External - discharge	**Viral:** watery **Bacterial:** pus	None	None	Watery or purulent
External - corneal appearance	Clear	Usually clear	Hazy	Change in clarity depends on cause
Intra-ocular pressure (IOP)	Normal	Normal	Very high	Normal
Treatment	**Viral:** observation, +/- warm compresses **Bacterial:** antibiotic drops or ointment qid x 4-5d	Steroid drops qid or more often Cyclopentolate 1% or Tropcamide 1% drops qid	Pilocarpine 2% drops qid to both eyes Refer to ophthalmologist, if possible, and as soon as possible.	If cornea not perforated, antibiotic drops 6-8 x per day If cornea is perforated, no drops or ointment. Protective shield, only. No pressure on eye. Refer to ophthalmologist if possible

Adapted with permission from: Vaughn D, Asbury T, Rieudanr-Eva P: General Ophthalmology, 1995

III. EYELID PROBLEMS
A. Hordeolum (stye)
1. **Cause** - infection (usually *Staph.*) of oil glands along edge of lid (Meibomian glands and glands of Zeis).
2. **Presentation** - red swelling along lid margin; a small localized abscess, mildly tender and painful.
   a. Internal hordeolum - abscess points on inner (conjunctival) side of lid.
   b. External hordeolum - abscess points along lid margin or on skin surface of lid.
3. **Treatment** - local heat (hot compresses) qid x 4-5d; careful surgical drainage (I&D) if pointing externally; oral antibiotics (e.g. tetracycline) if multiple and recurrent.
4. **Topical antibiotics** - useless.
B. Chalazion
1. **Cause** - lipogranuloma resulting from rupture of obstructed Meibomian gland; may follow a hordeolum as it resolves.
2. **Presentation** - initially similar or identical to a hordeolum. As the inflammation subsides there remains a round, non-tender and non-inflamed swelling near the lid margin.

3. Treatment - during inflammatory phase use local heat as above for hordeola. If <5mm usually resolves spontaneously over weeks to months.

4. Topical antibiotics - useless.

C. Blepharitis

  1. Cause - infection (usually *Staph.*) +/- seborrhea of lid margin.

  2. Presentation - redness of lid margin, +/- mild swelling, and +/- scales along lid margin or on eyelashes.

  3. Treatment - lid hygiene. Use warm compresses bid (AM and hs) + clean lid margins bid with dilute baby shampoo on cotton swab or fingertip + anti-dandruff shampoo for scalp prn. Often a life-long problem.

  4. Topical antibiotics - generally ineffective, but if inflammation is severe it may be worthwhile to add antibiotic eye ointment bid to the regimen.

D. Dacryocystitis

  1. Cause - obstruction of outlet of lacrimal sac into the nose, with resultant infection.

  2. Presentation

    a. Acute dacryocystitis - painful, tender, and red swelling of the lacrimal sac, occasionally with conjunctivitis, tearing, and discharge; most common in infancy. Gentle pressure on the sac may elicit purulent discharge from the lacrimal puncta.

    b. Chronic dacryocystitis, usually seen in adults, may present without inflammation.

  3. Treatment

    a. Infancy - systemic antibiotics mandatory (cloxacillin, amoxicillin/clavulanate, cefuroxime). Surgical drainage by an ophthalmologist may be helpful. After the infection clears, probing of the lacrimal duct may prevent recurrence.

    b. Adults - systemic antibiotics mandatory. (amoxicillin/clavulanate, if available). If very ill use cefazolin 1gm IV q8h. Investigate to find cause of obstruction (e.g. intra-nasal tumor). Surgery as appropriate to relieve obstruction.

  4. Topical antibiotics - generally add nothing to the regimen of systemic antibiotics.

E. Entropion and ectropion

  1. Causes

    a. Entropion (lid margin turns in) - usually caused by scarring. Trachoma is a very common cause in many developing countries.

    b. Ectropion (lid margins turns out) - may be caused by scarring (e.g. facial burns), or by muscle laxity in older people.

  2. Presentation

    a. Entropion - eye discomfort with foreign body sensation, conjunctival redness, tearing, and +/- corneal scarring.

b. Ectropion
   (1) Mild - eye discomfort and tearing.
   (2) Severe - inability to close eyes completely, with tearing, and corneal exposure +/- scarring.
3. Treatment depends on cause and severity of problem.
   a. Entropion - see trachoma below; surgery is usually required.
   b. Ectropion - plain antibiotic eye ointment at least qid prn for moisture. Surgery is usually required.

IV. CONJUNCTIVITIS
A. Viral conjunctivitis
1. **General** - more common in adults; often adenoviral. May occur in epidemics.
2. **Presentation** - vision normal, conjunctiva moderately red, scant watery discharge. Often bilateral but may be asymmetric.
3. **Pre-auricular lymph node** - usually present.
4. **Course** - self-limited but may last weeks. Highly contagious (e.g. by fomites), low morbidity.
5. **Treatment** - antibiotics and anti-viral agents are useless. Cool compresses prn for comfort. Patient must not share towel/wash cloth.
B. Ordinary bacterial conjunctivitis
1. **General** - more common in children.
2. **Presentation** - vision normal, conjunctiva markedly red, purulent exudate present. Often unilateral.
3. **Pre-auricular lymph node** - absent.
4. **Course** - self limited, lasts 1-2 weeks without treatment. Not very contagious, low morbidity.
5. **Treatment**
   a. Culture is unnecessary. Do Gram stain of palpebral conjunctival scraping if discharge is hyper-purulent and/or if GC is suspected.
   b. Treatment of ordinary (non-GC) bacterial conjunctivitis is with antibiotic eye drops or ointment (erythromycin, bacitracin, sulfacetamide, chloramphenicol, etc.) qid x 4-7 days.
   c. Warm compresses prn for comfort.
C. Adult gonococcal conjunctivitis
1. **General** - treat this as a potentially serious systemic disease.
2. **Presentation** - vision may be decreased because of very copious discharge or because cornea is directly infected. Usually unilateral; conjunctiva markedly red, hyper-purulent discharge, +/- conjunctival edema (chemosis). Cornea may perforate, leading to endophthalmitis and blindness. If seen in young children suspect abuse.
3. **Pre-auricular lymphadenopathy** - common, and may be prominent.
4. **Course** - may lead to blindness if untreated or inadequately treated. Patient may also have GC urethritis, pharyngitis, proctitis, septicemia. Look for other coincident STD's (*chlamydia*, HIV).

5. Treatment (see Chapter 1, VI, A)

    a. Consider hospitalization for systemic antibiotics

      (1) Ceftriaxone one gm IV/ IM followed by cefixime for 5 days.

      (2) Amoxicillin/clavulanic acid 3 gm as a stat dose orally followed by 500 mg tid for 7 days.

      (3) Ciprofloxacin 500 mg bid x 7-10d.

      (4) Continue IV treatment for at least 24 hrs after the patient is clinically improved, then complete 7-10 days of treatment with oral anti-gonococcal drug.

    b. Always treat for chlamydial co-infection.

    c. Investigate and treat sexual partners.

    d. Gentle saline irrigation prn to remove exudates. Gentamicin or penicillin ophthalmic drops q4-6h may be of some use.

D. Neonatal conjunctivitis

  1. General - still a possible cause of childhood blindness in developing countries. Etiologies include chemical (from silver nitrate used for prophylaxis), common bacteria (*Staph*), *Chlamydia, N. gonorrhoeae.*

  2. Presentation - highly variable, but often depends on causative agent.

    a. Chemical - scant watery discharge.

    b. Common bacteria - usually scant purulent discharge.

    c. *Chlamydia* - scant watery discharge, occurring 3-10 days after birth. May develop associated pneumonia.

    d. *N. gonorrhoeae* - starts 1-3 days after birth, may be hyperpurulent.

  3. Pre-auricular lymphadenopathy - absent.

  4. Course - depends on causative agent. *N. gonorrhoeae* can cause corneal perforation and blindness, as well as septicemia.

  5. Treatment

    a. Chemical - none.

    b. Common bacteria - as per ordinary bacterial conjunctivitis above.

    c. *Chlamydia* - erythromycin 50 mg/kg/day po x 14 days, or azithromycin 20 mg/kg/day x 3 days, plus tetracycline or erythromycin ointment qid x 14 days. Follow STD guidelines for mother and partners.

    d. *N. gonorrhoeae* - confirm with Gram stain, but if hyperpurulent treat as GC even without laboratory confirmation. Treat as a systemic disease with Aq. penicillin G 100,000U/kg/d IV in 4 divided doses x 7 d or ceftriaxone 25-50mg/kg/d IV x 7d. Gentle saline irrigation may be done prn to remove discharge. Some authors recommend gentamicin or penicillin ophthalmic drops. Treat mother and partners.

  6. To prevent neonatal conjunctivitis at birth, instill silver nitrate 1% drops, or erythromycin 0.5% ointment, tetracycline 1% ointment or povidone iodine 2-3% drops in both eyes.

E. Trachoma

  1. General

    a. Chronic conjunctivitis involving mostly the palpebral conjunctiva. It is the 2nd leading cause of blindness in the world.

    b. Children under age 10 years are a continually infected reservoir. Women are affected more than men, because they are the caregivers of infected children. Usually transmitted by flies.

    c. Environmental risk factors are as follows (5F's):

        (1) Flies

        (2) Filth (garbage attracts flies)

        (3) Feces (attracts flies)

        (4) Fingers

        (5) Fomites

2. Presentation - look at palpebral conjunctiva of upper lid. It appears red with many small follicles, later scarring with contraction and entropion. Trichiasis with corneal scars may occur.

3. Pre-auricular lymphadenopathy - none.

4. Course - chronic and repeated infections over years or decades.

5. Treatment - easiest regimen is tetracycline 1% ointment qid x 6 weeks. Azithromycin 1 g PO single dose (10 mg/kg for children <10 years) seems effective. Lid surgery required for entropion-trichiasis.

6. Prevention - break chronic re-infection cycle by improving sanitation and personal hygiene.

  F. Allergic conjunctivitis

    1. General - very common, often seasonal.

    2. Presentation - the two hallmarks are bilaterality and itching. There is mild redness, watery discharge.

    3. Pre-auricular lymphadenopathy - none.

    4. Course - recurrent as long as patient in contact with allergen. Usually low morbidity but if severe can cause corneal opacities.

    5. Treatment - separate patient from allergen. If mild, use cool compresses prn. If moderate, antihistamine drops (Vasocon A or Albalon-A) may help. If severe, prednisolone 1% drops qid x 14 days if cornea normal.

V. EYE TRAUMA

  A. Foreign body

    1. Conjunctival or corneal FB

      a. Treatment

        (1) Topical anesthetic drops to examine with magnification and good light. Try gentle irrigation with saline or lift off with sterile cotton swab moistened with antibiotic eye ointment.

        (2) If corneal and no luck with irrigation or swab, lift off with sterile needle held tangentially to corneal surface.

        (3) Instill antibiotic eye drops or ointment and patch the eye.

      b. Disposition - return next day for re-evaluation. Cornea should be back to normal.

2. Intra-ocular FB (or corneal/scleral laceration)
  a. Treatment
  (1) DO NOT instill any topical medications.
  (2) DO NOT apply any pressure to the eye.
  (3) DO NOT apply an eye patch.
  (4) Cover the eye with a protective shield.
  (5) Begin systemic antibiotics (ampicillin and gentamicin).
  (6) Administer tetanus toxoid prn.
  b. Disposition - consult ophthalmologist.
B. Hyphema (blood in the anterior chamber)
  1. Treatment
  a. Bed rest with head elevated x 5 days.
  b. Medications
  (1) Atropine 1% drops, 1 gtt bid x 5d.
  (2) Prednisolone 1% drops, 1 gtt qid x 5d.
  c. Observe for glaucoma (increased pain and redness); if present treat with acetazolamide (Diamox) 250 mg PO qid x 5d or more prn.
  d. Observe for repeat bleeding into the anterior chamber. If this occurs start the 5-day cycle again.
  2. Disposition - consult ophthalmologist if anterior chamber not obviously clearing after 5 days. (A clot may take a week or more to resolve, however).
C. Chemical injuries
  1. General
  a. Most dangerous are alkaline agents and dry cement powder which can cause blindness.
  b. Chemicals such as acids, soaps, glues, and petroleum products usually do not cause permanent damage.
  2. Treatment
  a. START IRRIGATION IMMEDIATELY with saline or water. Irrigate continuously for 30 minutes.
  b. Instill anesthetic drops if available; if not, irrigate without.
  c. Check pH if litmus paper is available. Stop irrigation when pH is neutral (7.4).
  d. Then, instill dilating drops, antibiotic drops or ointment. The eye may be patched for comfort.
  3. Disposition - consult ophthalmologist, if possible. Re-check in 24 hours.
D. Lid lacerations
  1. General - examine eyeball carefully to make sure there is no corneal or scleral laceration as well.
  2. Place 1ˢᵗ suture (e.g. 6-0 silk) at the lid margin, then suture the skin. Sutures do not need to be placed along the conjunctival surface.
  3. Administer tetanus toxoid prn.

VI. LEADING CAUSES OF BLINDNESS IN DEVELOPING COUNTRIES
A. Adults
1. Cataract
2. Trachoma
3. Glaucoma
B. Children
1. **Vitamin A deficiency (VAD)** - xerophthalmia (nutritional blindness)
   a. Almost exclusively in children under age 6 years, and especially under age 2 years.
   b. Develops in association with general malnutrition.
   c. Sudden keratomalacia (corneal melting) often precipitated by an acute febrile illness, e.g. measles.
2. **Measles keratitis**
   a. The measles virus may affect the cornea directly.
   b. The cornea may become secondarily infected by bacteria.
   c. Measles + VAD under age 2 years commonly leads to blindness.
3. **Traditional eye medications**, for example, ground up leaves, may be extremely caustic. They can cause severe corneal scarring or even destruction of the cornea. Use should be actively discouraged.

VII. OTHER EYE CONDITIONS REQUIRING URGENT ATTENTION
A. Bacterial orbital cellulitis
1. **General**
   a. Extremely serious infection of the orbit which may be complicated by cavernous sinus thrombosis and extension of the infection. May cause blindness or death.
   b. Occurs secondary to:
      (1) Sinusitis (by far the most common cause).
      (2) Spread of infection from adjacent structures, e.g. teeth.
      (3) Trauma to the orbit (penetrating injury, e.g. knife).
      (4) Post surgery of the eye, orbit, lacrimal duct.
2. **Pathogens**
   a. Most common pathogens are *S. aureus*, *Group A Streptococcus* and *Strep. pneumoniae*. S. aureus is the most common pathogen in adults. In children, where HiB vaccine is unavailable, *H. influenza* is an important pathogen.
   b. In the presence of trauma and/or crepitus, anaerobes including *Clostridia* should be considered.
   c. In diabetics - consider the possibility of gram negatives and invasive filamentous fungi (mucor, rhizopus).
3. **Presentation**
   a. Abrupt onset of orbital pain and headache, with fever and malaise.
   b. Leukocytosis with left shift may be present.
   c. Hallmark features are proptosis, decreased ocular motility, +/- decreased vision, +/-chemosis (edema of the conjunctiva).

    d. High morbidity or even fatality if untreated. Infection can spread to adjacent structures (eyeball, meninges, cavernous sinus, brain).

  4. Treatment - admit for aggressive high-dose parenteral antibiotic therapy.

    a. Where third generation cephalosporins are available, ceftriaxone 100 mg/kg/day (children) or 1 gram q12h (adults) can be used.

    b. Children <age 13 years - cefuroxime 150 mg/kg/day IV in 3 divided doses or ampicillin 200 mg/kg/day IV in 4 divided doses PLUS chloramphenicol 100 mg/kg/day PO in 4 divided doses.

    c. Adults - cefuroxime 1.5 g q8h or cefazolin 2 g q8h or cloxacillin 1 g IV q6h PLUS chloramphenicol 1 g PO q6h.

    d. Add metronidazole 7.5 mg/kg IV q6h or chloramphenicol for post traumatic cases or if crepitus is present.

    e. Observe closely for development of orbital abscess (increasing proptosis, continued high fever) which must be drained.

B. Proptosis (exophthalmos)

  1. Causes

    a. Bacterial orbital cellulitis - see above.

    b. Fungal orbital cellulitis - more indolent course than bacterial disease, but commonly fatal. Family *Mucoaceae* affects diabetics in ketoacidosis; *Aspergillus* affects otherwise healthy individuals. Treatment is with IV amphotericin B and aggressive surgical debridement.

    c. Orbital tumors - hemangioma, lacrimal gland tumors, lymphangioma, metastatic disease.

    d. Carotid-cavernous fistula - post blunt trauma or spontaneous.

    e. Leukemia with granulocytic sarcoma - especially in children.

    f. Burkitt's lymphoma - especially in tropics.

  2. Treatment - according to cause.

C. Herpes simplex ocular infection

  1. Blepharoconjunctivitis

    a. Red eye and lids with typical fever blisters; usually benign and self-limited.

    b. Treatment with observation or topical antiviral agent as below.

  2. Keratoconjunctivitis

    a. Red eye with decreased vision; fluorescein staining often shows dendritic (branching) lesion of cornea.

    b. Treatment with one of the following:

      (1) Acycloguanosine 3% ointment (Zovirax, acyclovir) 5x/day x 10-14 days.

      (2) Trifluridine 1% drops q 2h during waking day.

      (3) Iododeoxyuridine (IDU) 1% drops.

      (4) Adenine arabinoside (Vidaribine) 3% ointment., 0.1% drops.

D. Herpes zoster ophthalmicus (HZO)

1. Affects dermatome of cranial nerve 5, ophthalmic division. 50% of cases have ocular (eyeball) lesions, such as:
   a. Conjunctivitis - common
   b. Scleritis/episcleritis
   c. Keratitis (corneal involvement)
   d. Iritis
   e. Glaucoma
   f. Choroiditis
   g. Retinitis
   h. Optic neuritis
   i. Cranial nerve palsy
2. **Suspect immunodeficiency**, especially AIDS.
3. **Systemic treatment**
   a. Skin rash for <72 hours (one of the following):
      (1) Acyclovir 800 mg PO 5x/day x 7 d.
      (2) Famciclovir 500 mg tid x 7 d.
      (3) Valacyclovir 1 g PO tid x 7 d.
   b. Skin rash for >72 hours, and children
      (1) Warm compresses to skin lesions tid.
      (2) Antibiotic ointment to skin lesions tid.
   c. Pain medications if/as needed.
4. **Ocular treatment**
   a. Usually none required.
   b. If keratitis, uveitis, retinitis, optic neuritis, cranial nerve palsy, consult ophthalmologist or appropriate text.

E. **Non-healing corneal ulcer or impending perforation**
1. Microbial keratitis (MK) - infected corneal ulcer. All are very difficult to treat; most respond very poorly to topical medications.
   a. Bacterial corneal lesions heal very slowly and poorly, may progress to perforation and loss of the eye.
   b. Fungal lesions - common in developing countries. These do even worse, very commonly progress to perforation.
   c. Viral lesions may progress to scar but seldom perforate.
2. Perforation of cornea may also occur with vitamin A deficiency.
3. Surgical treatment where corneal transplant is not an option - conjunctival covering graft (Gunderson flap). Simple to perform - consult ophthalmologist or see appropriate text.

F. **Vitamin A deficiency and nutritional blindness**
1. **Xerophthalmia** - the ocular manifestations of vitamin A deficiency.
2. **General**
   a. Leading cause of childhood blindness in developing countries.
   b. Almost always affects children under age 6 years, and especially under age 2 years.

c. Occurs in context of generalized protein-energy malnutrition (PEM) plus a sudden febrile or systemic challenge, (e.g. diarrheal disease, and especially measles).

3. Presentation (not necessarily in this order):
   a. XN = night blindness.
   b. X1A = conjunctival dryness (xerosis) with Bitot spot(s).
   c. X2 = corneal dryness.
   d. X3A = corneal ulceration.
   e. X3B = keratomalacia (sudden melting of the cornea with perforation).

4. Treatment
   a. Children under age 6 years with xerophthalmia or corneal ulcers

Oral Vitamin A Dosing (IU)		
Day	Dose Age 1 Year & Older	Dose < Age 1 Year
1	200,000	100,000
2	200,000	100,000
7-28	200,000	100,000

   b. Children with measles, frequent diarrhea, frequent pulmonary infections, or severe malnutrition - PO vitamin A 200,000 IU age 1 year and older, 100,000 IU < age 1 year.

5. Prevention - children under age 6 years

Supplemental Vitamin A		
Group	PO Vitamin A (IU)	Frequency
Children < age 1 year	100,000	Q 4-6 months
Children age 1 year & >	200,000	Q 4-6 months
Mothers just post delivery	300,000	Once only
Pregnant women	10,000	QD x 2 weeks

   a. Encourage improved nutrition
      (1) Foods rich in vitamin A - liver, eggs, fish, milk, meat.
      (2) Foods rich in vitamin A precursors - red palm oil, carrots, spinach, sweet potatoes, mangoes, tomatoes, green beans.

CHAPTER 18

ENT

I. EAR

A. Otitis externa (swimmer's ear)

1. Clinical

a. Characterized by inflammation of the skin lining the external auditory canal, often secondary to trauma and/or infection.

b. Symptoms - pain when pulling on the tragus or pinna, itching and/or discharge.

c. Signs - edematous, erythematous external auditory canal with discharge.

2. Treatment

a. The most important thing is to gently clean the external ear canal by using cotton, suction or hydrogen peroxide irrigation.

b. The ear must be kept dry. Swimming should be avoided and care must be taken when bathing to keep water out of the ear.

c. The ear may be irrigated and cleansed with a mixture of alcohol 70-95% + acetic acid (1/3 vinegar, 2/3 alcohol) q 4 hr x 2-3 days.

d. Antibiotic + hydrocortisone otic drops (neomycin/polymyxin, aminoglycoside or ciprofloxacin) 3-4 drops bid or tid should be given for 7-10 days. A small wick of rolled up cotton may be inserted into the ear canal to facilitate entry of the medication. It should be changed or removed in 2-3 days.

e. If the TM cannot be seen or otitis media cannot be ruled out, oral antibiotics should be given as well (treat as for OME below).

3. Malignant otitis externa

a. Uncommon, but severe necrotizing external ear infection which may occur in diabetics and immunocompromised patients.

b. It is caused by *Pseudomonas* and can be fatal if untreated. May cause facial nerve paralysis.

c. Most patients should be treated in the hospital with IV antibiotics which cover *Pseudomonas*. Debridement of necrotic soft tissue may be necessary as well.

4. Fungal otitis externa

a. Should be suspected when "cotton fibers" with or without small black spores are visualized in the ear canal. Especially common in tropical, humid climates.

b. Treat with careful, thorough cleaning using cotton swabs, and then use clotrimazole 1% solution, nystatin, acetic acid or gentian violet (2% in 95% alcohol) 3-4 times a day for 1-2 weeks. Placement of a wick will help distribution of the medication.

B. Otitis media with effusion (OME)

1. Acute OME (purulent effusion)

a. General

(1) Characterized by inflammation of the middle ear.
(2) The most common bacterial infection in children, frequently recurrent.
(3) Most common in the first 3 years of life, but can occur at any age, including adults.
(4) Complications include TM perforation, acute mastoiditis, facial nerve paralysis, CNS infections. According to WHO, otitis media is the leading preventable cause of deafness in developing countries.
(5) Etiology - *S. pneumoniae, H. influenza, M. catarrhalis* and viral infections.

b. Clinical
(1) Symptoms -may include ear pain or pulling at the ear. Young infants may present with nonspecific symptoms such as fever, irritability, poor feeding and diarrhea. May be asymptomatic. Associated upper respiratory infection or allergic rhinitis is common in children.
(2) Signs - red, bulging TM with obscured landmarks. Purulent drainage suggests perforation.

c. Management
(1) Neonate (0-4 weeks) - full sepsis evaluation and admission for parenteral antibiotics is indicated due to high risk of associated sepsis or meningitis.
(2) >6 weeks of age
  (a) The question of whether to treat acute otitis media with antibiotics or not is a controversial issue in pediatrics at the present time, and local standards of care should be followed, if known. In 80% of uncomplicated patients, the infection resolves in a few days without antibiotic treatment. Complications are rare, but do occur, and might be prevented by giving antibiotics.
  (b) In general, it is reasonable to treat those patients who are systemically ill, have drainage from the ear, or those in whom follow-up is difficult. First line treatment is usually with amoxicillin 45-80mg/kg/d divided bid or tid x 5-10days. TMP/SMX 0.5cc/kg bid for 5-10days is also effective.
  (c) Resistant cases can be treated with amoxicillin/clavulanate (same dose as amoxicillin), clarithromycin 8mg/kg/dose bid x 10 days or azithromycin 10mg/kg x 1 dose, then 5mg/kg/d x 4 days.
  (d) Paracetamol (acetaminophen) or ibuprofen may be given for pain or fever. Auralgan (antipyrine, benzocaine, glycerin) is a topical anesthetic which may help with pain. Do not use if the TM is perforated or if there is discharge in the ear canal. Antihistamines and decongestants are usually not effective.

(e) If possible, recheck ears in 2-3 weeks. If effusion is present, but asymptomatic, recheck in 1-2 months.

2. Acute OME (serous effusion)

a. General

(1) Middle ear effusion results from eustachian tube obstruction. May be associated with a recent URI or with chronic eustachian tube dysfunction.

(2) Need to rule out allergic rhinitis, nasopharyngeal masses and sinusitis.

b. Clinical

(1) Signs - decreased hearing, +/ - pain.

(2) Symptoms - TM dull and immobile, +/- air bubbles, conductive hearing loss, Rinne negative.

c. Management

(1) Have patient "pop" ears by blowing hard against closed nose.

(2) Pseudoephedrine 60 mg. po qid.

(3) Myringotomy if symptoms persist more than 2 -4 weeks (and nasopharynx has been checked and is clear).

3. Chronic OME (serous or mucoid effusion)

a. General

(1) Common cause of delayed speech development in young children.

(2) May be due to partially treated acute OME. May be found in follow-up of a patient who has been treated for acute otitis media or as an incidental finding in an asymptomatic patient.

(3) Frequently seen in children with cleft palate.

b. Clinical

(1) Symptoms - decreased hearing, delayed speech.

(2) Signs - retracted, dull immobile, amber colored TM, conductive hearing loss, Rinne negative.

c. Management

(1) If the child is under 4 years of age, a trial of amoxicillin or TMP/SMX should be given for one month.

(2) If effusion persists for at least 3 months, the child will require myringotomy, preferably with a ventilation tube. This may improve hearing and prevent a delay in language development.

(3) Antihistamines, decongestants and steroids have no proven benefit.

C. Chronic suppurative otitis media

1. General

a. This is the most common cause of chronic draining ears. Hearing loss may be present.

b. Always associated with a TM perforation.

(1) Central perforations - involve the pars tensa, usually safe and will respond to local therapy.

      (2) Marginal perforations - perforation is in pars flaccida or at the edge of pars tensa, may be associated with a cholesteatoma (white epithelial debris in perforation or middle ear) and may not respond to local therapy.

      (3) Active - purulent discharge present.

      (4) Inactive - TM perforation present, but clean, dry and middle ear mucosa normal.

    c. Complications - hearing loss, vertigo, CNS infections.

    d. Etiology - *Pseudomonas, Proteus* and *Staph.* are the most common.

2. Clinical

    a. Symptoms - chronic foul smelling drainage, hearing loss, rarely vertigo.

    b. Signs - TM perforation, mucopurulent, foul smelling discharge, +/- granulation tissue, +/- whitish epithelial debris in middle ear or perforation, retracted TM.

3. Management

    a. Clean external canal with suction, by "dry mopping" using fluffy cotton twisted on a stick or irrigation with saline.

    b. Antibiotic otic or ophthalmic drops 3-4 drops bid. Would preferably use non-ototoxic drops such as the fluoroquinolones or chloramphenicol, but aminoglycosides have been used for decades without clinical proof of significant hearing loss. One can make ear drops by dissolving a 250 mg ciprofloxacin tablet in 25-50 cc of water. One can also use gentamicin or tobramycin ophthalmic drops.

    c. Patients must avoid contaminating ears with dirty water from washing hair or swimming.

    d. If there is profuse drainage, patient may need to wash ear with saline bid before using eardrops. They can make saline by using ½ teaspoon of salt in 1 cup of boiled water. Use a 10 cc syringe or small bulb syringe to irrigate the ear canal.

    e. Oral antibiotics are seldom needed.

4. Follow-up

    a. If ear dries up, patient must avoid contamination and retreat if drainage recurs. If available, refer for tympanoplasty.

    b. If drainage persists for six to eight weeks despite compliance and good therapy, patient has a high chance of having a cholesteatoma. This will require surgical therapy, probably a mastoidectomy. Patients with no treatment are at risk for mastoiditis and CNS complications.

D. Sudden sensorineural hearing loss

  1. Clinical - sudden onset of moderate to profound sensorineural hearing loss, usually unilateral. Seldom accompanied by vertigo. Usually felt to be viral etiology.

  2. Management - approximately 50% will recover with or without therapy. A 10 -14 day tapering course of prednisone may help some cases if

started in the first week. Vasodilators, diuretics, vitamins, ginseng etc. are of no proven value.
  E. Vertigo (see Chapter 10, IV, A, 2)

II. NOSE
A. Allergic rhinitis
  1. General - perennial allergic rhinitis is common in tropical countries. The most common causes are dust mites, mold and grasses. In temperate climates seasonal allergic rhinitis is more common.
  2. Symptoms - nasal obstruction, watery discharge, sneezing, nasal or pharyngeal itching and watery, red, itchy eyes.
  3. Signs - swollen pale bluish turbinates and discharge, which is usually clear.
  4. Management
    a. First generation antihistamines such as chlorpheniramine are cheap, but are sedating. Second generation antihistamines such as loratadine are more effective with less side effects. They are more expensive, but generics will soon be available.
    b. Nasal steroid sprays such as beclomethasone or fluticasone are very good, but expensive.
    c. Avoid triggers if known, as well as irritants such as smoke and dust.
B. Non-allergic rhinitis (vasomotor rhinitis)
  1. General - symptoms are similar to allergic rhinitis, but the etiology is unclear. Less responsive to therapy.
  2. Symptoms - mainly nasal obstruction and +/- nasal discharge. Nasal discharge in infants can cause nasal obstruction and interfere with breast-feeding and cause difficult breathing. The discharge may become thick, yellow and purulent in appearance. Unilateral purulent nasal discharge with odor in a child suggests foreign body.
  3. Signs - swollen pale turbinates with a cobblestone appearance to the mucosa.
  4. Management
    a. Adults - trial of nasal steroids and/or decongestants with or without antihistamines.
    b. Children - antihistamines and decongestants are not effective in young children. Parents should be advised to clear the nose if the discharge interferes with feeding in infants. Mucus may be moistened with saline nose drops, making suctioning more effective. Medicated nose drops should not be used.
    c. Supportive care includes good hydration and paracetamol (acetaminophen) for comfort.
C. Nasal polyps
  1. General - nasal polyps are associated with allergic rhinitis, asthma and/or sinus infections.

2. **Symptoms** - nasal obstruction and loss of smell.
3. **Signs** - pale yellowish grape-like masses coming from the middle meatus.
4. **Management**
   a. Trial of nasal steroid sprays, and 2-3 week tapering course of prednisone.
   b. Surgical removal if medical therapy fails.

D. **Acute sinusitis**
   1. **General** - sinusitis is inflammation of one or more paranasal sinuses. May occur as a sequela to a URI. With unilateral maxillary sinusitis one needs to consider a dental infection as etiology. Bacterial sinusitis is uncommon in younger children.
   2. **Symptoms** - purulent nasal drainage, pain over involved sinus, referred pain to teeth, eye or occiput, low grade fever. Cough may result from post-nasal drainage. Suspect in patient with symptoms of rhinitis which persist >10 days.
   3. **Signs** - erythema and swelling of turbinates, purulent, sometimes blood-tinged nasal discharge from middle meatus. May be tender to palpation over sinuses.
   4. **Management**
      a. Antibiotics for 2 weeks (first episode), 3 weeks if recurrent (amoxicillin, TMP/SMX, amoxicillin/clavulanate, cephalexin or clindamycin).
      b. Topical decongestant - ephedrine, phenylephrine or oxymetazoline (Afrin) nasal spray bid for a maximum of 5-7 days.
      c. Oral decongestant - pseudoephedrine (Sudafed) 60 mg tid in adults. Not recommended in children.
   5. **Complications**
      a. Serous otitis media.
      b. Periorbital cellulitis or abscess - swelling of periorbital area, proptosis and eye pain.
      c. CNS infections - meningitis, epidural, subdural or brain abscesses.
      d. Cavernous sinus thrombosis - absolute emergency. Patients will present with bilateral proptosis, chemosis, globe fixation and rapid loss of vision with pain and a severe headache. Patient will need IV antibiotics and heparin as well as treatment for the sinusitis. Bilateral eye findings and rapid progression of symptoms are what distinguish this from a periorbital abscess or cellulitis.

E. **Chronic sinusitis**
   1. **General** -sequela of acute sinusitis, or sinus ostium obstruction from polyps, allergies, etc.
   2. **Symptoms** - purulent nasal discharge, vague sinus pains, fatigue, bad breath and +/- nasal obstruction.
   3. **Signs** - purulent nasal discharge from the middle meatus or on the posterior pharyngeal wall, +/- swelling and erythema of the turbinates.

4. Management

a. Antibiotics - same as for acute sinusitis, but may need to treat for anaerobes adding metronidazole or using clindamycin and treating for 3-6 weeks.

b. Sinus irrigations.

c. In patients who fail 2-3 months of aggressive medical therapy, surgically opening the sinuses to facilitate drainage and restore ciliary function is indicated.

F. Epistaxis

1. General - 90% of epistaxis is minor and from the anterior septum. Less than 10% are from the lateral posterior or the superior part of the nose. Bleeding from these locations can be severe or even life threatening. Consider contributing factors such as coagulopathies, hypertension, uremia, trauma etc.

2. Symptoms - may vary from recurrent small amounts of bleeding to profuse large amounts in a short period of time. Usually they are unilateral.

3. Signs - look for the bleeding site. Decongest and anesthetize the nose with a spray or cotton soaked with ephedrine, phenylephrine or oxymetazoline combined with 4% Xylocaine (lignocaine). Will need a light source and suction.

4. Management

a. Septal - instruct patient on how to pinch nose and septum for five minutes. If bleeding site is visualized (usually a prominent vessel or an area of erosion which bleeds when touched) cauterize with silver nitrate stick/liquid or electrocautery.

b. Posterior bleed - place anterior nasal pack using strip gauze soaked in vaseline or antibiotic ointment. Layer in nose, packing tightly from posterior to anterior. If there is still bleeding use a posterior nasal pack. This can be done with a Foley catheter passed through the nose, fill bag with 5 cc of saline and pull tightly into posterior choana. Pull snugly as the anterior pack is being replaced and packed tightly against the Foley. If all else fails one can ligate the ipsilateral external carotid artery.

III. THROAT

A. Acute pharyngitis

1. Etiology

a. Most sore throats are due to viruses.

b. Antibiotics are indicated to treat suppurative complications of streptococcal pharyngitis (cervical adenitis, retropharyngeal and peritonsillar abscess) and to prevent acute rheumatic fever.

c. Streptococcal pharyngitis is uncommon in children under 2-3 years of age and rheumatic fever is rare in this age group. May occur in adults.

2. Diagnosis

    a. Clinical signs of streptococcal pharyngitis include tender, enlarged cervical lymph nodes, white pharyngeal exudate, and absence of rhinorrhea, conjunctivitis, and cough.

    b. Although clinical diagnosis is unreliable, rapid antigen tests and cultures are not readily available in developing countries. Most national rheumatic fever programs base treatment of suspected streptococcal pharyngitis on clinical signs.

3. Treatment

    a. Benzathine penicillin 600,000 units IM (< 20kg), 1.2 million units IM (> 20kg) as one dose.

    b. Pen VK 125mg po tid (< 20kg), 250mg po tid or 500mg po bid (> 20kg) x 10 days.

    c. Erythromycin is an alternative for penicillin-allergic patients. Cephalexin or cefuroxime can be used, if available. Sulfonamides are ineffective.

    d. Supportive treatment with warm salt water gargles, throat lozenges, and paracetamol (acetaminophen) for fever.

4. Suppurative complications

    a. Cervical adenitis - large, tender lymph nodes in the neck which persist after the sore throat has resolved. Anti-staphylococcal antibiotics may be necessary. Failure to respond to a normal 10 day course of antibiotics may indicate non-bacterial cause of node enlargement (such as tuberculosis) or need for surgical drainage.

    b. Peritonsillar abscess - see below.

    c. Retropharyngeal abscess - see below.

5. Differential diagnosis - includes acute infectious mononucleosis, which may also present with sore throat and fever. Fatigue is usually present as well. Examination may show exudative pharyngitis, lymphadenopathy, and hepatosplenomegaly. WBC may be low normal, with monocytes and abnormal lymphocytes.

B. Peritonsillar abscess

1. Symptoms - severe unilateral sore throat, +/- trismus, fever, history of recent sore throat.

2. Signs - unilateral tonsillar swelling with the tonsil being pushed towards the midline and with uvular deviation.

3. Management

    a. Use topical anesthesia and 20 gauge needle with 10cc syringe to aspirate superior and lateral to the tonsil. If pus is aspirated, perform I&D.

    b. Hospitalize and treat IV with the same antibiotics used for strep pharyngitis.

C. Chronic pharyngitis

1. Symptoms - dry scratchy throat with mild pain, heartburn, postnasal drip.

2. **Signs** - pharyngeal mucosa may appear dry and mildly erythematous. There may be some hypertrophied studding of lymphoid tissue on the posterior pharyngeal wall and one may note some exudate stuck to the mucosa.

3. **Etiology** - smoking, alcohol, inadequate water intake, voice abuse, gastroesophageal reflux disease (GERD), chronic postnasal drip from chronic sinusitis.

4. **Management**
   a. First, rule out serious disease such as a malignancy.
   b. Increase water intake.
   c. Recommend voice rest.
   d. Treat GERD with H-2 blockers or proton pump inhibitors.
   e. Treat sinusitis.

D. **Foreign bodies**

1. **Symptoms** - localized pain in the throat or lower neck area, odynophagia, history of swallowing a foreign body such as a fish bone or some other food product.

2. **Signs** - patient will localize the pain to a small area, pain on rocking the larynx, visualization of foreign body.

3. **Management**
   a. Careful examination of the oropharynx and hypopharynx, looking especially at the tonsil, base of tongue, vallecula and pyriform sinuses.
   b. If nothing is visualized a soft tissue lateral x-ray of the neck or barium swallow may be helpful.
   c. If nothing is found, the patient may be followed carefully (daily) for 2-3 days. If still symptomatic, direct laryngoscopy and esophagoscopy will be needed. An alternative is to do a CT scan of the neck, if available.

IV. NECK MASSES

A. **Deep neck abscess** - submandibular, parapharyngeal or retropharyngeal

1. **Symptoms** - fever, neck pain and swelling, +/- torticollis and/or trismus, history of sore throat or dental infections.

2. **Signs** - localized neck swelling, +/- skin erythema. The mass is seldom fluctuant.

3. **Management**
   a. Needle aspiration for pus. CT or neck x-ray may be helpful if available.
   b. I&D over maximum point of swelling, place Penrose drain.
   c. IV antibiotics to cover *Staph, Strep* and anaerobic bacteria (high dose penicillin, clindamycin, cephalosporins, metronidazole).

B. **Cervical tuberculosis**

1. **Symptoms** - slowly enlarging mass, sometimes with a draining fistula. Usually no fever. History of drinking unpasteurized milk or TB exposure.

2. **Signs** - mass may be firm to soft with minimal erythema. Multiple lymph nodes present.
3. **Management**
   a. Tuberculin skin test unless patient had BCG as a child.
   b. Chest x-ray, needle aspiration for AFB smear and culture or excision biopsy of mass will help make the diagnosis.
   c. Treat with anti-tuberculosis therapy.
4. **Differential diagnosis** - atypical mycobacterium is usually in young children and will present with a soft bluish-red mass over the parotid or submaxillary area. Diagnosis may be difficult to make, but treatment is surgical excision of mass. Sometimes just I&D, with curettage of the center will be adequate. Treating with oral anti-tuberculosis drugs is controversial and most people would not recommend this.

C. **HIV**
1. **Symptoms** - history of HIV with gradual soft enlargement of parotid glands.
2. **Signs** - generalized enlargement of parotid glands, without erythema or pain.
3. **Management** - observation. Surgical excision and/or biopsy are not necessary.

D. **Congenital**
1. **Thyroglossal duct cyst**
   a. Midline neck mass between hyoid bone and thyroid isthmus. Will move with swallowing and sticking out the tongue. May present as a midline neck abscess.
   b. Treatment is surgical excision using the Sistrunk procedure, which involves removing the mass in continuity with the center of the hyoid and a 1cm cuff of soft tissue to the base of the tongue.
2. **Branchial cleft cyst and/or fistula**
   a. Lateral neck mass or fistula along the anterior border of the sternocleidomastoid muscle between the ear lobule and clavicle.
   b. Management is surgical excision.

E. **Tumors**
1. **Benign**
   a. Masses of the thyroid, parotid, submaxillary gland, neuromas or carotid body tumor will present as firm palpable lesions.
   b. Management is excision.
2. **Lymphoma**
   a. Usually presents with multiple neck nodes, may be bilateral and may have an intraoral lesion, such as an enlarged tonsil or adenoid hypertrophy.
   b. Management is a lymph node biopsy and then appropriate chemotherapy.
3. **Malignant** (usually squamous cell carcinoma)

a. These patients will present with one or more "rock" hard lymph nodes in the cervical chain. Depending on the level, one may have a clue as to the primary site.

   (1) Nodes in the submaxillary triangle are usually from the lip or oral cavity.

   (2) Nodes in the upper cervical region are usually from the base of the tongue, tonsil, nasopharynx, pharyngeal walls, larynx or pyriform sinus.

   (3) Nodes in the mid-cervical chain are usually from the larynx, pyriform sinus, tongue or thyroid.

   (4) Nodes in the lower cervical chain (supra-clavicular) especially on the left side could be from the lung or GI tract.

b. Management

   (1) First try to find the primary site by examination and upper airway endoscopy.

   (2) Fine needle aspirate for cytology, if available, is very helpful.

   (3) Management consists of surgery and/or radiation therapy depending on the primary site and size of tumor.

CHAPTER 19

UROLOGY

I. URINARY TRACT INFECTIONS (see Chapter 14, section VII, A)
  A. Lower UTI in females
    1. Clinical
      a. Symptoms generally include dysuria, frequency, urgency, hesitancy and suprapubic pain. Fever is uncommon.
      b. The physical examination is usually unremarkable except for mild suprapubic tenderness. Physical examination should include a pelvic exam if the patient is at risk of STD's to evaluate for PID, cervicitis or vaginitis, which can give similar symptoms.
      c. Urinalysis (clean catch midstream or catheterized specimen) shows pyuria (>5 WBC's per high power field) and bacteriuria. Hematuria may also be present. On dipstick, the leukocyte esterase is usually positive.
      d. Leukocytosis is not usually present in UTIs confined to the lower tract.
    2. Uncomplicated cystitis may be treated with the following regimens:

Drug	Single Dose Treatment	Three Day and Standard Treatment Dosage
Amoxicillin	Not recommended	500mg q 8h or 875mg q12h
Amoxicillin-clavulanate	500mg	500mg q 8h or 875mg q12h
Cephalexin	2gm	500mg q 8h
Ciprofloxacin	250-500mg	250-500mg q 12h
Doxycycline	Not recommended	100mg q 12h
Nitrofurantoin	200mg	100mg q 12h
Norfloxacin	400mg	400mg q 12h
Sulfisoxazole	Not recommended	500mg - 1gm q 6h
Tetracycline	Not recommended	500mg q 6h
TMP/SMX	DS tablet	1 DS tab bid
Trimethoprim	400mg	100mg q 12h

      a. Single-dose therapy has a cure rate of 60-100%. It should only be used early in the course of infection. Avoid antibiotics with unacceptable resistance rates such as amoxicillin, tetracycline.
      b. Three-day course has a higher cure rate, and is the preferred treatment for uncomplicated cystitis in females. Be aware of local resistance patterns.
      c. Standard course with 7-10 days of therapy is preferred for complicated cystitis, recurrent disease, and previous treatment failures. Diabetics and pregnant women should be treated for 7 days. Dosage is the same as for the three day regimen.

    d. Lack of response to antibiotics suggests resistance. A culture should be done, if possible. If UTI recurs after treatment, upper tract infection may be present. Urine culture should be done, if possible, and treatment given for 2 weeks. Patients with persistent pyuria despite treatment, who are sexually active, should be treated for *Chlamydia* infection with a tetracycline. Those with pyuria but no bacteriuria should be evaluated for renal TB, with AFB smears of the urine.

3. Recurrent UTI

    a. Patients with frequent reinfection (>3/year) may be treated with prophylactic antibiotics after a standard treatment course is given.

    b. The following medications may be used: nitrofurantoin 50mg qd, trimethoprim 100mg qd, TMP/SMX 1 tab 3x/week or after coitus.

    c. Treat for 6 months. If reinfection occurs within 3 months after stopping therapy, give prophylaxis for 1-2 years.

    d. Recommend post-coital voiding.

4. UTI in pregnancy

    a. Many patients with bacteriuria early in pregnancy develop acute symptomatic pyelonephritis in later pregnancy. They are also prone to have low birth-weight infants.

    b. Treat all patients with significant bacteriuria (even if asymptomatic) and try to maintain sterile urine throughout pregnancy. Screening for asymptomatic bacteriuria is recommended during pregnancy and should be done at all pre-natal visits, if possible.

    c. Antibiotics which may be given safely in pregnancy include TMP/SMX (avoid in the last few weeks of pregnancy), ampicillin or amoxicillin, nitrofurantoin, cephalexin. Treat for 7-10 days and follow for recurrence.

5. Sterile pyuria

    a. Sterile pyuria is defined as the presence of >20 WBC per high power field in the absence of bacteriuria.

    b. Infectious organisms that may cause sterile pyuria, but are not recovered in routine culture include tuberculosis, *Chlamydia trachomatis, Neisseria gonorrheae*, Herpes simplex virus.

    c. Non-infectious causes include glomerulonephritis, acute and chronic interstitial nephritis, and nephrolithiasis.

B. Lower UTI in males

1. Clinical

    a. Symptoms are similar to those in females and include dysuria, frequency, hesitancy and dribbling. A careful sexual history is important. Ask specifically about the presence of a urethral discharge.

    b. Young males should be examined for urethritis, prostatitis and structural abnormalities. Elderly men need to be evaluated for bladder dysfunction, outflow obstruction and prostatitis.

    c. Divided urine collection may help localize infection in the male. The first voided 10cc is urethral, midstream is from the bladder and first 10cc voided after prostate massage (EPS) is prostatic.

  2. Acute cystitis

    a. Cystitis is uncommon in males. If recurrent, obtain an ultrasound or IVP and cystoscopy to evaluate.

    b. Treatment includes TMP/SMX, nitrofurantoin, amoxicillin/clavulanate or ciprofloxacin for 7-10 days.

  3. Acute urethritis - (see Chapter 1, VI)

C. Acute pyelonephritis

  1. Definition - acute infection of the upper urinary tract, often associated with bacteremia.

  2. Symptoms - flank or back pain, fever, chills, voiding symptoms, headache, nausea, vomiting and, occasionally, diarrhea. Pyelonephritis mimics many other illnesses and diagnosis is frequently incorrect.

  3. Signs - percussion tenderness of the affected kidney, leukocytosis with left shift, U/A with pyuria, WBC casts, bacteriuria.

  4. Management

    a. With mild symptoms, use oral agents (TMP/SMX, cephalexin, amoxicillin/clavulanate, ciprofloxacin, other newer quinolones) and treat as an outpatient for 2 weeks.

    b. If toxic, with high fever, chills, or hypotension, the patient needs hospitalization and parenteral therapy. May use ampicillin or cefazolin plus gentamicin. Treat with IV antibiotics until afebrile 1-2 days, then complete a 2 week course with oral antibiotics. Many other regimens also are effective for acute pyelonephritis.

    c. If fever persists after 3 days, look for obstruction or abscess (IVP or U/S).

II. PROSTATE DYSFUNCTION

  A. Prostatitis

  1. Acute bacterial prostatitis

    a. Symptoms - perineal, sacral or suprapubic pain, fever, and irritative voiding symptoms. Urinary retention, fever and chills may also be present.

    b. Physical exam - boggy, tender prostate on rectal exam. Do not perform prostatic massage in suspected acute prostatitis as this may induce bacteremia.

    c. Labs - pyuria, positive urine cultures. Blood cultures may be positive. Gram stain of urine will demonstrate the organism except where *Chlamydia* is the cause.

    d. Pathogens - *Neisseria gonorrheae, Chlamydia* in young, sexually active men <35 years. Gram negative bacilli (*E. coli, Klebsiella, Pseudomonas*) in older men.

    e. Management
      (1) Avoid urethral catheterization. For acute urinary retention place a suprapubic drainage tube.
      (2) If the patient looks septic, hospitalize for IV antibiotics (ampicillin + gentamicin). After afebrile for 24-48h, give oral antibiotics for 4-6 weeks (TMP/SMX or quinolones).
      (3) If not toxic, treat as an outpatient with TMP/SMX or a quinolone for a minimum of 4-6 weeks.
      (4) Young men should be treated for *N. gonorrheae* (aqueous penicillin G or ceftriaxone or ciprofloxacin, if available) and *Chlamydia* (doxycycline or azithromycin).

  2. Chronic bacterial prostatitis
    a. Low back and perineal discomfort, voiding symptoms with insidious onset, no systemic signs, normal prostate exam.
    b. Differential diagnosis includes urethral stricture, carcinoma in situ of the urinary bladder and chronic interstitial cystitis. Pass a 20F urethral catheter in males to rule out urethral stricture.
    c. Examination of prostatic secretions (EPS) shows inflammatory cells and occasionally bacteria. U/A has WBCs and bacteria, if secondary cystitis is present.
    d. Treatment
      (1) Sitz baths tid.
      (2) NSAIDs.
      (3) Alpha-adrenergic drugs (prazosin, terazosin, doxazosin, tamsulosin). Anticholinergic drugs are contraindicated.
      (4) It is difficult to achieve therapeutic antibiotic levels in the absence of inflammation. TMP/SMX or quinolones may be tried for 3 months for "cure".
    e. Treatment failure - parenteral aminoglycoside x 3d, then oral antibiotics. Low dose prophylactic therapy (TMP/SMX qhs, nitrofurantoin 100 mg qd) may be considered also. Radical TURP achieves "cures" in up to 30%.

B. Benign prostatic hypertrophy (BPH)
  1. Clinical
    a. Onset is after age 50 and rises with increasing age.
    b. Correlation between the size of the gland and symptoms is poor. Progression of symptoms is variable.
    c. Obstructive symptoms - decreased force and caliber of the urinary stream, hesitancy in initiating urination, retention, post-micturition dribbling, overflow incontinence.
    d. Irritative symptoms - dysuria, frequency, nocturia, urgency, hematuria.
    e. Prostate is usually enlarged on exam.
    f. U/A may show infection. BUN and creatinine may be elevated, if obstruction is long-standing.

2. Management

   a. Catheterize or use bladder ultrasound to check post-void residual in patients not already in retention.

   b. Measure serum creatinine.

   c. Treat or suppress infection with antibiotics.

   d. Alpha-blocking agents (prazosin, terazosin, doxazosin, tamsulosin) may improve symptoms for many patients, and delay the need for surgery.

   e. Surgical therapy

     (1) Cystoscopy should be done for patients not responding to medical therapy.

     (2) Transurethral resection of the prostate (TURP) improves voiding symptoms in the majority of patients. Complications include incontinence (1%), impotence (up to 5%), and retrograde ejaculation (>80%). Indications for TURP include uremia and/or hydronephrosis, acute or chronic urinary retention, bladder calculi, local or systemic sepsis, and symptoms highly bothersome to the patient.

C. Prostate cancer

  1. General

   a. Most common male cancer. Incidence increases with age. Increased rates for black men.

   b. Suggested by prostatic induration or focal nodules in the prostate on digital rectal examination.

   c. Early disease is asymptomatic. As the cancer enlarges, it may cause obstructive voiding symptoms and urinary retention. Metastases are to pelvic lymph nodes and bone, and may present with back pain or pathologic fractures.

   d. The rate of progression of disease is variable; many people do well for years.

  2. Laboratory

   a. Elevated serum acid phosphatase suggests metastatic disease.

   b. Prostate-specific-antigen (PSA), if available, is the most useful test for detecting and monitoring prostate cancer and monitoring response to treatment

INTERPRETATION OF PSA RESULTS		
Normal	<4ng/ml	-
Intermediate	4-10ng/ml	May have cancer
Elevated	>10ng/ml	Likely has cancer
Very elevated	>40ng/ml	Has cancer, likely metastatic

   c. Prostate biopsy

     (1) Trans-rectal needle biopsy establishes the diagnosis.

     (2) Often the cancer is detected in pathologic analysis of prostate material removed during TURP (up to 10%).

(3) Stages

    (a) Stage A - discovered incidentally during surgery for BPH.

    (b) Stage B - palpable on rectal exam; confined to the prostate.

    (c) Stage C - extends beyond the prostate, but confined within the pelvis.

    (d) Stage D - metastatic to pelvic lymph nodes and/or bone.

3. Treatment

a. Stages A and B - radical prostatectomy or radiation, if available.

b. Stage C - radiation combined with androgen deprivation or androgen deprivation alone (radiation therapy alone isn't very effective).

c. Stage D - androgen-deprivation therapy with orchiectomy, estrogen therapy (DES 3mg/d) or an LHRH agonist +/- antiandrogen. General consensus is to treat immediately. These patients have longer survival and less complications compared with those treated with delayed therapy.

III. ACUTE SCROTAL PAIN AND MASSES

A. Acute scrotal pain

1. Trauma

a. Should be apparent from the history.

b. Scrotal ultrasound may diagnose testicular disruption.

2. Orchitis

a. The prepubertal child has fever, chills, scrotal swelling and pain. Mumps is the usual cause in the younger child. Parotid swelling may be present and the serum amylase level elevated. Treatment is supportive. Sitz baths and scrotal support may help.

b. The postpubertal child with orchitis may also have urinary symptoms and penile discharge (gonorrhea). Treatment is Sitz baths, scrotal support, and antibiotics for gonorrhea.

3. Urolithiasis

a. Hematuria/associated flank pain.

b. Normal scrotal contents.

4. Hernia

a. An inguinal hernia is the protrusion of abdominal contents into the scrotum or inguinal region. Hernias occur in both males and females (more common in males).

b. Most are unilateral. Right-sided hernias are more common. May have inguinal, femoral or scrotal swelling.

c. If a hernia is reducible, it may be repaired electively.

d. If a hernia is not reducible, it is considered to be incarcerated. If incarceration is present in a child, there may be a history of vomiting, irritability and abdominal distension. On examination, a mass will be palpated in the scrotum or labia. It may be more obvious when the child is crying or straining. Adults with incarceration may also have vomiting and distension. There will be pain in the area of the hernia and a non-reducible mass.

e. If the hernia is unable to be reduced, it may become strangulated, with vascular compromise producing gangrene (worsened clinical state with tenderness of abdomen and hernia, tachycardia, leukocytosis). Immediate surgery is indicated.

5. Epididymitis

a. Sexually-transmitted form is associated with urethritis (*Chlamydia* or GC). Non-sexually-transmitted form results from retrograde spread of infection from the lower GU tract (UTI or prostatitis).

b. Symptoms include fever, irritative voiding symptoms, painful enlargement of the epididymis. Symptoms may follow acute physical strain, trauma or sexual activity. Urethral discharge may be present.

c. On examination, the scrotum is inflamed and very tender. Testes may also be enlarged and tender.

d. Lab may show leukocytosis with a left shift. U/A may demonstrate pyuria and/or bacteriuria.

e. Treatment
   (1) Bedrest until pain-free; ice (early) or heat (late).
   (2) Scrotal elevation and support helps relieve pain.
   (3) NSAIDs may be helpful.
   (4) If sexually active, treat for GC and *Chlamydia*. In older males, treat with TMP/SMX or quinolones for 21 days.
   (5) Hospitalize and look for abscess in patients with high fever and signs of toxicity. Treat with IV ampicillin and gentamicin.

6. Torsion of the testicle

a. Presents as sudden onset of pain with marked tenderness of the testis, generally in young males. Abdominal pain and nausea may be present.

b. Caused by twisting of the testis within the scrotal sac, with torsion of the spermatic cord. Rotation causes the epididymis to be anterior in the scrotum. The testis is elevated in the scrotum due to cord shortening.

c. Examination may show localized tenderness of the testicle. If torsion has been present for some time, the epididymis will also be swollen and tender. Differentiation of torsion from epididymitis may be difficult.

d. Management
   (1) This is a urologic emergency. The testicle needs reduction in 4-6 hours to prevent necrosis and loss of the testicle.
   (2) Manual detorsion should be attempted. Infiltrate the spermatic cord near the external inguinal ring with 5cc of 2% lidocaine. Counter-rotate the testicle (rotate right testicle counterclockwise, left testicle clockwise while standing below the patient's scrotum).

(3) If detorsion is unsuccessful, the patient needs immediate surgery. If detorsion is successful, orchiopexy may be done electively (should be bilateral).

B. Painless scrotal masses

1. Hydrocele

a. Collection of fluid between the two layers of the tunica vaginalis. Presents as a painless swelling in the scrotum. An accompanying hernia may or may not be present.

b. On examination, the hydrocele feels smooth and is nontender. Scrotal skin is normal. It may be differentiated from a hernia in the following ways: a hydrocele cannot be reduced, a hernia usually can; a hydrocele is translucent when transilluminated, a hernia is not; auscultation of the scrotum often reveals bowel sounds when a hernia is present but not when there is a hydrocele.

c. Hydroceles generally resolve in newborns. If accompanied by a hernia or if there is waxing and waning swelling (indicating a communicating hydrocele), surgical repair is necessary. In adults, hydroceles may become very large. Aspiration is inadequate, since fluid will always reaccumulate.

2. Varicocele

a. Engorgement of the internal spermatic veins above the testis. Almost always occurs on the left side.

b. Common in young males. Usually noted incidentally.

c. Causes swelling in the left scrotum with varicosities palpated above and separate from the testicle.

d. Should diminish in size or disappear when the patient is supine. It enlarges with Valsalva maneuver.

e. If painful, treat with firm scrotal support, or ligation of the internal spermatic vein.

f. Needs further evaluation if:

(1) Large or bilateral in adolescent or young adult.

(2) Infertility - 40% of men presenting with infertility have varicocele(s).

(3) New onset in male >30 years old.

(4) Right-sided without concomitant left-sided varicocele.

3. Spermatocele

a. Usually asymptomatic.

b. Firm mass superior to and separate from the testicle.

c. Ultrasound can help with diagnosis.

d. No treatment is necessary, unless symptomatic.

4. Undescended testicles

a. An undescended testicle is one that rides high in the scrotum or is not palpable. Undescended testes may be unilateral or bilateral. They are common in neonates. Orchiopexy is recommended if the testicle is still undescended by the age of 1 ½ - 2 years.

b. A retractile testis is normally descended but is intermittently retracted. It requires no therapy.

5. Testicular tumor

   a. Usually occurs in young adults (20-35 years). Cryptorchidism is an important risk factor.

   b. Presents as a solid, painless mass in the testis.

   c. Treatment following radical orchiectomy may include additional surgery, radiation, chemotherapy, and combinations of these modalities.

IV. PENILE ABNORMALITIES

1. Phimosis

   a. Foreskin cannot be retracted over the glans.

   b. Treat acutely by dorsal slit or circumcision.

2. Paraphimosis

   a. The foreskin has been left retracted behind the glans, resulting in painful engorgement and edema of the glans.

   b. Treatment - manual reduction, if possible, dorsal slit of constricting ring or circumcision.

3. Hypospadias

   a. Congenital anomaly of the urethral meatus, wherein it is located on the ventral aspect of the penis, scrotum or perineum. Urethral meatal stenosis and/or penile chordee may be associated with hypospadias. In the newborn, meatal stenosis could require meatotomy.

   b. May be electively repaired, in which case surgical correction of the anomaly(ies) is performed generally before age 3 years.

4. Priapism

   a. Pathologic prolongation of a penile erection associated with pain.

   b. May be caused by sickle cell disease, trauma, neoplasms, drugs.

   c. Treated with aspiration of intracorporal blood and intracavernous injection of alpha-sympathomimetics. Surgical drainage may be needed.

   d. Impotence not uncommonly results even if acute treatment is successful.

5. Squamous cell carcinoma of the penis

   a. Results from phimosis and poor hygiene.

   b. Presents with ulceration, foul-smelling discharge and firm mass under a phimotic foreskin.

   c. May have inguinal adenopathy from inflammatory response or metastasis.

   d. Treatment is partial or total penectomy, depending on extent of disease.

   e. Inguinal metastases may respond to methotrexate.

V. UROLITHIASIS

A. Clinical manifestations

1. Pain - usually of sudden onset, unilateral, severe and colicky, beginning in the flank, with radiation into the groin and/or genitalia. Frequently accompanied by diaphoresis, nausea and vomiting.
2. Physical examination may reveal costovertebral angle tenderness.
3. U/A will show microscopic or gross hematuria in most cases. BUN and creatinine not necessary. KUB may identify some stones. IVP is usually done to rule out obstruction and document the presence of stones. It may not be necessary in patients with a previous history of stones and typical findings on exam.

B. Management

1. **Acute episode**
   a. Hydration - may make the pain worse, especially if significant obstruction is present.
   b. Analgesics.
   c. Strain the urine to recover passed stones.
   d. Hospitalize if parenteral analgesics are required for persistent vomiting, suspected pyelonephritis and/or in the presence of high-grade urinary obstruction. Stones that are obstructing outflow or causing infection require bypass or removal.
   e. If the pain is mild, the patient may be followed as an outpatient until the stone is passed. Oral analgesics should be given (such as NSAIDs) or narcotics.

2. **Continuing care**
   a. All patients should increase their daily fluid intake to prevent development of further stones.
   b. More specific treatment depends on the stone composition.
      (1) Calcium stones - reduce calcium intake, can try thiazide diuretics.
      (2) Uric acid stones - alkalinization of urine (Shoals solution 20cc 2-3x/d or sodium bicarbonate). Allopurinol 300mg qd may be helpful also.
      (3) Triple phosphate stones (staghorn calculi) - occur with chronic infections. Clear/suppress UTI with antimicrobials, acidify the urine. Generally require removal.

VI. OTHER UROLOGIC PROBLEMS

A. Hematuria

1. **General**
   a. Microscopic - greater than 2-5 RBC/HPF on microscopic exam.
   b. Gross - visible, produces red discoloration of urine. Not all red urine is due to hematuria (see Chapter 6, section V, A, 6, e)
2. **Etiology**

a. Younger patients with transient low grade hematuria are more likely to have a benign etiology (menstruation, viral illness, exercise or mild trauma, transient unexplained hematuria). Serial specimens should be evaluated to R/O a persistent problem.

b. Patients with persistent or gross hematuria and older patients should undergo evaluation. Consider the following:

(1) Infection (UTI, schistosomiasis, tuberculosis).

(2) Upper tract pathology (trauma, stones, neoplasms, polycystic kidney disease).

(3) Lower tract pathology (prostate disease, endometriosis).

(4) Intrinsic renal disease (glomerulonephritis, esp IgA nephropathy).

(5) Sickle cell disease or trait.

(6) Coagulation disorders (ITP).

3. Evaluation

a. Review the history for:

(1) Symptoms of UTI.

(2) Acute flank pain suggesting stone disease.

(3) Persistent flank pain suggesting chronic problem (renal tumor).

(4) Symptoms of prostatic diseae.

b. Physical examination

(1) Vital signs - fever, hypertension.

(2) Abdominal exam - flank tenderness, renal mass.

(3) Skin rash, purpura, petechiae or joint swelling.

(4) GU exam - prostate enlargement, pelvic mass.

c. Urinalysis

(1) WBCs suggest infection (UTI, prostatitis).

(2) Significant proteinuria or RBC casts indicate glomerular disease.

(3) The three glass test can be used to compare three urine specimens (initial few ml of urine, mid-voiding specimen, last few ml of urine). These specimens can be evaluated as follows:

(a) Blood in the initial specimen suggests a urethral lesion (stricture or stenosis).

(b) Terminal hematuria may indicate a lesion in the posterior urethra, or bladder neck or trigone.

(c) Blood present in all three specimens indicates a lesion in the bladder or upper urinary tract.

(4) In endemic areas, look for Schistosoma eggs.

d. Look for upper tract lesions with IVP or renal ultrasound. Cystoscopic exam should be done in patients at increased risk for bladder cancer (age > 50 yrs, smokers).

B. Urinary incontinence

1. Etiology

a. Incontinence results from either failure to store urine, failure to empty the bladder, or a combination of these.

b. Both failure to store urine and failure to empty the bladder can be due to bladder dysfunction or outlet (sphincter) dysfunction.

2. Diagnosis

   a. History

     (1) Determine duration of symptoms (recent onset vs. chronic problem), irritative symptoms (urgency, nocturia, frequency), obstructive symptoms (straining, hesitancy, sensation of incomplete voiding), loss of control with coughing, sneezing, or straining, relation to fluid intake. Look for chronic medical problems (diabetes, neurologic disease).

     (2) Medications that affect bladder function (diuretics, tricyclic antidepressants, anticholinergics, beta blockers).

   b. Examination

     (1) Perform a thorough generalized examination including a neurologic examination to rule out systemic disease.

     (2) Males - evaluate for prostatic enlargement.

     (3) Females - evaluate for bladder or uterine prolapse, signs of estrogen deficiency, vesicovaginal fistula.

     (4) Pelvic neurologic abnormality - look for perineal sensory deficits, reflex abnormalities (bulbocavernosus reflex, anal sphincter tone).

     (5) Urinalysis to R/O infection.

     (6) Check for post voiding residual urine by doing straight catheterization. > 50 ml is abnormal.

     (7) Cystometrogram is not usually required. It can be used to determine volume where patient senses bladder filling (100-250 ml), non-urgent urge to void (250-350 ml), and detrusor contraction (400-550 ml). With urge incontinence, bladder contraction occurs with smaller volumes. With overflow incontinence, larger volumes are required to produce contraction.

3. Types of incontinence

   a. Transient functional incontinence usually has a definable, sudden onset, often with a discrete cause. Causes include (mnemonic "diapers"):

     (1) Drugs

     (2) Delirium or altered mental status

     (3) Infection

     (4) Atrophy of the vagina or urethra

     (5) Psychologic disorder, functional depression

     (6) Endocrine - hyperglycemia or hypercalcemia

     (7) Restricted mobility

     (8) Stool impaction

   b. Stress incontinence - in men, may be seen following prostate surgery. In women, occurs due to laxity in the pelvic floor allowing prolapse of the bladder or uterus. Results in small amounts of urine being lost with coughing, sneezing, or straining. Post void residual is small.

c. Urge incontinence (detrusor instability) - occurs secondary to neurologic disease resulting in increased motor tone in the bladder musculature, or bladder irritation secondary to infection or other cause. Symptoms of frequency and urgency occur. Post void residual is small.

d. Overflow incontinence - results from chronic outlet obstruction, especially in men with prostatic hypertrophy. Small volume, frequent urination occurs. Large post void residual is present.

e. Reflex incontinence - results from neurologic damage causing loss of sensation from the bladder and coordination of voiding reflexes.

4. Treatment

a. Address the underlying problem, if possible.

b. Alter fluid intake, modify chronic medications.

c. Avoid catheters, if possible. Use of incontinence pads and diapers is preferable - watch for skin breakdown.

d. Stress incontinence - in females, try estrogen replacement if atrophic vaginitis is present. Pelvic strengthening exercises may help.

e. Urge incontinence - imipramine 10-25 mg 1-4 times daily, oxybutynin 2.5-5 mg 1-4 times daily, or tolterodine 1-2 mg bid may be helpful. Give the lowest effective dose.

f. Overflow incontinence - decompress the bladder by catheterization and consider drugs to decrease sphincter tone (prazosin 2-20 mg/day, doxazosin 2-8 mg/day) or increase bladder tone (bethanechol 25-125 mg/day). Catheterization is required if post void residual volumes are large (> 300 ml).

CHAPTER 20

SURGERY

I. ACUTE ABDOMINAL PAIN
A. Evaluation
1. Severe abdominal pain in a previously healthy patient, which lasts longer than six hours is likely due to surgical disease.
2. Patients in some cultures may be very stoic, even in the face of tremendous pain. Their outward appearance may not accurately reflect the severity of their pain and significant surgical illness may not be suspected. Pain scales and knowledge of the culture may help to avoid misinterpretation of the patient's clinical condition. Also, patients who are HIV positive may present atypically and have a different differential diagnosis of disease than those who are not HIV positive.
3. Most surgeons recommend that analgesics be avoided as much as possible during the evaluation of abdominal pain. They may be given if the patient is extremely uncomfortable, once the decision to operate has been made, or if there is a delay in obtaining surgical consultation.
4. History
   a. Establish the time and acuteness of onset of symptoms.
   b. Determine the character, severity, location, and radiation of pain. Is it pleuritic, rather than abdominal?
   c. Is the patient nauseated, or has vomiting occurred? When was the last bowel movement? Was it normal? What is the relationship of these symptoms to the pain?
   d. Obtain a menstrual and sexual history (previous pregnancies and outcomes, last menstrual period - was it normal flow and duration?).
   e. Is the illness progressive? Has the pain been getting progressively worse?
   f. Is the patient known to be HIV positive? Are there other underlying medical problems?
5. Examination
   a. Record pulse, blood pressure, temperature and respiratory rate.
   b. Examine the heart and lungs for abnormalities.
   c. Inspect the abdomen (look for abdominal distension or hernias).
   d. Auscultate for bowel sounds (present, diminished, high pitched, rushes).
   e. Percuss and palpate the abdomen. Look for masses, tenderness, rigidity, guarding, or rebound.
   f. Perform a rectal exam. Look for tenderness, lateralization, masses or blood.
   g. Perform a pelvic exam. Look for vaginal discharge or bleeding, tenderness or pelvic masses.
B. General treatment
1. Make the patient NPO.

2. Insert a naso-gastric tube and connect to suction, if the patient is vomiting.

3. Begin IV fluids. Replace the patient's fluid deficit with NS or RL (may require several liters of fluid). Monitor intake and output (urine + suction) and give maintenance fluids plus replace ongoing losses.

4. Obtain a chest x-ray, flat and upright abdominal x-rays. Look for free air under the diaphragm, or the presence of air fluid levels in the small bowel.

5. Obtain CBC, U/A, and electrolytes, if available.

6. Re-examine the patient frequently if the diagnosis is unclear. Serial exams are key.

7. If no diagnosis can be made and the patient is in severe pain, abdominal exploration may be necessary.

C. Differential diagnosis

1. Peritonitis

a. Etiology (usually results from intra-abdominal pathology resulting in contamination of the peritoneal cavity)

    (1) Perforation of abdominal viscus - ruptured appendix, perforated peptic ulcer, typhoid perforation (distal ileum).

    (2) Gangrene of the bowel - secondary to volvulus, or intussusception.

    (3) Disseminated infection - PID, ruptured abscess.

    (4) Occasionally results from sepsis.

b. Clinical presentation

    (1) Inflammation of the peritoneum results in acute, severe pain. Vomiting is common. Abdominal distension, inability to pass gas and constipation may be present.

    (2) Examination - the patient is usually quiet, since movement increases the pain. Bowel sounds are diminished or absent. Distension may be present with a large amount of peritoneal fluid. Peritoneal signs are present (guarding, rigidity, rebound), as well as percussion tenderness over the area of inflammation. Fever, tachycardia, oliguria and tachypnea are signs of hypovolemia and sepsis, common in patients with neglected perforated viscus.

c. Evaluation and treatment

    (1) Begin general treatment as outlined above. Obtain baseline laboratory (CBC, electrolytes).

    (2) Fluid resuscitation is important if the patient is volume depleted.

    (3) Begin broad-spectrum antibiotics. Important organisms to cover are Gram (-) rods (*E. coli*), anaerobes (*Bacteroides*), and *Enterococcus*. Use broad coverage (ampicillin plus gentamicin, and chloramphenicol or metronidazole). Third generation cephalosporins are good but do not cover *Enterococcus*.

    (4) Urgent operative therapy aimed at determining the etiology, resecting and débriding necrotic bowel, and draining potential abscesses is mandatory.

2. Acute appendicitis

  a. Less common in developing countries.

  b. Clinical presentation

    (1) Typical presentation begins with periumbilical discomfort that shifts to the right lower quadrant and increases in intensity over several hours. Anorexia is almost always present. Minor nausea and vomiting may occur.

    (2) Classic physical findings include focal pain, guarding, and rebound tenderness in the right lower quadrant. Atypical findings may occur with retrocecal location of the appendix or late presentation. The diagnosis is based on clinical examination (reproducible, consistent RLQ tenderness).

    (3) Low-grade fever and leukocytosis or left shift are usually present. 10% of patients will have a normal CBC, however.

  c. Management

    (1) Timely appendectomy usually results in a good outcome.

    (2) Complications include localized abscess or peritonitis.

    (3) Advanced peritonitis is not required to justify surgical exploration. A "cold appendix" rate of 16% is reasonable for the developing world.

3. Bowel obstruction (mechanical obstruction)

  a. Causes

    (1) Common causes of small bowel obstruction are strangulated groin hernias, volvulus, intussusception, and adhesions. Occasionally, obstruction secondary to Ascaris may be seen.

    (2) Colonic obstruction is usually due to neoplasm or sigmoid volvulus. Diverticulitis may cause secondary obstruction from mesenteric edema. Diverticular disease is rare in developing countries, however. Sigmoid volvulus is occasionally the cause of obstruction in elderly patients (x-ray is diagnostic).

  b. Clinical presentation

    (1) Patients with bowel obstruction usually present with crampy, colic-like abdominal pain, vomiting (bilious or feculent), and abdominal distension. Also look for obstipation, and lack of flatus or passage of stool.

    (2) On examination, the patient may be volume depleted due to third spacing of fluid in the bowel. The abdomen is distended and tympanitic. Bowel sounds occur in rushes and are frequently high pitched. There are no peritoneal signs unless generalized peritonitis has developed. Abdominal tenderness is variable.

  c. Laboratory

    (1) Abdominal x-rays (plain film and upright) should be done on all patients with suspected bowel obstruction. They may differentiate small vs. large bowel obstruction, identify free air, or masses.

    (2) CBC and electrolytes should be measured, if possible.

    d. Management

      (1) Bowel strangulation with necrosis may occur if the obstruction is not promptly relieved. Abdominal pain increases and may be continuous. Bowel sounds are decreased or absent, abdominal tenderness is present. WBC may be increased with a left shift. Fever may be present.

      (2) Treatment of mechanical bowel obstruction is operation. Fluid resuscitation and NG drainage should be done prior to surgery. Broad-spectrum antibiotics should be given.

4. Paralytic ileus (adynamic ileus)

    a. Causes include sepsis, abdominal infections, electrolyte abnormalities, trauma.

    b. Clinical presentation

      (1) Patients usually present with abdominal distension. Pain is usually absent.

      (2) On physical examination, the abdomen is distended and there are decreased to absent bowel sounds. There are no peritoneal signs.

      (3) Abdominal x-ray shows dilated small bowel loops without colonic distension. Upright films show air-fluid levels.

      (4) May be difficult to distinguish from bowel obstruction.

    c. Management is usually non-operative with IV fluids, NG decompression and observation. Surgery is rarely necessary.

5. Peptic ulcer disease with perforation

    a. Prior history of ulcer symptoms is usually but not always present.

    b. Typical presentation includes the sudden onset of severe epigastric pain with the development of marked abdominal rigidity over several hours.

    c. Upright abdominal films show free air in 50% of cases. Pneumogastrography may be performed in equivocal cases, to document free air. This is done by insufflating 400-500cc of air into an NG tube in the stomach, after which it is clamped and an upright CXR is done. This usually will show free air that may not have been present on the routine abdominal x-ray, and confirms perforation.

    d. Prompt surgical repair of the perforation should be performed.

    e. Mortality remains high, especially with late presentation.

6. Gynecologic causes

    a. Ectopic pregnancy

      (1) Presentation

        (a) Suspect in any sexually active female with abdominal pain and positive pregnancy test. Almost always presents in the first trimester. History of prior PID is common.

        (b) There may be abnormal vaginal spotting or bleeding with a history of a recent missed or abnormal period.

        (c) Must differentiate from acute PID and spontaneous abortion.

      (2) Exam

(a) Abdominal exam may show lower abdominal tenderness.
(b) Pelvic exam may show blood in cervical os, cervical motion tenderness, tenderness and guarding on bimanual exam, and the presence of an adnexal mass in about one half of the patients.
(c) If the cervical os is dilated, with vaginal bleeding, spontaneous abortion is more likely.
(3) Diagnosis
(a) CBC - look for anemia.
(b) Pregnancy test. Quantitative serum ß-HCG is helpful, if available.
(c) Pelvic ultrasound may show the uterus to have a thickened endometrium without a yolk sac. An adnexal mass may be present.
(d) Aspiration of blood from the cul-de-sac confirms the diagnosis.
(4) Treatment
(a) Begin a large bore IV.
(b) Type and cross-match blood.
(c) If ruptured, monitor the patient closely for development of shock.
(d) Urgent exploration with salpingectomy is necessary.
(e) Perform autotransfusion if massive hemoperitoneum is present.
b. Ovarian torsion
(1) Sudden onset of severe pain on one side of the lower abdomen. Nausea and vomiting may be present.
(2) Pelvic exam shows tenderness of the ovary. Fever and leukocytosis may be present.
(3) Ultrasound is diagnostic, if available.
(4) Treatment is surgical.
c. Ruptured ovarian cyst
(1) Sudden onset of unilateral lower abdominal pain. Usually subsides within 12-24 hours.
(2) Ultrasound may show fluid in the pelvis.
(3) Hgb/Hct should be checked. Surgery is indicated only if bleeding is uncontrolled (persistent pain, decreasing hematocrit).
d. Dysmenorrhea
(1) Low abdominal cramping pain, often with diarrhea, that occurs just before and during menses. Especially common during initial menses at menarche.
(2) Usually improved with nonsteroidal antiinflammatory agents, such as ibuprofen.
7. Medical illnesses, such as acute cholecystitis or biliary colic, acute pancreatitis, acute gastritis, acute hepatitis and acute pyelonephritis may present with abdominal or flank pain. These are nonsurgical problems and can be treated with medical therapy. Acute pneumonia can

sometimes present with abdominal pain, especially in children. A pleuritic component to the pain, cough, rales and infiltrate on chest x-ray confirm the diagnosis.

II. BURNS
A. Classification (classified according to the depth of tissue injury)
1. **First degree burns** (sunburn)
   a. Injury involves superficial skin only (the epidermis).
   b. Characterized by pain and redness.
   c. Heals without scarring within a few days with peeling of superficial skin.
2. **Second degree burns**
   a. Injury extends deeper into the skin - through the epidermis into the dermis (involving nerve endings, hair follicles, blood and lymph vessels).
   b. Parts of the skin remain viable so spontaneous regrowth of the skin occurs.
   c. Considered "partial thickness" burns. They may be superficial, extending into part of the dermis, or deep, involving the deeper layers of dermis.
   d. Characterized by skin lesions that are erythematous, weeping, blistering, and painful.
3. **Third degree burns**
   a. Injury extends through the entire dermis, down to the subcutaneous fat.
   b. Considered "full thickness" burns. All skin elements are destroyed so that regrowth of skin is not possible.
   c. Characterized by skin that is dry, hard, inelastic, translucent, and painless.
   d. Healing occurs only by scarring, (ingrowth of tissue from the wound margins). Skin grafting often necessary.
B. Assessment
1. Estimate the extent of body surface area involvement, and the depth of skin injury.
2. Use the "rule of nines in adults" or "rule of sevens" in children. Use only areas of second and third-degree burns in the calculation.

ASSESSMENT OF EXTENT OF BURNS		
Anatomic Area	**Adults**	**Children**
Head	9%	28%
Right arm	9%	7%
Left arm	9%	7%
Anterior trunk	18%	14%
Posterior trunk	18%	14%

Assessment of Extent of Burns (continue)		
Anatomic Area	**Adults**	**Children**
Right leg	18%	14%
Left leg	18%	14%
Perineum	1%	2%

3. Evaluate for respiratory involvement. Burns of the oral mucosa and nasal passages or the presence of stridor may indicate smoke or heat damage to the respiratory system.
4. Evaluate for associated injuries (depending on the circumstances of the burn injury).

C. Management

1. In general, the following patients should be admitted to the hospital for treatment:
   a. All patients with third-degree burns of > 5% of the body.
   b. Adults with second-degree burns >20%.
   c. Children with second-degree burns >10%.
   d. When significant second- or third-degree burns involve the face, perineum, hands, fingers, feet or toes.
2. Initial first aid involves drenching the burn with cool water to prevent further tissue damage. Burnt clothing should be removed from the patient. If the burn area is limited, immerse the site in cold water for 30 minutes to reduce pain and edema. Try to avoid hypothermia, especially in young children, by keeping them warm and wrapping the burned area in clean dressings or material, such as linen.
3. Analgesics, such as morphine, should be given to relieve pain.
4. Closely observe the patient's cardiorespiratory status. Assess adequacy of the airway. In patients with facial burns, upper airway obstruction may occur within the first 48 hours after injury due to soft tissue swelling in the oral pharynx and vocal cords from exposure to hot gases. Intubation may be required.
5. Pulmonary injury is the major cause of death in burn patients. Give oxygen, if available.
6. Fluid management
   a. IV resuscitation is indicated if the burn is 10% or more of the body area of an infant, or 15% or more of that of an adult, regardless of burn depth.
   b. In severe burns, there are massive fluid shifts following burn injury and IV fluids are important in restoring intravascular fluid volume. If the patient is hypotensive, begin fluid resuscitation with normal saline. As blood pressure normalizes, fluids can be changed to D5/.45 NS.
   c. If the patient is suspected of being significantly acidotic, consider adding sodium bicarbonate to the IV fluids in a dose of 1-2 mEq/kg.
   d. During the first 24 hours following injury, when fluid losses are the greatest, the rate of fluid resuscitation can be gauged according to the

following formula: amount of IV solution = 4 cc/kg x % 2nd and 3rd degree burn. Give 1/2 of the fluid over the first 8 hours, then the remainder over the next 16 hours (calculated from the time of the burn).

   e. Fluid requirements in the second 24h are roughly 1/2 of the first 24h. Urine output should be maintained between 30-70ml/hr or 0.5-1ml/kg/hr. Assess fluid requirements regularly. Try to avoid fluid overload. Urine output is the best indicator of volume status.

   f. Potassium should not be added to IV fluids during the first 24 hours because large amounts are initially released from injured cells. Acidosis and renal failure may elevate potassium levels initially. After the first day, depending on urine output, renal function, and the condition of the patient, 20-30 mEq of potassium may be added to each liter of IV fluid.

7. Local care of wounds - débride eschar (non-viable skin) and cleanse with an antiseptic solution. Apply an antimicrobial cream, such as silver sulfadiazine, or Neosporin/Polysporin to the wounds prior to covering them with a sterile dressing. Adequate analgesia should be given prior to wound debridement.

8. Antibiotics are not routinely given to burn patients. If a wound infection develops, *staphylococcus, Pseudomonas* or Gram-negative rods are usually responsible. Broad spectrum antibiotics should then be given.

9. If not adequately immunized, tetanus antitoxin should be given in addition to tetanus toxoid.

10. Maintain nutrition with oral or NG feeding.

11. Succinylcholine should not be used in burn patients for up to 1 year after the burn.

12. Circumferential burns of the extremities or chest can create a tourniquet effect with vascular compromise or ventilatory compromise. Escharotomies to relieve the constrictive scar may be required.

13. Burn patients use a large amount of resources. Consider transfer to a larger medical center or burn center, if possible and if survival is likely. If the sum of the patient's age plus the percentage of surface area burned exceeds 90, the chances of survival are not more than 50% (and even less in the very old and very young). Burns involving the respiratory passages are more severe, also.

III. FRACTURES

A. Terminology and classification

1. Causation

   a. Traumatic - most fractures are caused by trauma, either direct or indirect.

   b. Pathological - fracture occurs through a bone already weakened by underlying disease.

   c. Stress - bone is fatigued by repetitive stress.

2. Anatomic location
   a. Fractures are usually categorized as being in the proximal, middle or distal third of a long bone.
   b. Other terms used to describe the location of a fracture are head, shaft, and base.
3. Direction of fracture lines
   a. Transverse - running perpendicular to the bone.
   b. Oblique - runs across the bone at an angle of 45-60 degrees.
   c. Spiral - has a torsional component to the fracture.
   d. Comminuted - more than two fragments present.
   e. Impacted - the fractured ends are compressed together.
4. Relationship of the fracture fragments to each other
   a. Alignment - relationship of the axes of the fragment of a long bone to one another. Alignment is described in degrees of angulation of the distal fragment in relation to the proximal fragment.
   b. Apposition - describes the relationship of the fractured ends to one another (partially apposed, displaced, distracted).
5. Stability
   a. Stable fracture - does not have a tendency to displace after reduction.
   b. Unstable fracture - tends to displace after reduction.
6. Associated soft tissue injury
   a. Simple (closed) - overlying skin remains intact.
   b. Compound (open) - overlying skin is broken.
   c. Complicated - associated with neurovascular, visceral, ligamentous or muscular damage. Intra-articular fractures are also complicated.
   d. Uncomplicated - only a minimal amount of soft tissue injury.
7. Joint injuries
   a. Dislocation - total disruption of the joint surfaces with loss of normal contact between the two bony ends.
   b. Subluxation - partial disruption of a joint with partial contact remaining between the two bones that make up the joint.
   c. Diastasis - disruption of the interosseous membrane connecting a syndesmotic articulation (as between the radius and ulna and fibula and tibia).
B. Clinical features
   1. Pain and tenderness are the most common presenting complaints in patients with a fracture. These symptoms are usually well localized to the fracture site, but can be more diffuse if there is significant associated soft tissue injury.
   2. Loss of normal function may be noted, but in patients with incomplete fractures, functional impairment may be minimal.
   3. Every patient with a suspected fracture needs a complete neurovascular examination.
   4. Blood loss is a common problem with fractures, and may be significant in those with multiple fractures or pelvic fractures. Average blood loss

in closed fractures is estimated as follows:
  a. Radius and ulna - 150-250cc
  b. Humerus - 250cc
  c. Pelvis - 1500-3000cc
  d. Femur - 1000cc
  e. Tibia and fibula - 500cc
C. Goals of fracture management
  1. Reduction - restoration of the displaced fragments to their anatomical position.
  2. Immobilization or fixation - retention of the fragments in the reduced position until union.
  3. Achievement of union.
  4. Restoration of function.
D. Initial evaluation
  1. Stabilize the patient. Assess the extent of other injuries.
  2. Evaluate for shock, especially with fractures of the pelvis and femur (large amounts of blood can be lost in these fractures). Start IV fluids, if necessary.
  3. Evaluate for spine injuries. If cervical spine injury is suspected, immobilize the neck with a cervical collar or sandbags until x-rays are taken or fracture otherwise ruled out.
  4. Examine the injured area. Look for pain, swelling, deformity, ecchymosis, instability, or crepitus.
  5. Check the injured extremity for neurovascular injury (pulses, capillary refill, motor and sensory nerve function).
  6. Splint the fracture to prevent further soft tissue injury and for pain relief. If an open fracture is present, cover the skin with a sterile dressing. Apply an ice pack to reduce swelling.
  7. Confirm the fracture with appropriate x-rays. The fracture should be seen in two views. Include the joint above and below the injury. Nondisplaced fractures occasionally are not seen initially but are seen on follow-up films taken 1-2 weeks later.
  8. If the mechanism of injury and physical findings are suggestive of fracture, but the x-rays appear negative, treat as for fracture.
E. Definitive treatment
  1. **Closed fractures**
    a. Reduce the fracture and apply plaster cast.
    b. Use adequate analgesia or ketamine anesthesia.
    c. If considerable swelling is present, consider splinting and elevation for 24-48 hours before applying cast.
    d. Teach the patient the signs of vascular compression (increased pain, numbness, tingling).
  2. **Open fractures**
    a. Perform immediate, thorough debridement and irrigation under appropriate anesthesia in the operating room. Do not do primary

closure of the wound.

b. Reduce the fracture.

c. Dress the wound with a sterile dressing and apply a splint. Check peripheral pulses.

d. Begin broad-spectrum IV antibiotics (cephalothin 2gm IV q6h, or cefazolin 1gm IV or IM q6-8 hours).

e. Give tetanus prophylaxis.

f. Inspect and dress the wound daily. Consider closure of the wound after 5-7 days, if it appears healthy. If not, wait 2-4 weeks and close it loosely or do skin grafting.

3. Traction

a. Indications

  (1) Where powerful muscles tend to cause shortening or angulation of the fracture (e.g. fracture of the femur).

  (2) Extremely unstable fractures (e.g. oblique fractures which tend to shorten).

b. Types

  (1) Skin - usually only used in children. Can use in adults for short periods of time.

  (2) Skeletal - use of Steinmann's pins to apply traction. In general 1/10 to 1/7 of the patient's body weight provides adequate traction.

F. Complications of fractures

1. Compartment syndrome

a. May develop after any trauma to extremity. Results in progressive vascular compromise with injury to nerves and muscles of the extremity.

b. Signs - severe pain especially on passive stretching of the muscle. Decreased or absent pulses, pallor or coolness of extremity, paresthesias or loss of motor function are late findings.

c. Treatment - when suspected, do emergency fasciotomy.

2. Gas gangrene

a. Occurs in contaminated traumatic wounds which have been closed after inadequate debridement. An anerobic clostridial cellulitis begins several days later.

b. Initial symptoms are pain and a "heavy" sensation in the affected area. Onset is gradual. Edema then develops with exudation of a thin dark fluid from the wound. The condition progresses rapidly with myonecrosis and increasing toxemia. Foul smelling gas is present in the wound.

c. Treatment is prompt surgical decompression and debridement. Penicillin 3 million units every 3 hours should be started. If PCN-allergic, tetracycline 2-4gm IV/day is recommended.

3. Osteomyelitis - see Chapter 1

4. Fat embolism syndrome

a. May result after major trauma, especially long bone fractures. Occurs in 19% of patients with major trauma. One third of the cases are mild and require no treatment.

b. Onset of symptoms is 4 hours to several days after injury (average 46 hours).

c. Major features are respiratory insufficiency, cerebral involvement and petechial rash. Minor features include fever, tachycardia, retinal changes, jaundice and renal problems.

d. Dyspnea and tachypnea are the earliest signs. Moist rales are heard over the whole lung field. Restlessness and confusion then follow and fever may be present. Petechiae appear over the anterior axillary area, neck, buccal mucosa and conjunctiva.

e. Chest x-ray shows a patchy infiltrate.

f. Treatment is respiratory support with oxygen. The injured part should be immobilized and no excessive motion permitted. Parenteral steroids may be helpful (methylprednisolone 30mg/kg IV).

G. Healing times for fractures

Average healing times of common fractures in adults	
Clavicle	3 weeks
Humerus	6 weeks
Elbow	6 weeks
Forearm	6 weeks
Wrist	6 weeks
Navicular	12-16 weeks
Hand	3-4 weeks
Pelvis (single)	3-4 weeks
Pelvis (2 or more rami)	6-8 weeks
Femur	16-20 weeks
Tibia	12 weeks
Ankle- (trimalleolar)	8 weeks
Foot	6 weeks

Compound fractures may take longer to heal. Femur fractures vary considerably in healing time. In older patients, consider shorter period of immobilization to decrease joint stiffness, e.g. - wrist.

IV. WOUNDS AND LACERATIONS

A. History

1. Review the mechanism of injury - laceration with a sharp object, blunt trauma, or bite wound.

2. Note the duration of time passed since the injury (risk of infection increases with time). Wounds less than 6 hours old can generally be sutured. Clean wounds on the face or scalp may be closed primarily up to 24 hours after injury.

3. Determine the patient's tetanus immunization status.

4. If due to animal bite, determine if the attack was unprovoked and the availability of the animal for observation for rabies.

B. Physical exam

1. Examine the wound carefully for:

   a. Significant bleeding - apply pressure until the wound can be explored. For uncomplicated scalp lacerations, wound closure usually controls bleeding.

   b. Contamination - dirty lacerations should be thoroughly explored, irrigated, and debrided, if necessary. For grossly contaminated wounds, consider delayed closure.

   c. Neurovascular status - assess in all patients with skin disruption. If deficits are found, consultation with a specialist is needed.

2. Assess for tendon involvement in injuries involving extremities. Assess potential for joint penetration.

3. Obtain x-rays before suturing if a foreign body or fracture is suspected.

C. Wound healing

1. Types of closure

   a. Primary closure (primary intention) - clean, minimally contaminated wounds can be closed with sutures, wound tapes or staples. Should be repaired within 6-8 hours after injury for best results and less chance of infection.

   b. Secondary closure (secondary intention) - skin ulcerations, abscesses, punctured, bites and partial-thickness abrasions should be left to heal by secondary intention. They are allowed to heal by granulation without sutures. Grafting can be done later, if necessary.

   c. Tertiary closure (delayed primary closure) - closure after being cleansed, debrided and observed for 4-5 days. This is for wounds which are too contaminated to close primarily, but do not have significant tissue loss.

2. Complications of wound healing

   a. Wound infection - most serious and most common complication of wound and laceration repair. Risk of infection is increased the more time elapsed from injury to cleansing and repair.

   b. Suture marks - increased by excessive suture tension. Sutures remaining in place for 14 days or longer uniformly leave suture marks. Sutures removed before 7 days never leave suture marks.

   c. Keloids are inappropriate accumulations of scar tissue that originate from a wound and extend beyond its original boundaries. Hypertrophic scars are excessively large, but remain confined to the original borders of the wound.

D. Laceration repair

1. General

   a. Be sure to have adequate equipment and supplies available.

   b. Arrange adequate lighting.

    c. Provide adequate anesthesia.

    d. Be sure the injury can be adequately cared for in the setting where you are working. Assess whether the patient should be taken to the operating room.

2. Anesthesia

    a. Most often use 1% lidocaine with or without epinephrine. Maximum dose of lidocaine is 4.5mg/kg (30cc of 1% solution in an adult).

    b. Do not use epinephrine on fingers, toes, penis, ears, tip of nose or with digital blocks.

    c. NaHCO3 can be added to lidocaine to decrease the pain of injection (9:1 lidocaine to bicarb dilution).

    d. TAC (tetracaine, adrenaline and cocaine), or TLE (tetracaine, lidocaine, epinephrine) may be used topically in children (don't use near mucous membranes or on ear, nose, penis).

    e. Allergic reactions to local anesthetics - uncommon with the newer amide anesthetics (lidocaine, mepivacaine and bupivacaine). More common with the older ester solutions (procaine and tetracaine). If the allergy-causing drug is an ester, it can be substituted with an amide. Diphenhydramine has similar properties to standard local anesthetics. 50mg (1cc) can be diluted in a syringe with 4cc of NS to produce a 1% solution which can be used for local infiltration. It is more painful than lidocaine.

    f. For large wounds, consider general anesthesia.

3. Wound cleansing

    a. Wound cleansing solutions

       (1) Povidone-iodine (Betadine) - bactericidal. Scrub contains a detergent which may be toxic to wound tissues. The 10% solution when diluted to a 1% concentration, can be used for wound cleansing.

       (2) Chlorhexidine (Hibiclens) - bactericidal. Excellent for hand washing. Contains detergent which may be toxic to tissues.

       (3) Nonionic surfactants (Shur-Clens, Pharma Clens) - cleansing properties of soap, but no antibacterial activity. Not toxic to tissues, including the eye. Good for use on the face.

       (4) Hexachlorophene (pHisoHex) - bacteriostatic. Good for hand washing, but not often used anymore for wound cleansing.

       (5) Quaternary ammonium compounds (Zephiran) - not effective, shouldn't be used.

       (6) Hydrogen peroxide - weak antibacterial effect. Can delay healing. Use only to clean wounds encrusted with blood.

    b. Wound area hair removal - shaving may increase the wound infection rate. On the scalp, hair may be clipped with scissors. Hair should never be shaved or clipped on the eyebrow.

    c. Foreign material should be removed by direct visualization and with irrigation. 90% of glass can be seen on x-ray.

d. Scrubbing within the wound should be done only in those wounds with visible contaminants, since it can increase the potential for tissue damage. Wound irrigation is the most effective way to remove debris and reduce bacterial counts on the wound surface. Use of a 35cc syringe attached to a 19-gauge catheter is recommended.

4. Wound closure

a. Suture types

(1) Absorbable - gut, chromic gut, Dexon, Vicryl.

(2) Non-absorbable - nylon, silk, polypropylene, Dacron.

b. Needle types

(1) Cutting - used in skin suturing.

(2) Round - used in most areas other than skin.

c. Suture material and removal times (general guidelines)

	Suture size	Removal time
*Scalp	4-0, 5-0	7 days
Face	5-0, 6-0	3-5 days
Nose, ear	6-0	3-5 days
Chest, abdomen	4-0, 5-0	7-10 days
Extremities (not over joints)	4-0, 5-0	7-10 days
Extremities (near joints)	4-0, 5-0	10-14 days
Foot, toe	3-0, 4-0	12-14 days

5. Prophylactic antibiotics (with initial IV/IM dose at the time of wound repair) should be considered for the following wounds:

a. Complex or mutilating wounds, especially of the hand or foot.

b. Grossly contaminated wounds.

c. Lacerations in areas of lymphedema.

d. Extensive lacerations of the ear and its cartilage.

e. Suspected penetration of bone, joints or tendons.

f. Amputation injuries.

g. Presence of diabetes or immunosuppression.

E. Specific lacerations

1. *Scalp

a. Even small scalp lacerations can cause significant bleeding, even leading to hypovolemia and hypotension. If bleeding cannot be controlled with direct pressure on the wound, immediate repair using large bites, is indicated. Use of lidocaine with epinephrine may also reduce bleeding.

b. Interruptions of the galea should be closed separately with absorbable suture (4-0 chromic or Vicryl). This is especially important in the frontal area, since the frontalis muscle is anchored to the galea in this area. Closure of the galea also helps prevent infection.

2. Forehead

a. Lacerations perpendicular to dermal creases will leave a more visible scar than those that are parallel.

      b. Place as few dermal absorbable sutures as possible.

      c. Complex lacerations with jagged edges, large flaps and tissue defects are likely to cause large scars. Consider obtaining surgical consultation.

      d. Facial sutures should be removed in 3-5 days to prevent suture marks.

3. Eyebrow

      a. Should never be shaved.

      b. Débride with extreme caution.

      c. Laceration must be carefully aligned.

4. Eyelid

      a. Lacerations interrupting the lid margin, those involving the medial edge of the lid, through-and-through lacerations or those involving muscle should be referred for repair, if possible.

      b. Careful inspection of the eye is necessary to rule out hyphema, corneal abrasion or foreign bodies.

5. Cheek

      a. May result in injury to the facial nerve, parotid duct or parotid gland.

      b. Lacerations extending into the oral cavity should be repaired in two layers: the oral cavity laceration should be repaired first with 5-0 chromic gut or Vicryl, the wound re-irrigated and the skin closed with 6-0 nylon. Prophylactic antibiotics may be given (Pen VK 250-500mg po qid x5d or erythromycin if PCN-allergic).

6. Nose

      a. Septal hematoma should be looked for and incised or aspirated.

      b. If nasal packing is placed, antibiotics are recommended (amoxicillin or TMP-SMX) x 3-5d.

      c. Avulsions, mutilating injuries of the skin or cartilage or amputations of the nose need referral to a plastic surgeon for best results.

7. Ear

      a. Debridement should be very conservative. No cartilage should be left exposed.

      b. Through-and-through lacerations require a layered closure (use 6-0 Vicryl for the cartilage and 5-0 or 6-0 nylon for medial and lateral skin).

      c. Hematomas should be evacuated.

      d. When cartilage is involved or a hematoma has been drained, antibiotic prophylaxis is recommended (dicloxacillin, cephalexin, amoxicillin/clavulanate, erythromycin).

8. Lips

      a. Alignment of the vermilion border is essential.

      b. In a vertical through-and-through laceration involving the orbicularis oris muscle, the muscle is first approximated using 5-0 chromic or Vicryl sutures. Then the vermilion border is aligned and the remainder of the laceration repaired.

    c. Consider antibiotics for lacerations that extend into the oral cavity (Pen VK or erythromycin).

    d. Tooth fragments need to be looked for in the wound if teeth are chipped or absent.

9. Oral cavity

    a. Superficial lacerations <1-2cm don't require closure.

    b. Small lacerations of the tongue do not need closure. Those that gape widely, actively bleed, are flap shaped or involve muscle should be sutured. 4-0 chromic or Vicryl can be used. Sedation may be required, especially in children.

    c. Adults should rinse their mouths with half-strength hydrogen peroxide after meals and at bedtime.

    d. Prophylactic antibiotics (Pen VK, erythromycin x 3-5d) are recommended if sutures are placed.

F. Hand injuries and infections

1. Examination of the hand

    a. Should include visual inspection of the wound and thorough functional testing of nerves and tendons.

    b. X-rays should be done to evaluate for fracture and foreign body.

    c. Nerve testing

        (1) Radial nerve - extension of the wrist and fingers. Test motor function by having the patient dorsiflex the wrist and fingers against resistance. Test pure radial nerve sensory function in the first web space.

        (2) Ulnar nerve - ability of the fingers to spread and close. Test motor function by having the patient adduct his fingers against an object. Test pure ulnar sensory function at the tip of the fifth digit.

        (3) Medial nerve - wrist flexors, thumb opposition. Test motor function by having the patient oppose the thumb with the tip of the little finger against resistance. Test pure median nerve sensory function at the tip of the index finger.

    d. Explore the wound to visualize tendons and do functional testing for both extensor and flexor tendons. Keep in mind the position of the hand at the time of injury.

2. Avulsions and partial amputations

    a. Any fingertip avulsion with <1cm area of tissue loss can be allowed to heal spontaneously.

    b. Larger avulsions or those with bone exposure can be closed if adequate soft tissue is present. Otherwise, skin grafting may be required. Antibiotics should be given if bone is exposed.

    c. For severe crush injuries, amputation of the distal phalanx may be necessary.

3. Nail injuries

a. Subungual hematomas should be evacuated by nail trephination (use cautery, #18 needle or #11 blade). Nail removal should be considered if the nail is partially avulsed, torn or deformed. Nail bed lacerations should be repaired, if present. Subungual hematomas with associated fractures do not need to be treated with antibiotics.

b. Nail bed lacerations should be repaired using 5-0 or 6-0 absorbable suture. The nail should be replaced under the eponychium for temporary splinting purposes. Nonadherent dressing material can also be used (keep in place for 7-10 days).

4. **Tendon lacerations**

a. Flexor tendon lacerations can be repaired primarily up to 3 weeks post injury. These are difficult to do, and should be referred to a hand surgeon, if available.

b. Extensor tendons are more easily repaired and can be done by non-specialists. Use 4-0 nonabsorbable suture in a figure-eight pattern.

c. If a tendon is more than 50% transected, it should be repaired. Lesser injuries can be treated with splinting.

d. A plaster splint should be placed on the palmar surface of the hand and wrist after tendon repair and kept on for 3 weeks. Close follow-up is important.

e. Patients with tendon lacerations should be treated with oral antibiotics (cephalosporin, cloxacillin or clindamycin) for 5-7 days.

5. **Infections**

a. Tenosynovitis

(1) Serious infection of the tendon sheaths of the palm. Prompt treatment is necessary to prevent permanent hand dysfunction.

(2) Treat with adequate surgical drainage, IV antibiotics and postoperative elevation of the hand.

b. Paronychia

(1) Infection of the eponychium, associated with a collection of pus between the eponychium and the nail root.

(2) Usually due to *Streptococcus pyogenes* or *Staphylococcus aureus*.

(3) Drain by inserting a #11 blade between the eponychium and the nail plate, elevating the eponychium. Following drainage, the patient should soak the finger in warm, soapy water twice a day and apply a band-aid.

(4) Antibiotics are unnecessary if the pus is completely drained and there is no surrounding cellulitis. If there is, a cephalosporin or clindamycin can be given for 7 days.

c. Felon

(1) Infection with a collection of pus in the pulp space of the fingertip. The finger pad is swollen and very tender.

(2) Caused by same organisms as a paronychia.

(3) If untreated, may result in necrosis or osteomyelitis.

(4) Drain by making a longitudinal incision directly through the finger pad on the volar surface of the digit. Keep the incision open with a small wick. This can be removed after 48 hours and the patient can then begin soaking the finger.

(5) Antibiotics should be given (cephalosporin or clindamycin).

V. BITE WOUNDS AND INFECTIONS

A. General

1. Dog bites are the most common bites in the US, and probably in other countries as well, followed by cats and humans.
2. The most common complication is infection. Wounds that penetrate deep structures (bones, joints, tendons, vessels, nerves or viscera) are at high risk of infection. Bites to the hand are also at high risk.
3. General management of bite wounds
   a. Cleanse
   b. Irrigate with at least 250cc of normal saline.
   c. Debridement of devitalized tissue and wound edges, if necessary.
   d. Ensure tetanus immunization.
   e. Assess need for rabies immunization.
   f. Treat high risk wounds with prophylactic antibiotics for 3-5 days.
   g. Re-evaluate high risk wounds in 24 hours, others in 48 hours.
   h. Wounds which are already infected at the time of initial evaluation should also be treated with cleansing, debridement and antibiotics (first dose IM or IV).
4. Wound closure
   a. Primary closure of animal bites is controversial.
   b. In general, wounds which can be safely sutured after cleansing are those on the face, scalp, trunk or proximal extremities.
   c. Wounds at risk of infection, such as human bites, cat bites, and hand wounds, are best left open with delayed primary closure at 48-72 hours.
5. Antibiotic therapy
   a. Punctures and high risk bite wounds should be treated prophylactically with amoxicillin/clavulanate, if available. Cephalosporins, penicillin or cloxacillin are reasonable alternatives. Prophylactic antibiotics should be given for 3-5 days.
   b. Infection that develops rapidly (within 12-24 hours after the bite) is usually due to *Pasteurella multocida*. Penicillin G, amoxicillin/clavulanate or cephalosporins are most effective. For patients with PCN allergy, doxycycline +/- clindamycin is effective in adults and TMP/SMX +/- clindamycin in children.
   c. Human bite infections often involve *Eikenella corrodens, which is* sensitive to penicillin, ampicillin and cephalosporins. Amoxicillin/clavulanate is effective in covering Eikenella, as well as Staph.

B. Dog bites

1. Most common on the extremities. In young children, facial lacerations are common.

2. *Pasteurella multocida* causes wound infections within 24 hours with prominent pain and swelling and a serosanguinous, grayish exudate. Other common bacteria found in dog bite wounds are *Enterobacteria, Pseudomonas, Staph. aureus, Bacillus subtilis* and *Strep viridans.*

3. *Capnocytophaga canimorsus* causes sepsis, gangrene, purpura and coagulopathy 7-14 days after dog bites in some patients (especially those who are immunosuppressed or have no spleen). This is a Gram-negative bacillus which responds to penicillin G.

C. Cat bites and scratches

1. Higher incidence of infection than dog bites (about 29% become infected). Cat scratches are bacteriologically similar to cat bites.

2. Organisms include *Pasteurella multocida, Streptococcus viridans,* other strains of streptococcus, *Staphylococcus aureus* and *Bacteroides.*

3. Cat bites should generally be left open. Prophylactic antibiotics are indicated.

4. Established infections should be treated as above.

D. Cat-scratch disease

1. Caused by a Gram-negative organism transmitted by scratch, lick or bite of cats most commonly, occasionally dogs.

2. Patients with cat-scratch disease are not initially ill-appearing. After 3-10 days, a tender papule develops at the site of the scratch. After 2 weeks, regional lymphadenopathy, fever, malaise and headache develop.

3. Spontaneous resolution occurs in a few weeks to months. There is controversy over whether antibiotics are needed or not. Doxycycline and rifampin, ciprofloxacin and erythromycin are all effective.

E. Human bites

1. Most common pathogens are *Streptococcus* and *Staphylococcus aureus. Eikenella corrodens,* an anerobe, is common in human bite infections, especially those with a long interval between injury and treatment.

2. Bites to the hand are common, especially the "clenched fist" injury which occurs when a person strikes someone in the mouth. The teeth often penetrate the joint space or tendon sheath of the MCP joint and are at high risk of infection.

3. Management

   a. Patients with deep or full thickness human bites to the hand should receive IV/IM antibiotics (cefazolin, ceftriaxone), wound cleansing and hospital admission or close outpatient follow up.

   b. Patients with human bite infections more than 24 hours old should have exploration and drainage, as well as antibiotics.

VI. SNAKE BITE
A. Local manifestations
1. Local swelling usually begins immediately, reaching a maximum in 2-3 days.
2. Pain may be present, but is usually mild. Rarely, injectable analgesics are needed.
3. Bleeding may occur at the site of the bite and into the affected extremity.
4. Local tissue necrosis may occur depending on the amount and type of venom. Sloughing of necrotic tissue and secondary infections (including osteomyelitis) occur in subsequent weeks and months.

B. Systemic manifestations
1. Shortness of breath, tachycardia, hyperventilation, and chest pain are virtually always due to fear associated with the snakebite.
2. The onset of systemic manifestations is variable (from 1/2 to 24 hours).
3. Cardiovascular abnormalities (hypotension, shock, ECG changes, pulmonary edema) may occur as a direct cardiovascular effect of the venom, or secondarily due to vasodilatation and hypovolemia (from capillary leak and bleeding).
4. Spontaneous hemorrhage may occur secondary to DIC, thrombocytopenia, and effects on vessel walls. Checking for the presence of non-clotting blood is a useful bedside test.
5. Neurotoxicity is produced by alteration of neuromuscular junction function. This may lead to respiratory failure as a result of paralysis of respiratory muscles.
6. Other problems include rhabdomyolysis and impaired renal function.

C. Management
1. Pre-hospital treatment
   a. Reassure the patient.
   b. Immobilize the affected limb (apply an ace or crepe wrap firmly over the involved extremity). Other forms of local treatment (incisions, suction, tourniquets, etc.) have not proven beneficial.
   c. For spitting cobra venom in the eyes, wash the eyes with large amounts of water.
   d. Local pain can be controlled with paracetamol or acetaminophen (aspirin may exacerbate hematological problems). For severe pain, use pethidine or pentazocine SQ or IV (avoid IM injections).
   e. If the patient is vomiting, aspiration precautions should be observed. Antiemetics may also be used.
   f. For hypotension/bronchoconstriction, give epinephrine (1mg/ml) 0.5cc SQ.
2. Definitive treatment
   a. Remove the tourniquet or compressive dressing. Elevate the limb.
   b. Débride the necrotic tissue from the involved area. Apply appropriate dressings. Observe for signs of infection.

    c. Closely observe the patient for:
      (1) Progressive swelling in the involved extremity - measure the circumference.
      (2) Monitor vital signs closely - watch for signs of shock, or respiratory depression.
      (3) Observe for abnormal bleeding, follow the Hgb.
      (4) Observe urine output for development of renal failure.
    d. Early use of antibiotics is not indicated. If necessary later, cover for Gm (-) rods, anaerobes, and Clostridia.

3. Antivenin use
    a. Indications for antivenin
      (1) Any signs of systemic envenoming listed above for up to 72 hours after the bite.
      (2) Usefulness of antivenin to prevent local necrosis is less certain. When marked swelling of an extremity occurs within four hours of being bitten, antivenin should be given.
    b. Administration
      (1) Dilute the antiserum in saline.
      (2) Begin the infusion slowly, and observe the patient closely for reaction. Increase the rate, and complete the infusion over 1-2 hours.
      (3) Children are given the same dose as adults.
      (4) Antivenin is contraindicated in the presence of known allergy, except in life-threatening bites. Serum sensitivity tests are unreliable. Consider premedicating the patient with epinephrine. Treat allergic reactions aggressively. For mild reactions (urticaria, nausea), give antihistamines. For severe reactions (bronchospasm, hypotension), give SQ epinephrine. Have a syringe of epinephrine available when the infusion is started.
      (5) If the patient does not improve after the first infusion, consider repeating the dose.

4. The effects of snake venom are complex, with some types of venom producing more than one effect. Attention should be paid both to the local and systemic effects of the bite.

VII. TRAUMA - (Printed with permission from The Advanced Trauma Life Support Course - American College of Surgeons)
  A. Initial care
    1. Primary survey - identify life-threatening conditions, treat simultaneously.
      A - Airway - maintain an adequate airway by lifting the chin, removing airway secretions, and inserting an oral or nasal airway. Maintain control of the cervical spine.
      B - Breathing and ventilation - use high flow oxygen, if necessary

support with bag ventilation. Intubate the patient, if necessary. If the airway cannot be secured and maintained secondary to upper airway trauma, perform a cricothyroidotomy.

C - Circulation with hemorrhage control - control hemorrhage. Evaluate the patient for shock (see below). Insert two large bore IV catheters. Begin crystalloid administration. If shock is present, give 1-2 liters of fluid or 20 ml/kg in children.

D - Disability - neurologic status. Evaluate using the Glasgow Coma Scale (see below), and observe the patient closely for changes in neurologic status.

E - Expose - undress the patient.

2. **Secondary survey** - re-evaluate the patient.
   a. Review the history, including mechanism of injury, and time of last meal.
   b. Monitor the vital signs.
   c. Perform a detailed physical exam looking for abnormalities in each region (head, neck, chest, abdomen, extremities, and neurologic exam).

3. Draw blood for appropriate laboratory testing - CBC, at a minimum.
4. Provide definitive care for all injuries.
5. Document injuries and treatment.

B. Shock

1. Definition - any abnormality of the circulatory system that results in inadequate organ perfusion.
2. Pathophysiology
   a. Progressive vasoconstriction occurs in response to blood loss. Tachycardia is the earliest sign.
   b. Hypoperfusion results in metabolic acidosis (lactic acidosis).
   c. Treat with oxygen, fluids and blood.
3. Types of shock
   a. Hemorrhagic - the most common type in trauma patients.
   b. Cardiogenic - cardiac dysfunction may result from cardiac contusion, tamponade, or tension pneumothorax. Myocardial infarction is uncommon.
   c. Neurogenic - not associated with head injury. Spinal cord injury may result in hypotension due to loss of sympathetic tone.
   d. Septic - unusual initially, but may occur within hours of injury, especially with abdominal injuries.
4. Classification and management of hemorrhagic shock

Classification and Management of Hemorrhagic Shock				
	Class I	**Class II**	**Class III**	**Class IV**
Blood loss (ml)	up to 750 ml	750-1000	1500-3000	2000 or more
Blood loss (%BV)	up to 15%	15-30%	30-40%	40% or more
Pulse rate	< 100	> 100	> 120	140 or higher
Blood pressure	normal	normal	decreased	decreased
Pulse pressure	normal or increased	decreased	decreased	decreased
Capillary refill test*	normal	positive	positive	positive
Respiratory rate	14-20	20-30	30-40	> 35
Urine output (ml/hr)	30 or more	20-30	5-15	negligible
CNS-Mental status	slightly anxious	mildly anxious	anxious & confused	confused-lethargic
Fluid replacement (Three for one rule)**	crystalloid	crystalloid	crystalloid + blood	crystalloid + blood

*Capillary refill test - depress fingernail, normal color returns within 2 seconds (not valid in hypothermic patients).
**Three for one rule - blood loss may require 300 ml of fluid replacement for each 100 ml of volume lost. Monitor the patient closely to avoid over and under replacement.

C. Chest trauma
1. General
    a. Perform primary assessment and resuscitation as above.
    b. Maintain adequate oxygenation using supplemental oxygen.
    c. Deal with immediately life-threatening injuries first before dealing with other problems.
    d. Most life-threatening chest injuries can be adequately managed with an appropriately placed chest tube.
2. Types of chest injuries
    a. Simple pneumothorax
      (1) Defined as the presence of air in the pleural space.
      (2) Diagnosed by finding hyperresonance on percussion of the chest and decreased breath sounds on the involved side of the chest. Expiratory chest x-ray shows displacement of lung from the chest wall.
      (3) Treatment is insertion of a chest tube and connection to a bottle with underwater seal.
    b. Tension pneumothorax
      (1) Results from increased intra-thoracic pressure as a result of a "one way valve" air leak into the pleural cavity.
      (2) Causes shifting of the heart and mediastinum away from the side of the pneumothorax, with compromise of cardiac and pulmonary function.

(3) Treatment is immediate decompression by insertion of a needle into the pleural space in the second intercostal interspace, then insert a chest tube.

c. Open pneumothorax - "sucking chest wound"
  (1) Results from large injuries to the chest wall with a persistent opening into the pleural space and free air movement in and out of the pleural space with respiration.
  (2) Treatment is covering the wound with an occlusive dressing (Vaseline gauze). The dressing is taped on only three sides to allow air to escape during expiration. A chest tube may also be placed at a second site.

d. Massive hemothorax
  (1) Greater than 1500 ml of blood in the pleural space.
  (2) Usually results from penetrating injury of the chest with injury to the major vessels.
  (3) Treatment is rapid volume expansion and transfusion. Consider autotransfusion. Usually requires emergent thoracotomy.

e. Rib fractures
  (1) Motion of the rib cage produces pain, the most common problem. Splinting of the chest wall may result in atelectasis and lung infection.
  (2) Fracture of ribs 1-3 usually indicates severe trauma. Look for other associated injuries.
  (3) Suspect when local tenderness, pain on palpation, and crepitus are present. Confirm with chest x-ray.
  (4) Treatment is adequate analgesia. Taping and rib belts are not recommended.

f. Pulmonary contusion
  (1) Produces hypoxia secondary to lung injury. Looks similar to ARDS.
  (2) Intubation and ventilation are required if respiratory failure occurs.

g. Flail chest
  (1) Results from severe chest wall trauma, with multiple rib fractures resulting in paradoxical chest wall movement during respiration. Hypoxia is multifactorial, but mainly results from the underlying pulmonary contusion.
  (2) Diagnosis is made by recognizing the presence of multiple rib fractures on exam or x-ray, and the presence of respiratory failure.
  (3) Treatment is oxygen. Use care when administering fluids to avoid overhydration. Intubation and ventilation are frequently required.

h. Cardiac injury
  (1) Cardiac tamponade

(a) Usually secondary to penetrating injuries, less commonly due to blunt trauma. Significant tamponade may be produced by small amounts of blood in an acute setting.

(b) Look for increased venous pressure, decreased arterial blood pressure, and muffled heart tones. Check for a pulsus paradoxus (decrease in systolic blood pressure of > 10 mm Hg with inspiration), or Kussmaul's sign (a raise in venous pressure with inspiration).

(c) Treatment is pericardiocentesis via a subxiphoid approach. Use a #16-18 gauge 6 inch needle + plastic catheter. Watch for an injury pattern on ECG monitor. Insert the needle to the left of the xiphoid process, and aim at the tip of the left scapula. Removal of small amounts (15-20 ml) of blood may be helpful.

(2) Myocardial contusion - suspect in the setting of chest trauma with ECG abnormalities (ST segment changes, bundle branch block), cardiac arrhythmias (atrial or ventricular), or myocardial enzyme elevation. Close observation with cardiac monitoring is required.

i. Subcutaneous emphysema - results from injury to the airway or lung with dissection of air into the subcutaneous tissues. No specific treatment is indicated.

D. Abdominal trauma

1. **History** - look for time and mechanism of injury (blunt or penetrating trauma).

2. **Physical exam**
   a. Perform a careful exam looking for abdominal pain, tenderness, or rigidity.
   b. Look for signs of hypovolemia - tachycardia, hypotension, and shock.
   c. The patient must be fully undressed.
   d. Inspect the abdomen, chest, and back for signs of trauma.
   e. Auscultate the abdomen for presence of bowel sounds and the chest for breath sounds.
   f. Percuss the abdomen for tenderness, or areas of dullness.
   g. Palpate the abdomen for signs of peritoneal irritation - tenderness, guarding, rebound tenderness.
   h. Perform a rectal exam for presence of blood, palpable fractures, displacement of the prostate.

3. **Lab** - CBC + amylase.

4. **Management**
   a. Stabilize the patient as outlined above.
   b. Insert:
      (1) If the patient is in shock at least one or two large-bore IVs.
      (2) Foley catheter - look for adequate urine output and bleeding. A suprapubic catheter should be used if scrotal or urethral trauma is suspected, or the prostate is displaced.
      (3) Nasogastric tube - look for bleeding.

c. Obtain abdominal x-rays - chest, flat and upright abdominal films. Look for free air under the diaphragms.

d. Consider peritoneal lavage if the diagnosis is unclear (>95% accurate for intra-abdominal injury)

(1) Insert a small catheter into the peritoneal cavity.

(2) Aspirate for free blood - more than 10-20 cc is positive.

(3) Infuse one liter of IV fluid (NS or LR).

(4) Turn the patient side to side to ensure adequate mixing.

(5) Lower the IV container to drain fluid from the peritoneal cavity.

(6) The lavage is positive if > 100,000 RBCs or 500 WBCs/mm are present in the fluid.

5. Definitive treatment

a. Alert patient, benign examination - observation.

b. Unclear diagnosis - do peritoneal lavage

(1) If negative, observation.

(2) If positive, abdominal exploration.

(3) Patients with unexplained hypotension or blood loss, or overt peritoneal irritation should undergo laparotomy.

(4) At laparotomy, look for injury to bowel, liver, spleen, pancreas, retroperitoneal hematoma.

c. Penetrating abdominal trauma - look for:

(1) Wounding agent - stab wounds cause intraabdominal injury in 30-40% of cases, gunshot wounds cause injury in > 90% of cases.

(2) If the abdominal pain is stable, no peritoneal signs are present, perform local wound exploration, and peritoneal lavage. If peritoneal cavity is penetrated or lavage is positive, perform laparotomy.

(3) If shock, or peritoneal signs are present, perform exploratory laparotomy.

(4) If gunshot wounds penetrate the peritoneum, perform exploratory laparotomy.

E. Head trauma

1. Obtain a detailed history of the injury; especially identify the type of trauma.

2. Monitor the vital signs (hypertension with bradycardia may reflect increasing intracranial pressure).

3. Physical exam

a. Assess pupillary function - response to light should be brisk. Pupils should be equal within 1 mm in size.

b. Look for lateralized extremity weakness - abnormality suggests intracranial mass lesion.

c. Glasgow coma scales - perform serially. Decrease in the score of more than 2 points indicates deterioration.

Glasgow Coma Scale		
Best motor response	Obeys	M 6
	Localizes	M 5
	Withdraws	M 4
	Abnormal flexion - decorticate posture	M 3
	Extensor response - decerebrate posture	M 2
	No movement	M 1
Verbal response	Oriented	V 5
	Confused	V 4
	Inappropriate words	V 3
	Incomprehensible sounds	V 2
	None	V 1
Eye opening	Spontaneous	E 4
	To speech	E 3
	To pain	E 2
	None	E 1

   d. Definitions
- (1) Coma - the absence of eye opening, inability to follow commands, and lack of word verbalization (E 1, M 1-5, V 1).
- (2) Severe head injury - GCS of ≤ 8.
- (3) Moderate head injury - GCS of 9-12.
- (4) Minor head injury - GCS of 13-15.

4. Types of head injury
   a. Skull fractures
- (1) Presence of a fracture identifies a patient at high risk for intracranial hematoma. Fractures are not always associated with severe intracranial injury.
- (2) Types of fractures
  - (a) Linear non-depressed - requires no specific treatment.
  - (b) Depressed - evaluate for underlying brain injury. Bone fragment should be elevated if depressed more than the thickness of the skull.
  - (c) Open - directly communicates with brain through the dura. Bone fragments should be removed or elevated, and dura closed.
  - (d) Basal skull fractures - diagnosis is made by the presence of CSF leaking from the ear or nose, ecchymosis in the mastoid area, or in the periorbital area.

   b. Diffuse brain injuries - occur with rapid head acceleration and deceleration, producing diffuse brain dysfunction.
- (1) Concussion - injury that results in brief neurological dysfunction (confusion, amnesia, or loss of consciousness). The patient complains of headache, dizziness, nausea but has no localizing signs. There is no specific treatment, but the patient should be

closely observed for the following 24 hours for development of additional neurologic problems.
    (2) Diffuse axonal injury (closed head injury) - resembles a severe concussion. Deep coma is present which lasts for days to weeks. Decorticate or decerebrate posturing may be present. Autonomic dysfunction with fever, hypertension, or sweating may be present. CT scan shows no mass lesion. Mortality is up to 50%.
  c. Focal injuries - severe injury to a small local area.
    (1) Contusion - frequently are associated with concussions. Location is near the area of impact or on the opposite side of the brain. CT scanning is necessary to distinguish from concussion. Diagnosis is important because of the possibility of neurological progression from edema or bleeding. Herniation and brain stem dysfunction may occur. Alcoholic patients are more likely to develop bleeding late.
    (2) Intracranial hemorrhage - presentation is variable due to the site and rapidity of bleeding. CT scanning is necessary to localize the site of bleeding.
      (a) Epidural hemorrhage - usually results from laceration of a dural artery (middle meningeal artery). Presents with an initial loss of consciousness, followed at times by a lucid period. A secondary loss of consciousness then occurs, followed by development of hemiparesis of the side opposite the injury, with a dilated pupil on the side of injury. Treatment is emergent surgery to remove the hematoma.
      (b) Acute subdural hematoma - common injury resulting from tearing of veins in the subdural area. Prognosis is poor from associated brain injury. Treatment is emergent surgery to evacuate the hematoma.
      (c) Subarachnoid hemorrhage - produces bloody CSF and meningeal irritation. Other symptoms include sudden severe headache, loss of consciousness, seizures. Treatment includes bed rest, stool softeners, and analgesics. Blood pressure is controlled to keep the systolic pressure < 140 mmHg. Administration of a calcium channel blocker (nimodipine 60 mg q 4 hours) may decrease the incidence of cerebral vasospasm.
      (d) Brain hemorrhage and laceration - types include intracerebral hematoma, impalement injuries, and bullet wounds. Treatment requires definitive neurosurgery.
5. Treatment of increased intracranial pressure
  a. Avoid overhydration.
  b. Steroids - dexamethasone 4-8 mg IV q 6 hours.
  c. Diuretics - mannitol 1gm/kg or furosemide 40-80mg IV.
  d. Induced hypocapnia - probably most helpful. Requires intubation and hyperventilation . Maintain the pCO_2 at 26-28 mmHg.

The growth chart

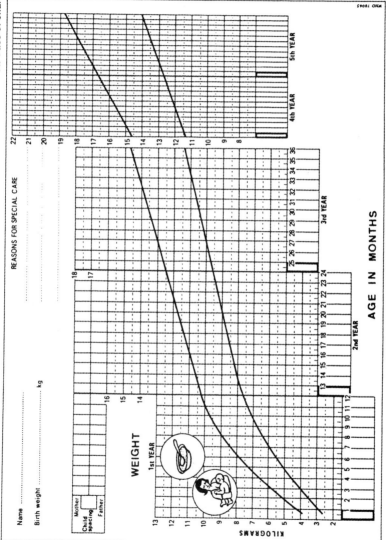

GROWTH CHART

Health centre | **Child's No.**

Child's name

Date first seen | **Birthday**

Mother's name | Registration No.

Father's name | Registration No.

Where the family lives (address)

BROTHERS AND SISTERS

Year/birth	Boy/Girl	Remarks	Year/birth	Boy/Girl	Remarks

IMMUNIZATIONS

TUBERCULOSIS Vaccine (BCG) - Date :

DIPHTHERIA, WHOOPING COUGH, TETANUS Vaccine (DPT)

Date : 1 dose   2 dose
       3 dose

POLIOMYELITIS Vaccine (OPV)

Date : 1 dose   2 dose
       3 dose

MEASLES Vaccine-Date :

OTHER Vaccines (specify with date) :

APPOINTMENTS

Has the mother had her tetanus vaccine?

Date: 1st dose   2nd dose

Repeat dose

Fig. 12. WHO prototype growth chart (reverse)

WHO 78066

World Health Organization. *The Growth Chart: A tool for use in infant and child heath care.* Switzerland, 1996.

432

NCHS/WHO normalized reference values for weight-for-height and weight-for-length

Boys' weight (kg)					Length[a] (cm)	Girls' weight (kg)				
-4 SD	-3 SD	-2 SD	-1 SD	Median	Median	Median	-1 SD	-2 SD	-3 SD	-4 SD
1.8	2.1	2.5	2.8	3.1	49	3.3	2.9	2.6	2.2	1.8
1.8	2.2	2.5	2.9	3.3	50	3.4	3.0	2.6	2.3	1.9
1.8	2.2	2.6	3.1	3.5	51	3.5	3.1	2.7	2.3	1.9
1.9	2.3	2.8	3.2	3.7	52	3.7	3.3	2.8	2.4	2.0
1.9	2.4	2.9	3.4	3.9	53	3.9	3.4	3.0	2.5	2.1
2.0	2.6	3.1	3.6	4.1	54	4.1	3.6	3.1	2.7	2.2
2.2	2.7	3.3	3.8	4.3	55	4.3	3.8	3.3	2.8	2.3
2.3	2.9	3.5	4.0	4.6	56	4.5	4.0	3.5	3.0	2.4
2.5	3.1	3.7	4.3	4.8	57	4.8	4.2	3.7	3.1	2.6
2.7	3.3	3.9	4.5	5.1	58	5.0	4.4	3.9	3.3	2.7
2.9	3.5	4.1	4.8	5.4	59	5.3	4.7	4.1	3.5	2.9
3.1	3.7	4.4	5.0	5.7	60	5.5	4.9	4.3	3.7	3.1
3.3	4.0	4.6	5.3	5.9	61	5.8	5.2	4.6	3.9	3.3
3.5	4.2	4.9	5.6	6.2	62	6.1	5.4	4.8	4.1	3.5
3.8	4.5	5.2	5.8	6.5	63	6.4	5.7	5.0	4.4	3.7
4.0	4.7	5.4	6.1	6.8	64	6.7	6.0	5.3	4.6	3.9
4.3	5.0	5.7	6.4	7.1	65	7.0	6.3	5.5	4.8	4.1
4.5	5.3	6.0	6.7	7.4	66	7.3	6.5	5.8	5.1	4.3
4.8	5.5	6.2	7.0	7.7	67	7.5	6.8	6.0	5.3	4.5
5.1	5.8	6.5	7.3	8.0	68	7.8	7.1	6.3	5.5	4.8
5.3	6.0	6.8	7.5	8.3	69	8.1	7.3	6.5	5.8	5.0
5.5	6.3	7.0	7.8	8.5	70	8.4	7.6	6.8	6.0	5.2
5.8	6.5	7.3	8.1	8.8	71	8.6	7.8	7.0	6.2	5.4
6.0	6.8	7.5	8.3	9.1	72	8.9	8.1	7.2	6.4	5.6
6.2	7.0	7.8	8.6	9.3	73	9.1	8.3	7.5	6.6	5.8
6.4	7.2	8.0	8.8	9.6	74	9.4	8.5	7.7	6.8	6.0
6.6	7.4	8.2	9.0	9.8	75	9.6	8.7	7.9	7.0	6.2
6.8	7.6	8.4	9.2	10.0	76	9.8	8.9	8.1	7.2	6.4
7.0	7.8	8.6	9.4	10.3	77	10.0	9.1	8.3	7.4	6.6
7.1	8.0	8.8	9.7	10.5	78	10.2	9.3	8.5	7.6	6.7
7.3	8.2	9.0	9.9	10.7	79	10.4	9.5	8.7	7.8	6.9
7.5	8.3	9.2	10.1	10.9	80	10.6	9.7	8.8	8.0	7.1
7.6	8.5	9.4	10.2	11.1	81	10.8	9.9	9.0	8.1	7.2
7.8	8.7	9.6	10.4	11.3	82	11.0	10.1	9.2	8.3	7.4
7.9	8.8	9.7	10.6	11.5	83	11.2	10.3	9.4	8.5	7.6
8.1	9.0	9.9	10.8	11.7	84	11.4	10.5	9.6	8.7	7.7

SD: standard deviation score (or Z-score). Although the interpretation of a fixed percent-of-median value varies across age and height, and generally the two scales cannot be compared, the approximate percent-of-median values for -1 and -2 SD are 90% and 80% of median, respectively (Gorstein J et al. Issues in the assessment of nutritional status using anthropometry. *Bulletin of the World Health Organization*, 1994, 72:273–283).

[a] Length is measured for children below 85 cm. For children 85 cm or more, height is measured. Recumbent length is on average 0.5 cm greater than standing height; although the difference is of no importance to individual children, a correction may be made by subtracting 0.5 cm from all lengths above 84.9 cm if standing height cannot be measured.

Continued on next page.

Boys' weight (kg)					Height[a] (cm)	Girls' weight (kg)				
−4 SD	−3 SD	−2 SD	−1 SD	Median		Median	−1 SD	−2 SD	−3 SD	−4 SD
7.8	8.9	9.9	11.0	12.1	85	11.8	10.8	9.7	8.6	7.6
7.9	9.0	10.1	11.2	12.3	86	12.0	11.0	9.9	8.8	7.7
8.1	9.2	10.3	11.5	12.6	87	12.3	11.2	10.1	9.0	7.9
8.3	9.4	10.5	11.7	12.8	88	12.5	11.4	10.3	9.2	8.1
8.4	9.6	10.7	11.9	13.0	89	12.7	11.6	10.5	9.3	8.2
8.6	9.8	10.9	12.1	13.3	90	12.9	11.8	10.7	9.5	8.4
8.8	9.9	11.1	12.3	13.5	91	13.2	12.0	10.8	9.7	8.5
8.9	10.1	11.3	12.5	13.7	92	13.4	12.2	11.0	9.9	8.7
9.1	10.3	11.5	12.8	14.0	93	13.6	12.4	11.2	10.0	8.8
9.2	10.5	11.7	13.0	14.2	94	13.9	12.6	11.4	10.2	9.0
9.4	10.7	11.9	13.2	14.5	95	14.1	12.9	11.6	10.4	9.1
9.6	10.9	12.1	13.4	14.7	96	14.3	13.1	11.8	10.6	9.3
9.7	11.0	12.4	13.7	15.0	97	14.6	13.3	12.0	10.7	9.5
9.9	11.2	12.6	13.9	15.2	98	14.9	13.5	12.2	10.9	9.6
10.1	11.4	12.8	14.1	15.5	99	15.1	13.8	12.4	11.1	9.8
10.3	11.6	13.0	14.4	15.7	100	15.4	14.0	12.7	11.3	9.9
10.4	11.8	13.2	14.6	16.0	101	15.6	14.3	12.9	11.5	10.1
10.6	12.0	13.4	14.9	16.3	102	15.9	14.5	13.1	11.7	10.3
10.8	12.2	13.7	15.1	16.6	103	16.2	14.7	13.3	11.9	10.5
11.0	12.4	13.9	15.4	16.9	104	16.5	15.0	13.5	12.1	10.6
11.2	12.7	14.2	15.6	17.1	105	16.7	15.3	13.8	12.3	10.8
11.4	12.9	14.4	15.9	17.4	106	17.0	15.5	14.0	12.5	11.0
11.6	13.1	14.7	16.2	17.7	107	17.3	15.8	14.3	12.7	11.2
11.8	13.4	14.9	16.5	18.0	108	17.6	16.1	14.5	13.0	11.4
12.0	13.6	15.2	16.8	18.3	109	17.9	16.4	14.8	13.2	11.6
12.2	13.8	15.4	17.1	18.7	110	18.2	16.6	15.0	13.4	11.9

SD: standard deviation score (or Z-score). Although the interpretation of a fixed percent-of-median value varies across age and height, and generally the two scales cannot be compared, the approximate percent-of-median values for −1 and −2 SD are 90% and 80% of median, respectively (Gorstein J et al. Issues in the assessment of nutritional status using anthropometry. *Bulletin of the World Health Organization,* 1994, 72:273–283).

[a] Length is measured for children below 85 cm. For children 85 cm or more, height is measured. Recumbent length is on average 0.5 cm greater than standing height; although the difference is of no importance to individual children, a correction may be made by subtracting 0.5 cm from all lengths above 84.9 cm if standing height cannot be measured.

World Health Organization. *Management of severe malnutrition: a manual for physicians and other senior health workers.* England, 1999.

Composition of Mineral and Vitamin Mixes

Mineral Mix Solution	
Substance	**Amount**
Potassium chloride	89.5gm
Tripotassium citrate	32.4gm
Magnesium chloride	30.5gm
Zinc acetate	3.3gm
Copper sulfate	0.56gm
Sodium selenate	10mg
Potassium iodide	5mg
Water to make	1000ml

The above solution can be stored at room temperature. It is added to ReSoMal or liquid feed at a concentration of 20ml/litre.

Vitamin Mix	
Vitamin	**Amount per litre of liquid diet**
Water-soluble	
Thiamine (vitamin B1)	0.7mg
Riboflavin (vitamin B2)	2.0mg
Nicotinic acid	10mg
Pyridoxine (vitamin B6)	0.7mg
Cyanocobalamin (vitamin B12)	1µg
Folic acid	0.35mg
Ascorbic acid (vitamin C)	100mg
Pantothenic acid (vitamin B5)	3mg
Biotin	0.1mg
Fat-soluble:	
Retinol (vitamin A)	1.5mg
Calciferol (vitamin D)	30µg
a-tocopherol (vitamin E)	22mg
Vitamin K	40µg

Preparation of F-75 and F-100 Diets

Using dry skimmed milk		
Ingredient	**Amount**	
	F-75	**F-100**
Dried skimmed milk	25grams	80grams
Sugar	70grams	50grams
Cereal flour	35grams	-----
Vegetable oil	27grams	60grams
Mineral mix	20ml	20ml
Vitamin mix	140mg	140mg
Water to make	1000ml	1000ml

Using whole dried milk		
Ingredient	**Amount**	
	F-75	**F-100**
Whole dried milk	35grams	110grams
Sugar	70grams	50grams
Cereal flour	35grams	-----
Vegetable oil	17grams	30grams
Mineral mix	20ml	20ml
Vitamin mix	140mg	140mg
Water to make	1000ml	1000ml

Using fresh cows' milk		
Ingredient	**Amount**	
	F-75	**F-100**
Fresh cows' milk	300ml	880ml
Sugar	70grams	75grams
Cereal flour	35grams	-----
Vegetable oil	17grams	20grams
Mineral mix	20ml	20ml
Vitamin mix	140mg	140mg
Water to make	1000ml	1000ml

To prepare the F-75 diet, add the milk, sugar, cereal flour and oil to some water and mix. Boil for 5-7 minutes. Allow to cool, then add the mineral mix and vitamin mix and mix again. Make up the volume to 1000ml with water.

To prepare the F-100 diet, add the milk, sugar and oil to some warm boiled water and mix. Add the mineral mix and vitamin mix and mix again. Make up the volume to 1000ml with water.

A multivitamin supplement can be given instead of the vitamin mix. Alternatively, a combined mineral and vitamin mix for malnourished children is available commercially and can be used in the above diets.

The F-75 formula contains 75kcal and 0.9g protein/100ml
The F-100 formula contains 100kcal and 2.9g protein/100ml

Formulary

Drug Name	Dosage
acetazolamide (Diamox) 250 mg tab	250-1000 mg PO daily in divided doses
acyclovir 200 mg caps, 250 mg inj	HSV - 200 mg 5x/day HZV - 800 mg 5 x/day
albendazole 200 mg tab	Adult: 400 mg as single dose. Child - same dose
albuterol (salbutamol) 2, 4 mg tab, 0.5 mg/ml inj, 100 mcg/dose inhaler	Adults: 2-4 mg PO tid. SQ/IM/IV: 250-500 mcg q 4 hrs prn. Pediatric dosage: 0.1 mg/kg/dose PO tid. Nebulized: 2.5-5 mg qid; Inhaler: 1-2 puffs qid.
allopurinol (Zyloprim)100 mg tab	300-800 mg/day PO in divided doses
aminophylline 100 mg tabs, 250 mg/amp inj	Loading dose: 5 mg/kg over 15-20 min. Maintenance: 10-20 mg/kg/day in divided doses q 6-8 hours.
amitriptyline (Elavil) 25 mg tab	Initially: 50-75 mg/day; max: 150-300 mg/day, usually given as single dose at HS
amoxicillin (Amoxil, Polymox) 250 mg tab, 125 mg/5 ml susp	Adults: 250-500 mg PO q 8 hrs Child: 20-50 mg/kg/day PO in divided doses q 8 hrs
amoxicillin/clavulanate 250-875/125 mg tab	Adult: 500-875 mg q 12 hrs. Child: 20-40 mg/kg/day in divided doses q 8 hrs
ampicillin inj	Adult: 500 mg-2000 mg IV q 4-6 hrs Child: 100-400 mg/kg/day in divided doses q 4-6 hrs
arthemether 80 mg/amp inj	3.2 mg/kg IM stat, 1.6 mg/kg q24h until able to take oral meds.
artusenate 50 mg tab or IV	PO - 4 mg / kg daily x 5-7 days, IV - 2 mg/kg stat, 1 mg/kg at 12 hours, 1 mg/kg daily until oral Rx possible
aspirin 100-500 mg tab	Analgesia: 325-650 mg q 4-6 hrs; Anti-inflammatory: 2.4-3.6 gm/day increased gradually to 3.6-5.4 gm/day. Child: 60-90 mg/kg/day
atenolol (Tenormin) 50, 100 mg tab	25-100 mg PO q day
atropine 1 mg inj	0.01 mg/kg/dose IM q 4 hrs prn; max: 0.4 mg/dose
beclomethasone 50, 250 ug per dose	1-4 puffs q 6 hrs
benzathine penicillin 2.4 mu/vial inj	Adult: 1.2-2.4 mu IM (duration 2-4 wks) Child: <27 kg 300,000-600,000 u, larger child 900,000 u
benzylpenicillin (penicillin G) inj	Adult: up to 24 mu/24 hrs IV in divided doses q 2-4 hrs Child: 62,500-400,000 u/kg/day in divided doses q 4-6 hrs
biperiden 2 mg tab	For Parkinson's Dz - 1 mg PO tid-qid, max 16 mg/day
bisacodyl (Dulcolax) 5 mg tab	5-15 mg PO daily prn; rectally: 10 mg suppository prn
bupivacaine 0.25%	Max: 60 ml of solution
calcium gluconate 10% 10ml	1 amp slow IV push (max 50 mg/min - ½ ml of 10% sol)
calcium lactate 300 mg tab	800-1500 mg/day

Formulary (continued)

Drug Name	Dosage
captopril (Capoten) 25, 50 mg tabs	25-50 mg PO tid (begin at 6.25 or 12.5 mg bid)
carbamazepine (Tegretol) 100, 200 mg tab	Initially: 100-400 mg PO in 1-2 doses, increased to 600-1200 mg/day in divided doses. Max 2 gm/day
carbimazole 5 mg tab	30-60 mg/day until euthyroid, then 5-15 mg/day
cefixime 200 mg tab	Adult: 400 mg/day divided q 12-24 hrs Child: 8 mg/kg/day divided q 12-24 hrs
cefotaxime	Adult: 1-2 gm IM/IV q 6-8 hrs Child: 50-75 mg/kg IM/IV q 6-8 hrs
ceftriaxone 250 mg/amp	Adult: 1-2 gm q day IV Child: 50-100 mg/kg IV/IM divided 1-2 doses
cefuroxime 250 mg/amp	Adult: 0.75-1.5 g IM/IV q 8 hrs Child: 50-100 mg/kg/d IM/IV divided q 8 hrs
chloramphenicol 250 mg tab, 125 mg/5ml Susp, 1 Gm inj	Adult & Child: 50-100 mg/kg/24 hrs IV/PO (not IM) in divided doses q 6 hrs Max 4 gm/d. PO and IV administration achieve equivalent blood levels Neonates: 25mg/kg/24 hrs
chloroquine 100 mg tab, 200 mg/5 ml inj	Treatment: 10 mg/kg PO initially, then 5 mg/kg in 6 hrs and daily times two days. Prophylaxis: 300 mg or 5 mg/kg weekly (dose calculated as base). Parenteral: 5-10 mg/kg IM or very slowly IV (watch for hypotension), then 5 mg/kg IM or IV q 12 hours until oral drugs can be given or to a total of 25mg/kg.
chlorpheniramine (Chlor-Trimeton) 4 mg tab	Adult: 4 mg PO q 4-6 hrs Child: 0.4 mg/kg/day
chlorpromazine 25 mg tab, 50 mg/2 ml inj	0.5-2 mg/kg/dose q 4-6 hrs
chlorpropamide (Diabinese) 250 mg tab	100-500mg/d 1x/d. Max 750mg per day
cimetidine (Tagamet) 200 mg tab	300 mg IM/IV q 6 hrs; 2-400mg bid; maintenance: 400-800 mg hs
ciprofloxacin 250, 500 mg tab	250-750 mg bid
clindamycin (Cleocin) 150 mg caps, inj	Adult: 150-450 mg PO qid, 300-900 mg IV q 6 hrs Child: 25-40 mg/kg IV/IM in divided doses q 6-8 hrs
clofazimine 50, 100 mg tab	Antileprotic - 300 mg PO monthly supervised + 50 - 100 mg/day unsupervised
clonidine (Catapres)	0.1-0.3 mg PO bid
clotrimazole (Mycelex, Gyne-Lotrimin) 1% Cream	Topical - 1% cream applied bid; Vaginal - 100 mg tabs at hs x 7 days or 500 mg hs x 1 dose
cloxacillin 250 mg tab, 250 mg/vial inj	Adult: 250-500 mg PO/IM/IV q 4-6 hrs Child: 50-100 mg/kg/day in divided doses q 6 hrs

Formulary (continued)

Drug Name	Dosage		
codeine 30 mg tab	Adult: 15-60 mg q 4 hrs PO/IM Child: up to 1 mg, 3 mg/kg/day PO/IM given 4 hrs prn		
colchicine tab 0.6 mg tab, inj	0.6mg PO or IV q 1-2 hours. Max of 4 mg/24 hrs		
dapsone 25, 50, 100 mg tab	Antileprotic - 100 mg/day PO		
dehydroemetine	0.5-0.75 mg/kg (90 mg max) IM q 12 hours		
dexamethasone (Decadron) 5 mg/ml inj	Up to 0.5 mg/kg/day		
diazepam (Valium) 5 mg tab, 10 mg/2 ml inj	0.1-0.2 mg/kg/dose given q 6-12 hrs		
diethylcarbamazine (Banicide) 50 mg tab	See Filarial protocol, chapter 1, section VIII		
digoxin 0.25 mg tab, 0.5 mg/ml inj (Note: 1 ug = 0.001 mg)	Digitalizing dose		Maintenance dose
premature	20 ug/kg		5 ug/kg
newborns	30 ug/kg IM or IV		20-30% of digitalizing dose
< 2 year	35-60 ug/kg PO or 30-50 ug/kg IM or IV		10-15 ug/kg PO or 8-12 ug/kg IM or IV
> 2 year	10-40 ug/kg PO or 8-30 ug/kg IM or IV		2.5-9 ug/kg PO or 8-12 ug/kg IM or IV
adult	usual dose = 1 mg		max. maint. Dose = 0.5 mg
diphenhydramine (Benadryl) 50 mg tab	Adult: 25-50 mg PO q 4-6 hrs IM or po Child: 4-6 mg/kg/day		
dopamine 40 mg/ml inj	Initially 1-5 mcg/kg/min up to 50 mcg/kg/min. Max standard concentration: 400 mg/500 ml D5-W = 800 mcg /ml		
doxycycline (Vibramycin) 100 mg tab	100-200 mg/d PO in 1-2 doses Malaria prophylaxis: 100 mg daily		
enalapril (Vasotec)	1.25 mg IV q 6 hrs; 2.5-40 mg PO q day or bid		
ephedrine 30 mg tab, 50 mg/amp inj	Adults: 15-60 mg PO or IM 3-4 times daily Child: up to 3 mg/kg/day SQ in divided doses q 4-6 hrs		
epinephrine 1 mg/ml inj	0.01mg/kg/dose; max: 1 mg/dose; continuous infusion: 1-4 mcg/min (1mg/250 ml solution = 4 mcg/ml)		
ergonovine 0.5 mg tab, 0.5 mg/amp inj	0.5 mg IM prn or 0.5-1 mg PO qid		
ergotamine 2mg tab	For migraine: 1-2 at onset of headache max 4 tabs in 24 hours or 10 tabs/wk		
erythromycin (Eryc, E-Mycin, EES) 250 mg tab	Adult: 250-500 mg PO q 6 hrs Child: 30-50 mg/kg/day divided into 4 doses		
ethambutol 100-400 mg tab	Adult: 15-25 mg/kg (Max 2.5 gm/day) Child above age 5 yrs: 15-25 mg/kg		

Formulary (continued)

Drug Name	Dosage
ethinylestradiol 0.1 mg	Estrogen replacement: 1-2 tabs daily
ferrous sulfate 200 mg tab	2-300 mg tid
fluconazole 100, 200 mg cap	100-200 mg daily
folic acid 5 mg tab	1-2 mg daily
furosemide (Lasix) 40 mg tab, 20 mg/ml inj	0.5-2 mg/kg/dose IV q6-8h; 20 - 120 mg PO 1-2 times daily
gentamicin 80 mg/2 ml inj	Adult: 1-1.7 mg/kg IM/IV q 8 hrs or 5-7 mg/kg as single dose Child: 1.5-2.5 mg/kg IM/IV q 8 hrs
gentian violet	0.25-2% solution applied 2-3 times daily
glibenclamide (glyburide, Diabeta, Micronase) 5 mg tab	1.25-20mg/d 1-2x/d. Max 20mg per day
glycerin suppositories	one as needed
griseofulvin (Fulvicin, Grifulvin) 125, 250 mg tab	Adult: micronized - 500-1000 mg/day PO in 1-4 doses Child: 10 mg/kg/day in divided doses; ultramicronized - 330-750 mg/d
haloperidol (Haldol) 5 mg tab, 5 mg/ml inj	2.5-20 mg/day in 2 divided doses 2-10mg IM Initially, then 1-5 mg q 4-6hrs PRN
heparin 5000 u/ml inj	Intermittent dosing: loading - 10-20,000 u SQ then 8-10,000 u q 8 hrs; Continuous infusion: load - 80 u/kg then 18 u/kg/hr continuous infusion adjust dose based on PTT
hydralazine (Apresoline) 25 mg tab, 20 mg/amp inj	5-20 mg IM or IV slowly q 4-6 hours or 10-50 mg PO qid
hydrochlorothiazide 25, 50 mg tab	2-3mg/kg/d PO in 1-2 doses; 12.5-100mg/d
ibuprofen (Motrin, Advil) 200-400 mg tab	Adult: 400-800 mg qid; max: 3200 mg/day Child: 20-40 mg/kg/day
indomethacin (Indocin) 25 mg tab	25-50 mg tid-qid Child: 3 mg/kg/day; max: 200 mg/day
ipratropium	Adult: 2 inhalations 4 x daily Child 3-12 yrs: 1-2 inhalations 3 x daily
iron dextran (Imferon) 50 mg/ml inj	See Anemia protocol, Chapter 8, section I
isoniazid 100, 300 mg tab	Adult: 5-10 mg/kg (300 mg) Child: 10-15 mg/kg (300 mg)
isosorbide dinitrate 5 mg tab	5-40 mg PO bid-tid
ivermectin 3, 6 mg tab	0.15 mg/kg PO as a single dose (in adults usually 6 mg)
ketamine (Ketalar) 50 mg/ml inj	IM: 4-13 mg/kg (av-10 mg/kg) produces 12-25 min anesthesia; IV: 1-4.5 mg/kg (av-2 mg/kg) produces 5-10 min anesthesia
ketoconazole (Nizoral) 200 mg tab	200-400 mg PO daily
levodopa 250 mg + carbidopa 25 mg (Sinemet)	Initially: 125 mg 3-4 x daily, increased to 750-1500 mg daily in divided doses (calculated as levodopa).

Formulary (continued)

Drug Name	Dosage
levothyroxine 100 mcg tab	0.025-0.3 mg/day
lidocaine (Xylocaine) 1%, 2%, 2% cEpi	max: 3 mg/kg/dose
loperamide 2 mg tab	2 tabs initially followed by 1 tab after each loose stool (max 8 tabs per day)
Lugol's solution	1-5 drops tid
mag trisilicate/al hydroxide tab	1-2 PO qid and prn
magnesium SO4 15% sol, 10 ml amps, inj	See pre-eclampsia protocol, chapter 15, section XIII
magnesium trisilicate Liq	15 ml PO qid and prn
mebendazole 100, 500 mg tab	100 mg PO bid X 6 doses (> 2yrs)
medroxyprogesterone (Provera, Depo-Provera) 5 mg, 150 mg/ml	Dysfunctional uterine bleeding: 5-10 mg/day x 5-10 days Contraception: 150 mg IM q 3 months
mefloquine (Lariam) 250 mg tab	Treatment: 20 mg/kg PO (up to 1.5 Gm) as a single dose or divided into two doses 6-8 hrs apart. Prophylaxis: 250 mg weekly
metformin (Glucophage) 500 mg tab	500 mg bid - 850 mg tid. Max 2550 mg per day
methyldopa (Aldomet) 250 mg tab	250-500 mg PO bid/tid
metoclopramide (Reglan) 10 mg tab	10 mg PO/IM/IV ac and hs; antiemetic in cancer chemotherapy: 1-2 mg/kg/dose q 4-6 hrs prn
metronidazole (Flagyl) 250 mg tab, 500 mg Vag tab, 500 mg/100 ml inj	Adult: 250-750 mg PO tid or 15 mg/kg IV as a loading dose, then 7.5 mg/kg q 6 hrs Child: 10-30 mg/kg/day in divided doses q 6-8 hrs
morphine 10 mg/amp inj	Adult: IM: 5-15 mg q 4 hrs; IV: ½ IM dose Child: 0.1-0.2 mg/kg/dose SQ/IM q 4 hrs
multivitamins tab	1 q day
niclosamide 500 mg tab	Adults: 2 Gms chewed well as a single dose Children: 11-34 kg - single dose of 1 Gm
nifedipine (Procardia) 10 mg cap	20-30 mg PO tid
nitroglycerin 0.5 mg tab	1 tablet sublingual q 5 min x 3; IV drip - 5-50 mcg/min
nitroglycerin ointment (2% Oint)	½ - 1" q 8h
norethisterone 5 mg tab	5-10 mg tid. See Chapter 16
noscapine 15 mg tab	Adult: 15mg - 30mg every 4 - 6 hours Child: ½ the adult dose
nystatin (Mycostatin) 500,000 U Oral tab, 100,000 U Vag tab	Adult: 400-600,000 u PO qid Child: 200,000 u qid Vaginal: 100,000 u 1-2 times daily
omeprazole 20 mg tab	20-40 mg daily
oxytocin 10 u/ml inj	See chapter 15, section XVI

Formulary (continued)

Drug Name	Dosage
paracetamol (acetaminophen) 100-500 mg tab, 125/5 ml Liq	Adult: 0.5-1 gm q 4-6 hrs, max: 4 gm/day, max. long term: 2.6 gm/day Child: 10-15 mg/kg/dose q 4-6
pentazocine (Talwin) 30 mg/ml inj	Adult: 30 mg IV or up to 60 mg IM q 3-4 hrs, max: 360 mg/day Child: up to 1 mg/kg/dose IM
pethidine (meperidine, Demerol) 50, 100 mg tab,100 mg/2 ml inj	Adult & Child: IM 0.5-2 mg/kg q 4 hrs; IV: 0.5-1 mg/kg/dose
phenobarbital 50, 100 mg tab, 200 mg/2 ml inj	Adult: IV loading dose: 15-20 mg/kg. Maintenance: 60-180 mg/day PO as single dose Child: 5-8 mg/kg/day
phenoxymethyl penicillin (Pen V) 250 mg tab	Adult: 250-500 mg PO q 6 hrs Child: 50-100 mg/kg/day
phenytoin (Dilantin) 100 mg tab	Loading dose: 15-20 mg/kg IV. Maintenance: 5 mg/kg or 300-600 mg/day in 1-2 doses
piperazine 300 mg tab	75 mg/kg PO daily (max 3.5 gm)
potassium chloride 500 mg tab	Up to 40 mEq/day (500 mg = 6.75 mEq)
praziquantel 150, 600 mg tab	40-60 mg/kg total dose given in 2-3 doses in one day
prednisone 5 mg tab	Up to 2 mg/kg/day in divided doses
primaquine 7.5, 15 mg tab	15 mg (base) daily for 14-21 days
probenecid (Benemid) 500 mg tab	500 mg PO bid initially, up to 2 gm daily
procaine penicillin inj	600,000-2,400,000 u IM 1-2 times daily Max 8.8 mu/d Child 25-50,000 u/kg IM daily as single dose
procaine penicillin/penicillin G (BIPEN) inj	60-100,000 u/kg IM q 12 hrs
progesterone 25 mg/ml inj	25-50 mg as a single dose
proguanil (Paludrine) 100 mg tab	Prophylaxis: 100-200 mg/day
promethazine (Phenergan) 25 mg tab, 50 mg/2 ml inj	Adult: 25-50 mg IM or PO Child: 0.5-1 mg/kg/dose q 4-6 hrs
propantheline (Pro-Banthine) 15 mg tab	15 mg qid PO ac and hs max 120 mg/day
propranolol (Inderal) 40 mg tab	20-120 mg PO bid
pyrazinamide 500 mg tab	15-30 mg/kg, >50 kg: (2 gm), <50 kg: (1.5 gm) Child: 15-30 mg/kg (max: 2 gm)
quinine 200,300 mg tab, 600 mg/2 ml inj	25-30 mg/kg/day IV/PO in divided doses q 8 hrs (adult: 650 mg PO q 8 hrs) Child: same
reserpine 0.1, 0.25 mg tab	0.05-0.25 mg PO q day
rifampicin 150, 300 mg tab	10 mg/kg, >50 kg: 600 mg, <50 kg: 450 mg Child: 10-20 mg/kg (max: 600 mg)
spectinomycin 2 gm inj	For gonorrhea: 2 gm IM

Formulary (continued)

Drug Name	Dosage
spironolactone (Aldactone) 25 mg tab	50-200 mg PO in 1-2 doses Max 400 mg/d
streptomycin 1 Gm inj	Adult: 10-15 mg/kg, 500-1000 mg 5 times/wk Child: 20-30 mg/kg (1 gm)
sulfadoxine/pyrimethamine (Fansidar)	3 tablets as a single dose
testosterone inj	Short acting: 25-50 mg 2-3 x weekly long acting prep: 50-400 mg q 2-4 weeks
tetracycline 250 mg tab	250-500 mg PO q 6 hrs
thiabendazole 500 mg tab	25 mg/kg PO q 12 hrs; max 3 gm/d
tinidazole (Fasigyn) 500 mg tab	1-2 gm daily in 1-2 doses Child 50-60 mg/kg/day in 1-2 doses
triamcinolone 40 mg/ml inj	20-40 mg per injection, effect lasts 1-4 weeks
trimethoprim/sulfa SS 80/400 mg, DS 160/800 mg Susp 200/40 mg/5 ml (TMP/SMX, Co-trimoxazole, Bactrim)	160 mg PO q 12 hrs calculated as trimethoprim content Adult IV dose and Child IV/PO: 8-10 mg/kg/day in divided doses 2-4 times daily calculated as trimethoprim content
valproic acid (Depakene, Depakote) 200, 500 mg tab	Initially: 15 mg/kg/day in divided doses (usually 600 mg) PO, increased gradually to 20-30 mg/kg/day in divided doses (1-2 gm/day)
verapamil 40 mg tab verapamil SR (Isoptin, Calan Verelan)	40-120 mg bid/tid 120-480 mg PO q day
vitamin A 50,00 U tab	In acute deficiency states: 200,000 U daily x 2 days
vitamin B complex tab	1 daily
vitamin B 6 (pyridoxine) 50 mg tab	Up to 50 mg tid
vitamin B 12 1000 mcg/ml inj	1000 mcg monthly
vitamin C 200 mg tab	50-250 mg/day
vitamin E tab	75 IU daily
vitamin K 10 mg/ml inj	10 mg IM/SQ daily
warfarin (Coumadin) 5 mg tab	1-10 mg PO daily as determined by prothrombin time

Christian Mission Organizations

Africa Inland Mission International (AIM)
PO Box 178, Pearl River, NY 10965
Phone: 1-800-254-001   Fax: 845-735-1814
www.aim-us.org

Agape Medical Center - Russia
Rt. 9 Box 13-D, Manchester, KY 40962
Phone: 606-598-8888 Fax: 606-598-7179
www.agaperu.org

AIRO Ministries
PO Box 842, Petoskey, MI 49740
Phone: 616-347-7494
airo@nmo.net

American Baptist Churches Board of International Ministries
PO Box 851, Valley Forge, PA 19482
www.internationalministries.org

American Missions Hospital
PO Box 1 Manama, Baharain Arabian Gulf
Phone: +973-253-447 Fax: +973-234-194
ddoenitz@amh.org.bh

Baptist Medical & Dental Mission International
P.O. Box 608 Petal, MS 39465-0608
Phone: 601-544-3586 Fax: 601-544-6508
www.bmdmi.org

Baptist Mid-Missions
7749 Webster Road, Cleveland, OH 44130-8011
Phone: 440-826-3930 Fax: 440-826-4457
www.bmm.org

Belize Medical Missions
PO Box 1600 Centralia, IL 62801
Phone: 618-533-2873 Fax: 618-533-9489
www.belizemissions.com

Bethany Crippled Children Hospital of Kenya
391 Carrie Cres, Kinston Ontario, Canada K7M5X7
Phone: 613-384-0064 Fax: 613-384-9386
gis@post.queensu.ca

Bethel Christian Retreat
Box 1491 Newport PO, Manchester, Jamaica
Phone: 876-965-7453 Fax: 876-965-7454
bethel@cwjamaica.com

Bible Literature International (BLI)
625 E. North Broadway, Columbus, OH 43214-4133
Phone: 614-267-3116 Fax: 614-267-7110
www.bli.org

Blessings International
5881 S. Garnett Road, Tulsa, OK 74146
Phone: 918-250-8101 Fax: 918-250-1281
www.blessing.org/home.html

Calvary Ministries International
1343 E. Mel Curry Road, Bloomington, IN 47408
Phone: 812-334-6141 Fax: 812-331-3233
cmo@psci.net

Catholic Medical Mission Board, Inc.
10 West 17th St, New York, NY 10011
Phone: 800-678-5659
www.cmmb.org

Catholic Network of Volunteer Service
1410 Q St NW, Washington, DC 20009
Phone: 202-332-6000
www.cnvs.org

CBInternational
1501 W. Mineral Street Littleton, CO 80120-5612
Phone: 800-487-4224 Fax: 720-283-2250
www.cbi.org

Change A life International
3977 Rockmart Highway, Cedartown, GA 30125
Phone: 770-684-7107 Fax: 770-684-4925
jmorgan@changealifeint.org

Children's Medical Ministries
707 Hunters Mill Lane, Evington, VA 24550
Phone: 434-665-8451 Fax: 804-528-1052
smizenerm@aol.com

Chosen, Inc
3638 West 26th Street Erie, PA 16506
Phone: 814-833-3023 Fax: 814-833-4091
CHOSEN4Jay@aol.com

Christian Community Health Fellowship
PO Box 23429, 3812 W. Ogden Ave, Chicago, IL 60623
Phone: 773-843-2700 Fax: 773-542-0468
www.cchf.org

Christian Connection for International Health
1817 Rupert Street, McLean, VA 22101
Phone: 703-556-0123 Fax: 703-917-4251
martinrs@aol.com

Christian Medical & Dental Associations (CMDA)
P.O. Box 7500 Bristol, TN 37620
Phone: 423-844-1000 Fax: 423-764-1417
www.cmdahome.org

Christian Pharmacists Fellowship International (CPFI)
P.O. Box 1717, Bristol, TN 37621-1717
Phone: 423-764-6000 Fax: 423-764-4490
www.cpfi.org

CMF International
P.O. Box 501020, 5525E. 82nd Street
Indianapolis, IN 46250-6020
Phone: 317-578-2700 Fax: 317-578-2827
www.cmfi.org

COIMEA (Commission on International Medical Education Affairs)
- Now known as Medical Education International (MEI)
PO Box 7500, Bristol, TN 37620
Phone: 423-844-1000 Fax: 423-844-1017
www.cmdahome.org

(The) Cornerstone Foundation
135 Main Street, Suite 308, Biloxi, MS 39530
Phone: 228-435-7800 Fax: 228-435-7800
cornerstone@ametro.net

Dream Weaver Medical Foundation
1816 Prospector Avenue, Suite 102 Park City, UT 84060
Phone: 435-658-1188 Fax: 435-658-1155
www.dwfoundation.org

Domestic Mission Commission
Christian Medical & Dental Associations (CMDA)
P.O. Box 7500 Bristol, TN 37620
Phone: 423-844-1000 Fax: 423-844-1017
dmc@cmdahome.org

Evangelical Free Church Mission
901 E. 78th Street, Minneapolis, MN 55420-1300
Phone: 800-745-2202
www.efcm.org

Evangelism Task Force
P.O. Box 1494, Waycross, GA 31502
Phone: 912-285-0779 Fax: 912-285-8959
www.etforce.org

Fellowship of Associates of Medical Evangelism (FAME)
PO Box 34800, Indianapolis, IN 46234
Phone: 317-272-5937 Fax: 317-272-5940
www.fameworld.org

Fellowship of Christian Physician Assistants
4 Grieb Court, Wallingford, CT 06492-2637
Phone: 203-284-0780
www.fcpa.net

Global Health Outreach (GHO)
Christian Medical & Dental Associations (CMDA)
P.O. Box 7500 Bristol, TN 37620
Phone: 423-844-1000 Fax: 423-764-1417
www.cmdahome.org

Good Samaritan Clinic (World Impact)
3701 E. Thirteenth Street, Wichita, KS 67208-2077
Phone: 316-688-5020 Fax: 316-682-1880
fmclean@kscable.com

HCJB World Radio
PO Box 39800, Colorado Springs, CO 80949-9800
Phone: 719-590-9800 Fax: 719-590-9801
www.hcjb.org/healthcare

Health Care Ministries
521 W. Lynn Street, Springfield, MO 65802
Phone: 417-866-6311 Fax: 417-866-4711
www.healthcareministries.org

Health Outreach to the Middle East
6422 Winter Stone Houston, TX 77084
Phone: 281-856-7461 Fax: 281-856-7452
hometxus@yahoo.com

Health Teams International
10056 Applegate Lane, Brighton, MI 48114
Phone: 810-229-9247 Fax: 810-229-4336

Heart to Heart International
401 South Clairborne, Suite 302, Olathe, Kansas 66062
Phone: 913-764-5200 Fax 913-764-0809
www.hearttoheart.org

In His Image Family Practice Residency and Medical Missions Program
7600 S. Lewis Avenue, Tulsa, OK 74136
Phone: 918-493-7816 Fax: 918-493-7867
www.inhisimage.org

International Aid and Medical Equipment Services
17011 W. Hickory St, Spring Lake, MI 49456
Phone: 616-846-7490 Fax: 616-846-9431
www.internationalaid.org

International Foundation of Hope
PO Box 60219, Colorado Springs, CO 80960
Phone: 719-226-5110 Fax: 719-226-5381
www.ifhope.org

International Medical Assistance (IMA)
PO Box 255, ADA, MI 49301
Phone: 616-682-0408 Fax: 616-682-0413
www.ima-missions.org

International Mission Board SBC
PO Box 6767, Richmond, VA 23230-0767
Phone: 804-219-1000 Fax: 804-254-8980
www.imb.org

International Service Fellowship (InterServe/USA)
PO Box 418 Upper Darby, PA 19082-0418
Phone: 610-352-0581 Fax: 610-352-4394
www.interserve.org/usa

Jamkhed International Foundation
PO Box 291, Carrboro, NC 27510
Phone: 919-929-0650
www.jamkhed.org

Jericho Road Foundation
9642 S. Hoyne, Chicago, IL 60643
Phone: 708-206-0010 Fax: 708-206-0020
williamcrevier@aol.com

Josh McDowell Ministry
P.O. Box 131000, Dallas TX 75313-1000
Phone: 972-907-1000
www.josh.org

Lifeline Christian Mission
184 Old County Line Road, Westerville, Ohio 43081
Phone: 614-794-0108 Fax: 614-794-0109
www.lifeline.org

Loma Linda University and Medical Center
11060 Anderson St, Magan Hall, Loma Linda, CA 92350
Phone: 909-824-4420 Fax: 909-478-4116
www.llu.edu

(The) Luke Society
2204 S. Minnesota Ave., Suite 200, Sioux Falls, SD 57105-3712
Phone: 605-373-9686 Fax: 605-373-9711
www.lukesociety.org

Lumiere Medical Ministries
209 W. Second Avenue, Gastonia, NC 28054
Phone: 704-868-3703
LMMhaiti@carolina.rr.com

MAP International
2200 Glynco Parkway, PO Box 215000, Brunswick, GA 31521-5000
Phone: 800-225-8550
www.map.org

Medical Ambassadors International
PO Box 576645, Modesto, CA 95357-6645
Phone: 888-403-0600 Fax: 209-571-3538
www.med-amb.org

Medical Benevolence Foundation
PO Box 770636, Houston, TX 77215-0636
Phone: 800-547-7627 Fax: 281-590-3699
www.mbfoundation.org

Medical Education International (MEI)
- Formerly known as COIMEA (Commission on International Medical Education Affairs)
PO Box 7500, Bristol, TN 37620
Phone: 423-844-1000 Fax: 423-844-1017
www.cmdahome.org

Medical Ministry International
P.O. Box 1339, Allen, TX 75013-0022
Phone: 972-727-5864 Fax: 972-727-7810
www.mmint.org

Medical Strategic Network
PO Box 2052, Redlands, CA 92373
Phone: 909-797-2549
www.gomets.org

Mercy Ships
PO Box 2020, Garden Valley, TX 75771-2020
Phone: 903-939-7000 Fax: 903-882-0336
www.mercyships.org

Mexican Medical Ministries
251 Landis Avenue
Chula Vista, CA 91910-2628
Phone: 619-420-9750 Fax: 619-420-9570
www.mexicanmedical.com

Mission Society for United Methodist
6234 Crooked Creek
Norcross, GA 30092-3106
Phone: 770-446-1381 Fax: 770-446-3044
www.msum.org

MSI Professional Services
PO Box 670541, Cincinnati, OH 45267-0541
Phone: 513-558-0516 or 513-558-0543
www.msiprofessionalservice.org

Nazarene Health Care Fellowship
6401 The Paseo, Kansas City, MO 64131-1213
Phone: 877-626-4145 Fax 816-333-2948
www.nazcompassion.org

New Life International, Inc
6764 S. Bloomington Trail, Underwood, IN
47177
Phone: 812-752-7474 Fax: 812-752-5233
www.missionsalive.org

New Missions
PO Box 2727, Orlando, FL 32802-2727
Phone: 800-937-4248 Fax: 407-240-1962
www.newmissions.org

**North American Baptist Conference
International Missions Department**
1 South 210 Summit Ave, Oakbrook Terrace, IL
60181-3994
Phone: 630-495-2000 Fax: 630-495-3301
www.nabconference.org

Northwest Medical Teams
PO Box 10
Portland, OR 97207-0010
Phone: 503-624-1008 Fax: 503-624-1001
www.nwmedicalteams.org

Nurses Christian Fellowship
P.O. Box 7895
Madison, WI 53707-7895
Phone: 608-274-4823 Fax: 608-274-7882
www.ncf-jcn.org

Oasis Hospital
PO Box 1016 Al Ain, Abu Dhabi, United Arab
Emirates
Phone: 971-372-21251 Fax: 971-372-22007
www.oasishospital.org

Pan-African College of Christian Surgeons
76 Stuart St, Victory 3, Kingston, Ontario
K7L2V7 Canada
Phone: 613-548-3232 Fax: 613-548-2514
poearuda@kgh.kari.net

Presbyterian Church in America (PCA)
1700 North Brown Road, Lawrenceville, GA
30043
Phone: 678-825-1000 Fax: 678-825-1001
www.pcanet.org

Presbyterian Church USA
100 Witherspoon Street, RM. 3429A,
Louisville, KY 40202
Phone: 502-569-5573 Fax: 502-569-8039
www.pcusa.org

Project Compassion
11315 Rancho Bernardo Road, San Diego, CA
92127
Phone: 858-485-9694 Fax: 619-819-4011
www.projectcompassion.org

Project MedSend
PO Box 1098, Orange, CT 06477-7098
Phone: 203-891-8223
www.medsend.org

Red Bird Mission and Clinic
HC 69 Box 700, Beverly, KY 40913
Phone: 606-598-3155 Fax: 606-598-3151
www.rbmission.org

Romanian American Mission (RAM)
3894 Georgetown Road
Frankfort, KY 40601
Phone: 502-695-4050 Fax: 502-695-0594
www.ram-christian.org

Samaritan's Purse
PO Box 3000, Boone, NC 28607
Phone: 828-262-1980 Fax: 828-266-1048
SIM-USA
1838 Goldhill Road, Fort Mill, SC 29708
Phone: 803-802-7300 Fax: 803-548-0885
www.sim.org

Supplies Over Seas (SOS)
101 West Chestnut St.
Louisville, KY 40202-1881
Phone: 502-589-2001 Fax: 502-581-9022
www.suppliesoverseas.org

TEAM
P.O. Box 969, Wheaton, IL 60189-0969
Phone: 630-653-5300 Fax: 630-653-1826
www.teamworld.org

Team Expansion
3700 Hopewell Road
Louisville, KY 40299
Phone: 502-297-0006 Fax: 502-297-9823
www.teamexpansion.org

TECH - Technical Exchange for Christian Healthcare
PO Box 904, Mentor, Ohio 44061-0904
Phone: 440-354-4777 Fax: 440-354-4777
www.techmd.org

Touched Twice Ministries (The Clinic)
P.O. Box 8121, Louisville, KY 40207
Phone: 877-503-3193 Fax: 877-503-3193
www.touchedtwice.org

United Methodist Fellowship of Health Care Volunteers
475 Riverside Drive, New York, New York 10115
Phone: 1-800-862-4246
gbgm-umc.org

Vellore Christian Medical College Board (USA), Inc
475 Riverside Drive, Suite 243, New York, NY 10115
Phone: 212-870-2640 Fax: 212-870-2173
www.vellorecmc.org

Vision International Alliance
416 W Chestnut Avenue, Suite 206, Monrovia, CA 91016
Phone: 626-305-9076 Fax: 626-305-0387
www.viamission.org

Volunteers in Medical Missions
PO Box 756, Seneca, SC 29679
Phone: 864-885-9411
www.vimm.org

Whitecross Medical Missions Corp
2400 Holloway Road, Louisville, KY 40299
Phone: 502-261-0700 Fax: 502-261-0701
www.whitecrossmmc.org

World Gospel Mission (WGM)
3783 State Road 18 E, PO Box 948, Marion, IN 46952-0948
Phone: 765-664-7331 Fax: 765-671-7230
www.wgm.org

World Medical Mission
Box 3000, Boone, NC 28607
Phone: 828-262-1980
www.samaritan.org

Worldwide Lab Improvement, Inc
10046 Shuman St, Portage, MI 49024
Phone: 269-323-8407 Fax: 269-323-2030
www.wwlab.org

World Vision International
800 West Chestnut Avenue, Monrovia, CA 91016-3198
Phone: 626-303-8811 Fax: 626-301-7786
www.wvi.org

World Witness (Associate Reformed Presbyterian Church)
1 Cleveland St, Ste 220, Greenville SC 29601
864-233-5226
Phone: 864-233-5226
www.worldwitness.org

Other Mission Organizations

Albert Schweitzer Institute for the Humanities
275 Mount Carmel Avenue, Hamden, CT 06518
Phone: 203-582-3144 Fax: 203-582-8478
www.schweitzerinstitute.org

American Refugee Committee
430 Oak Grove St, Suite 204, Minneapolis, MN 55403
Phone: 612-872-7060 Fax: 612-607-6499
www.archq.org

Child Family Health International
953 Mission Street, Suite 220, San Francisco, CA 94103
Phone: 415-957-9000 Fax: 501-423-6852
www.cfhi.org

Children's HeartLink
5075 Arcadia Ave, Minneapolis, MN 55436-2306
Phone: 952-928-4860 Fax: 952-928-4859
www.childrensheartlink.org

Doctors of the World - USA, Inc.
375 West Broadway, 4th Floor, New York, NY 10012
Phone: 212-226-9890
www.doctorsoftheworld.org

Doctors without Borders USA
6 E. 39th St., 8th floor, New York, NY 10016
Phone: 212-679-6800 Fax: 212-679-7016
(212)   679-7016
www.doctorswithoutborders.org

Flying Physicians Association
PO Box 677427, Orlando, FL 32867
Phone: 407-359-1423 Fax: 407-359-1167
www.fpadrs.org

Health Volunteers Overseas
PO Box 65157, Washington, DC 20035
Phone: 202-296-0928 Fax: 202-296-8018
www.hvousa.org

International Medical Corps
11500 W Olympic Blvd, Suite 280, Los Angeles, CA 90064
Phone: 310-826-7800 Fax: 310-442-6622
www.imc-la.com

International Rescue Committee
122 East 42nd Street, New York, NY 10168
Phone: 212-551-3000
www.theirc.org

Operation Smile
6435 Tidewater Drive Norfolk, VA 23509
Phone: 757-321-7645 Fax: 757-321-7660
www.operationsmile.org

Orbis International
520 Eighth Avenue, 11th Fl, New York, NY 10018
Phone: 646-674-5500 Fax: 646-674-5599
www.orbis.org

Peace Corps
1111 20th Street NW, Washington, DC 20526
Phone: 1-800-424-8580
www.peacecorps.gov

Project Hope
255 Carter Hall Lane, Millwood, Virginia, 22646
Phone: 540-837-2100
www.projecthope.org

Medicine and Equipment Agencies

See previous contact information on:
➢ Chosen
➢ Global Health Ministries
➢ International Aid
➢ MAP International
➢ World Medical Mission

Also:
Interchurch Medical Assistance
PO Box 429, 500 Main St, New Windsor, MD 21776
Phone: 410-635-8720 Fax: 410-635-8726

King Benevolence Fund
1119 Commonwealth Ave, Bristol, VA 24201
Phone: 276-466-3014 Fax: 276-466-0955